American
Physicians
in the
Nineteenth
Century

WILLIAM G. ROTHSTEIN

American Physicians in the Nineteenth Century

FROM SECTS TO SCIENCE

THE JOHNS HOPKINS UNIVERSITY PRESS

BALTIMORE AND LONDON

Originally published in hardcover, 1972
Softshell Books edition, 1992

The Johns Hopkins University Press
701 West 40th Street
Baltimore, Maryland 21211-2190
The Johns Hopkins Press, Ltd., London

Library of Congress Catalog Card Number 77-186517
ISBN 0-8018-4427-4 (pbk.)

TO MY PARENTS

CONTENTS

PREFACE TO THE 1992 EDITION   xv

PREFACE   xxi

PART I.   METHOD OF ANALYSIS AND COLONIAL ANTECEDENTS

CHAPTER 1.   PLAN OF ANALYSIS   3

INTRODUCTION   3

MODEL OF ANALYSIS   8
THE BODY OF MEDICAL KNOWLEDGE   9;   EARNING OF
LIVELIHOOD   10;   THE INSTITUTION OF THE INDEPENDENT
PRACTITIONER   12;   PROFESSIONAL SOCIETIES   15;
MEDICAL SCHOOLS   18;   LICENSING   20;   MEDICAL SECTS   21;

OTHER CONSIDERATIONS   24

CHAPTER 2.   PROLOGUE: THE COLONIAL PERIOD   26

MEDICAL PRACTICE IN THE COLONIAL PERIOD   26
CINCHONA BARK   28;   INOCULATION AND VACCINATION   29;
BOTANICAL MEDICINE   32

THE OCCUPATIONAL ROLE OF THE PHYSICIAN   34

MEDICAL LICENSING   37

PART II.   THE REGULAR PROFESSION IN THE FIRST HALF OF THE NINETEENTH CENTURY

CHAPTER 3.   MEDICAL PRACTICE AMONG PHYSICIANS   41

THE BASIS OF MEDICAL THERAPEUTICS   41
BLOODLETTING   45;   PURGATIVES AND EMETICS   49;
OTHER THERAPIES   52

DISEASE IN EARLY NINETEENTH CENTURY AMERICA   55
ENDEMIC DISEASES 56;   EPIDEMIC DISEASES 58

CONCLUSION   61

CHAPTER 4. MEDICAL SOCIETIES AND
MEDICAL LICENSING   63

THE DEVELOPMENT OF EXCLUSIVE MEDICAL SOCIETIES   63
RELATIONS AMONG PHYSICIANS 63;   LOCAL MEDICAL
SOCIETIES 64;   STATE MEDICAL SOCIETIES 68;
GROWTH OF LOCAL AND STATE SOCIETIES 70

MEDICAL LICENSING LEGISLATION   72
LICENSING IN THE COLONIAL PERIOD 72;   THE ENACTMENT
OF LICENSING LEGISLATION 74;   CONTENT OF THE
LICENSING LAWS 76;   LICENSING BOARDS AND REGULAR
PHYSICIANS 79

REGULATION OF THE CONDUCT OF MEMBERS OF
MEDICAL SOCIETIES 80
FEE BILLS 81;   CODES OF ETHICS 82

SCIENTIFIC ACTIVITIES OF MEDICAL SOCIETIES   84

CHAPTER 5. MEDICAL EDUCATION   85

APPRENTICESHIP   85

MEDICAL SCHOOLS   87
THE INCEPTION OF MEDICAL SCHOOLS 87;   THE CURRICULUM
OF MEDICAL SCHOOLS 88;   THE PROLIFERATION OF
MEDICAL SCHOOLS 93;   COMPETITION AMONG
MEDICAL SCHOOLS 96;   THE ROLE OF THE MEDICAL SCHOOL
IN THE PROFESSION 97
CONCLUSION   100

CHAPTER 6. RELATIONS BETWEEN MEDICAL SCHOOLS AND
MEDICAL SOCIETIES   101

THE REACTIONS OF PHYSICIANS TO THE MEDICAL SCHOOLS   101

THE CONFLICT OVER LICENSING   104

MEDICAL SCHOOLS AND THE SUPPLY OF PHYSICIANS   108

THE FOUNDING OF THE AMERICAN MEDICAL ASSOCIATION   114

PART III.   THE REBELLION AGAINST THE
            REGULAR MEDICAL PROFESSION

CHAPTER 7.   THE THOMSONIAN MOVEMENT   125

             The Sectarian Nature of Regular Medical Practice   125

             Samuel Thomson and the Botanical Movement   128
             thomson's *New Guide to Health* 131;   thomson's
             organization 140;   the professional botanical
             practitioners 141;   the institutionalization of
             thomsonism 142;   medical licensing and the
             thomsonian movement 144;   botanical medical
             colleges 146

             The Thomsonian Movement and Regular Physicians   146

             Conclusion   150

CHAPTER 8.   THE RISE OF HOMEOPATHY   152

             The Discovery of the Homeopathic Law   152

             Homeopathy in American Medical Practice   158
             the state of public opinion 158;   the appeal of
             homeopathy 159;   early homeopathic physicians 161;
             the reaction of regular physicians to homeopathic
             physicians 165

             Homeopathy and the American Medical Association   170
             homeopathy and the ama code of ethics 170;   other
             aspects of the ama code of ethics 173

PART IV.   THE INSTITUTIONALIZATION OF MEDICAL SECTS

CHAPTER 9.   THE THERAPEUTICS OF THE REGULAR SECT
             AFTER THE CIVIL WAR   177

             The Decline of Heroic Medicine   177
             attacks on heroic therapy by regular physicians 177;
             the demise of heroic therapeutics 181;   therapeutic
             nihilism 183

             The New Vigorous Therapy   186
             antipyretics 187;   analgesics 190;   tonics 194

CHAPTER 10. STRATIFICATION AND SPECIALIZATION IN
THE REGULAR MEDICAL PROFESSION
AFTER THE CIVIL WAR 198

DEVELOPMENTS IN MEDICAL SOCIETIES 198
THE AMERICAN MEDICAL ASSOCIATION 198; STATE AND
LOCAL MEDICAL SOCIETIES 201; ELITE MEDICAL
SOCIETIES 201

SOCIAL STRATIFICATION IN THE MEDICAL PROFESSION 204

SPECIALIZATION IN THE MEDICAL PROFESSION 207
THE DEVELOPMENT OF MEDICAL SPECIALTIES 207; REACTIONS
OF GENERAL PRACTITIONERS TO SPECIALIZATION 209;
RELATIONS BETWEEN GENERAL PRACTITIONERS AND
SPECIALISTS 211; SPECIALTY MEDICAL SOCIETIES 212;
THE CONGRESS OF AMERICAN PHYSICIANS AND SURGEONS 214

CHAPTER 11. THE ECLECTIC SECT: SUCCESSOR TO
BOTANICAL MEDICINE 217

THE ORIGINS OF ECLECTICISM 217

THE DEVELOPMENT OF ECLECTIC THERAPEUTICS 221

INSTITUTIONAL DEVELOPMENTS IN THE ECLECTIC SECT 225

THE DISTINCTIVENESS OF THE ECLECTIC SECT IN THE
MEDICAL PROFESSION 228

CHAPTER 12. THE HOMEOPATHIC SECT 230

THE STRUGGLE WITH THE HOMEOPATHIC QUACKS 230

HOMEOPATHY'S BREAK WITH REGULAR MEDICINE 232

THE SUCCESS OF HOMEOPATHY 234

HOMEOPATHIC MEDICAL INSTITUTIONS 236

THE CONFLICT OVER HAHNEMANN'S LAWS 239
MEDICAL SOCIETIES 239; MEDICAL SCHOOLS 241;
THE DOMINANCE OF THE LOW-DILUTIONISTS 242

HOMEOPATHS AND REGULAR THERAPIES 243

PART V. THE RISE OF SCIENTIFIC MEDICINE

CHAPTER 13. THE BEGINNINGS OF SCIENTIFIC MEDICINE:
SURGERY 249

SURGERY BEFORE ANESTHESIA   249

ANESTHESIA AND SURGERY   250

BACTERIOLOGY AND ANTISEPTIC SURGERY   253

ANTISEPTIC SURGERY AND THE NON-REGULAR SECTS   259

CHAPTER 14.   BACTERIOLOGY AND THE MEDICAL
PROFESSION   261

SCIENTIFIC PRECURSORS OF BACTERIOLOGY   261

THE DEVELOPMENT OF BACTERIOLOGY   263

THE REACTIONS OF PHYSICIANS TO BACTERIOLOGY   265
TUBERCULOSIS 267;   DIPHTHERIA 272;   HOMEOPATHIC
AND ECLECTIC PHYSICIANS AND BACTERIOLOGY 278;   OTHER
EFFECTS OF BACTERIOLOGY ON PHYSICIANS 279

CHAPTER 15.   DEVELOPMENTS IN MEDICAL EDUCATION
AFTER THE CIVIL WAR   282

THE AMA AND MEDICAL SCHOOLS   283

CHANGES IN MEDICAL EDUCATION   285

DIFFERENCES AMONG MEDICAL SCHOOLS   288

THE DEATH OF COMMERCIAL MEDICAL EDUCATION   292

CHANGES IN THE HOMEOPATHIC AND ECLECTIC SCHOOLS   294
CONVERSION OF HOMEOPATHIC SCHOOLS TO REGULAR
SCHOOLS 296

CHAPTER 16.   THE DEATH OF SECTARIAN MEDICINE   298

CONFLICT BETWEEN REGULAR AND HOMEOPATHIC PHYSICIANS   298

THE MEDICAL SOCIETY OF THE STATE OF NEW YORK AND
THE CODE OF ETHICS   301

PATTERNS OF COOPERATION AMONG MEDICAL SECTS   305
THE REVIVAL OF MEDICAL LICENSING 305;   PUBLIC
HEALTH 310;   ADMISSION OF NON-REGULAR PHYSICIANS TO
REGULAR MEDICAL SOCIETIES 313

THE ATTACK ON THE CODE OF ETHICS   314

THE REORGANIZATION OF THE AMA   316
STRUCTURAL REORGANIZATION 318;   REVISISON OF THE

CODE OF ETHICS 320; REACTIONS OF THE STATE AND
LOCAL SOCIETIES 322

CONCLUSION 323

APPENDIX I. FOUNDING DATES OF IMPORTANT LOCAL
AND STATE REGULAR MEDICAL SOCIETIES
IN SELECTED STATES BEFORE THE
CIVIL WAR 327

APPENDIX II. MEDICAL LICENSING LEGISLATION IN
SELECTED STATES BEFORE THE
CIVIL WAR 332

APPENDIX III. SOURCES OF CITATIONS GIVEN IN
APPENDICES I and II 340

APPENDIX IV. ENUMERATIONS OF PHYSICIANS,
1850–1900 344

INDEX 347

TABLES

IV.1   Pre-Civil War Local Medical Societies Designated as State Medical Societies   70

IV.2   Inception of Stable Medical Societies in States Heavily Settled by 1840   71

V.1   Regular Medical Schools Providing Instruction on a Degree-Granting Basis, by Year, 1770–1860   93

V.2   Graduates of Medical Schools in the United States, 1769–1868   98

VI.1   Medical Students with Bachelors of Arts Degrees at Selected Medical Schools, 1870   113

X.1   Presidents of the American Medical Association by Type of Practice, 1860–1899   212

X.2   Date of Founding of National Specialty Medical Societies, 1864–1902   213

XIII.1   Mortality from Major Amputations at the Massachusetts General Hospital, 1822–60   252

XV.1   Medical Schools, Students, and Graduates, by Sect, 1850–1920   287

XV.2   Length of Course of Medical Schools, 1875–99   288

XV.3   Changes in Number of Medical Schools, 1900–1910   294

XVI.1   Sectarian Composition of State Medical Licensing Agencies ca. 1900   308

XVI.2   Appellate Court Decisions in Malpractice Suits, 1794–1930   325

PREFACE TO THE 1992 EDITION

I FIRST BECAME interested in nineteenth-century medicine because I wanted to answer a specific question: What do physicians do when they cannot treat patients successfully? The nineteenth century seemed an opportune period for such a study because at its beginning physicians could do very little for patients and at its end the first major steps toward useful treatment had been taken. My approach focused on nineteenth-century medical care from the viewpoint of the patient, not from the customary perspective of a historian trying to discover the antecedents of modern medicine.

As I found and described it, medical care in the nineteenth century consisted largely but not totally of symptomatic treatments that seldom did good and often did harm. Physicians knew little about disease or human biology, but their ignorance did not produce self-restraint. Instead, they pursued an aggressive and often ill-considered attack on illness using every weapon in the medical armamentarium, despite the urgings of a small number of physicians for greater reliance on the healing powers of nature.

This was my introduction to a timeless issue in medicine, which concerns the merits of active versus expectant or conservative modes of treatment. I subsequently discovered that the debate over this dilemma did not subside as medical care became more scientific in the twentieth century. It remains a pivotal issue today in the treatment of the multitude of diseases, ranging from the common cold to many fatal disorders, which cannot be cured but can only be palliated by medical care.

As a sociologist, I also found the nineteenth century intriguing because it was the period when American medicine became a profession. In my view, a profession has five characteristics. It can be defined as (1) a means of earning a livelihood (2) through the application to the needs of the public (3) of a complex and abstract body of knowledge (4) that is shared by members of the profession and (5) is accepted by the public.

Nineteenth-century physicians had little difficulty establishing themselves in a vocation that served the public and demonstrating that medical knowledge was sufficiently abstract and complex to make formal medical education essential for a well-trained physician. They were, however, unable to agree on the content of the body of medical knowledge, as shown by their disagreements over heroic therapy and homeopathy early in the century and over the germ theory at its end. Groups of physicians were also unable to convince the public to accept their definition of the body of medical knowledge by permitting them to determine who could practice medicine. State legislatures steadfastly refused to grant exclusive licensing privileges to any group of physicians until the end of the century. Even when regulatory licensing was finally adopted, the legislatures maintained the right to practice of the major sects.

When I began my research, I anticipated that the problem of acceptance of the body of medical knowledge would be resolved by physicians first arriving at their own consensus on its content and then convincing the public to accept it. To my surprise, I found that while this pattern was followed for some innovations in medicine, in others the public took the lead and the profession followed. For example, antiseptic surgery was first adopted by many physicians and then accepted by the public, but many public health components of bacteriology were accepted first by a few eminent physicians and the public and later adopted by most physicians. The public also played the dominant role in the rejection of much useless medical knowledge, including heroic therapy and homeopathy.

Reciprocity between physicians and the public in adopting medical knowledge continues today. For example, many aspects of the new public health movement, including the value of exercise and proper diet and the perils of smoking, were adopted by the public before being accepted by most physicians.

Once I understood the long and arduous struggle of physicians to be recognized as professionals, I realized that their status has never stopped changing. Specialization has so fragmented modern medicine that physicians today share only a limited part of the body of medical knowledge. In some respects the medical profession has retrogressed from the unity that was developing at the end of the nineteenth century. Certainly no single organization today plays a role in the medical profession comparable to that of the American Medical Association early in the twentieth century.

I also found that American medicine developed many of its most distinctive features, especially its free-wheeling capitalistic nature, in the nineteenth century. Unlike European physicians, American physicians have always been eager to establish profit-making medical enterprises, such as hospitals and medical schools in the nineteenth and early twentieth centuries and clinics and laboratories today.

The entrepreneurial spirit of the American medical profession has affected modern medicine in many ways. One way has been the reluctance of American physicians to give government a significant role in providing health care to paying or insured patients. Another has been competition and conflicts among physicians. For example, community physicians and the faculty members of medical schools in their communities have always been at odds over who should care for paying patients.

Medicine became increasingly scientific over the course of the nineteenth century, and yet I was struck by the importance of nonscientific factors in the evolution of medical care. The structure of our hospitals, ambulatory care facilities, and medical schools has been determined more by our culture and social and economic structure than by medical science. Similarly, the lack of a scientific understanding of such treatments as smallpox vaccination, quinine, and antiseptic surgery did not prevent their adoption in the nineteenth century and does not prevent the adoption of comparable innovations today. Physicians then as now adopted treatments because they and their patients found them useful. In many cases, the widespread adoption of treatments provided the impetus for scientific research to better understand them.

Thus my research on nineteenth-century medicine, which began as an effort to examine several specific issues, served as a most enlightening form of self-education. I learned that nineteenth-century medicine did not disappear; it evolved into modern medicine. I hope the reader will have the same realization.

RECENT DEVELOPMENTS IN THE HISTORY OF MEDICINE

What kind of research has been done on American medicine in the nineteenth century since this study was written? The major development has been a new orientation toward medical history that places greater emphasis on the social aspects of medical care and less on the internal dynamics of the medical profession and medical science. It focuses on the development of health care institutions such as hospitals and dispensaries, the medical care received by various groups in the population, the roles of health care providers such as nurses and midwives, the involvement of government in health care through public health and other programs, and the history of social issues such as abortion, sexually transmitted diseases, and the use of narcotic drugs. While this new research has greatly enlarged our understanding of the history of medicine, most of it concerns issues that became significant only at the end of the nineteenth century. Thus, these studies extend rather than supplant the research in this book.

The major area in which the findings of this book have been revised by subsequent research concerns medical education in the nineteenth century. While this book emphasized the proprietary and profit-making aspects of nineteenth-century medical schools, my subsequent research has revealed that the faculty members of medical schools were the nation's leading physicians and provided the best possible education for their students. My work and that of other scholars also found that medical education extended beyond medical schools to include classroom and clinical instruction at hospitals, dispensaries, and private courses. (These findings and many other developments in American medicine up to the present are described in William G. Rothstein, *American Medical Schools and the Practice of Medicine: A History* [New York: Oxford University Press, 1987].)

Although most recent research in the history of medicine has opened impressive new vistas in the field, a few trends have been less satisfactory. I tried to demonstrate in this book that the state of medical care in any era depends fundamentally on the body of medical knowledge used by health care providers and accepted by the public. I also endeavored to show that the patterns of adoption of new developments in medicine were complex and often lengthy processes that depended on a host of scientific, social, economic, and institutional factors.

Recent medical historians who have pursued the social aspects of medical history have tended to de-emphasize the relationship between medical knowledge and medical care. For example, nursing developed at a time when physicians could no longer provide by themselves the full range of care required by new developments in medicine and surgery. Yet few studies of nursing history have explained exactly how nurses cared for patients and for what conditions the public considered professional nursing to be superior to lay nursing. Similarly, the growing number of hospitals at the end of the century provided care for particular diseases and injuries, but few studies have explained why patients preferred hospital care in some diseases and home care in others or analyzed the impact of these preference on hospitals and health care providers.

A second problem has been the assumption that most important medical innovations have been so decisive that they should have been adopted immediately, and, based on this assumption, the criticism of those who failed to adopt them. I tried to show in this book that even great innovations are rife with contradictions and uncertainties when they are introduced. For example, the early literature on diphtheria antitoxin, which was a momentous advance in the treatment of a deadly disease, was filled with unconvincing and often flawed research by supporters of the antitoxin and persuasive arguments and plausible statistics by its opponents. As I read this literature, I found myself sympathizing with the many physicians who were confused and unclear about how to proceed. Hindsight is a poor guide to the study of medicine in any historical period.

Students interested in exploring recent research in all aspects of the history of medicine, which now includes many historical studies of the twentieth century, should consult the *Bibliography of the History of Medicine,* the most comprehensive listing of publications in the field. It contains listings by subject and by author of books, journal articles, and other types of publications that cover all historical periods and all areas of the world. It is published in annual and five-year cumulative editions by the National Library of Medicine and is available in nearly all health sciences libraries and many college and university libraries.

Two scholarly journals that publish numerous articles on the history of American medicine are the *Bulletin of the History of Medicine* and the *Journal of the History of Medicine.* Many other medical journals and some historical journals also publish articles in the field.

The Use of This Book as a Text

Chapter 1 of *American Physicians in the Nineteenth Century* is intended to provide a theoretical framework for issues in the history of medicine, and is addressed primarily to scholars. Students surveying the history of nineteenth-century medicine may therefore want to begin their reading of this book with Chapter 2, "Prologue: The Colonial Period." Chapter 1 may then be read as a conclusion.

PREFACE

THE STUDY of the history of medicine has three major focuses—the body of medical knowledge, the state of health of the populace, and the physicians who used medical knowledge to treat patients—each of which can be the subject of detailed historical analysis. Medical historians traditionally have taken as their focal point the body of medical knowledge, and particularly the growth and development of scientifically valid medical knowledge. A second, less common, focus is the study of the state of health of the populace, by means of such topics as epidemiology and public health.[1] The third focal point is the actual behavior of physicians and their institutions; this approach has been used in the numerous biographies of individual physicians and individual medical institutions, but less often in studies of medical institutions generally or of physicians as members of a profession.

This study is a history of nineteenth-century physicians as an occupational group. It focuses on their medical knowledge, their institutions, and their relations with patients. Its perspective is thus somewhat different from that used by most medical historians. Developments in medical science during the nineteenth-century that had no practical significance for the nineteenth-century physician will not be examined here, regardless of their significance for the twentieth-century physician. Conversely, medical knowledge which the nineteenth-century physician accepted and used will be examined in detail, even though the twentieth-century physician has rejected most of it. Epidemics, public health, patient care, and other questions of similar significance will be examined in this study only in terms of their significance for the nineteenth-century physician. Furthermore, this study will not emphasize the attitudes and beliefs of the few outstanding

[1] George Rosen, "People, Disease and Emotion," *Bulletin of the History of Medicine* 41 (1967): 9.

leaders of the profession who have been the subject of so much biographical research, but rather will examine the behavior of the majority of the professionally trained physicians. Thus, this study differs in several important respects from most others in the history of medicine.

At the same time, however, it should not be thought that the physicians described in this study constituted the lower ranks of the profession. No one who has read the comments of the leaders of the profession about their least competent colleagues or who has perused the truly third-rate medical journals of the period—of which there were many—can avoid feeling astonished at the abysmal ignorance, bizarre practices, and general incompetence of the lower ranks of the profession. The physicians described in this study were, if anything, above average as a group: they attended the better medical schools, read the best medical journals, belonged to medical societies, were acquainted with new discoveries, and in general constituted the bulwark of the reputable medical profession of the nineteenth century.

The writer has benefited from the assistance of numerous persons in the process of writing this book. His colleague, Dr. Benjamin Kleinberg, kindly read and commented on several chapters of the manuscript. His library research was aided by the cordial and sympathetic cooperation of the inter-library loan staff of the library of the University of Maryland Baltimore County, particularly Miss Suzanne Kemp, Mrs. Virginia Loovis, and Mrs. Marjorie Davis. The staff of the library of the Medical and Chirurgical Faculty of Maryland, especially the librarian Mrs. Elizabeth Sanford, were most helpful and considerate. The writer also made extensive use of the William H. Welch Library of the Medical Institution of Johns Hopkins University, and would like to express his appreciation to its staff. The manuscript was typed by Mrs. Laura Justus and others to whom the writer is indebted. Miss Kathleen Coogan cheerfully and patiently assisted the writer in several time-consuming tasks. Mrs. Linda Vlasak often went far beyond her role as copy editor and provided the writer with encouragement and much valuable assistance. Last, the writer would like to thank all his colleagues who took such sincere interest in the study and gracefully tolerated the writer's preoccupation with it.

PART I METHOD OF ANALYSIS
AND COLONIAL ANTECEDENTS

SOCIOLOGY AT PRESENT faces two opposite dangers—the danger of becoming ultra-theoretical and the danger of becoming ultra-empirical. The first is the danger of losing itself in abstract and meaningless generalizations about society in general. Society with a big S is as misleading a fallacy as History with a big H.... The other danger is ... the attempt to avoid generalization and interpretation by confining oneself to so-called "technical" problems of enumeration and analysis [which] is merely to become the unconscious apologist of a static society. Sociology, if it is to become a fruitful field of study, must, like history, concern itself with the relation between the unique and the general. But it must also become dynamic—a study not of society at rest (for no such society exists), but of social change and development. For the rest, I would only say that the more sociological history becomes, and the more historical sociology becomes, the better for both. Let the frontier between them be kept wide open for two way traffic.

EDWARD HALLETT CARR

CHAPTER 1 PLAN OF ANALYSIS

INTRODUCTION

IN RECENT YEARS, historical analysis—the study of social phenomena over a period of time, rather than simply the study of the social phenomena of a previous time—has become uncommon in sociological research, despite its long and distinguished tradition in the discipline.[1] This trend is unfortunate for several reasons. Historical analysis provides the sociologist with a major variable lacking in much sociological research: time. The examination of events over time enables the sociologist to move beyond simple correlations toward the search for causes that is, hopefully, the goal of sociological exploration. Historical analysis is of particular value to the sociologist studying institutions. It enables him to analyze institutions, not as static entities, but as variables changing in response to changes in more basic social forces. Extended historical analysis permits institutional changes to be related not only to proximate causes but also to more fundamental social forces which manifest themselves over relatively long periods of time. Thus the student of institutional behavior in particular can find in historical research a suitable vehicle for the analysis of institutional change in a broader social context.

At the same time, the sociological analysis of institutional behavior has much to contribute to historical research. The historian as well as the sociologist can benefit from the advantages of the study of institutions: their reflection of the needs and interests of their members, their significance for interpersonal and intergroup relations, and their mediating role between the individual and the larger society. The

[1] For a similar observation, see Barrington Moore, Jr., *Political Power and Social Theory* (Cambridge, Mass.: Harvard University Press, 1958), p. 123. The epigraph for Part I is taken from Edward Hallett Carr, *What is History?* (New York: A. Knopf, 1962), pp. 83–84.

state of institutions—particularly over moderately long periods of time —is a manifestation of the needs and interests of their members, who would not invest their resources, time, effort, and commitment without obtaining correspondingly valuable personal returns. If men are dissatisfied with the state of their institutions, they will alter or, in the extreme case, abandon them. They will not burden themselves indefinitely with institutional forms whose personal costs are not compensated by commensurate personal benefits. Furthermore, men seeking social change or engaged in social conflict are likely to rely on institutions (especially formal institutions) which can mobilize and multiply individual or unorganized effort. Thus, an examination of salient institutions is likely to reveal much about social change and social conflict in any period. The study of institutional behavior is advantageous not only because men prefer organized effort in certain situations, but also because institutional behavior is readily accessible to the researcher. Institutional behavior manifests itself in legal codes, institutional organization and composition, relations among institutions or between institutions and the state, and in the rise and fall of institutions. These substantive and methodological advantages make institutional behaviorism valuable for historical as well as sociological research.

This study is a historical analysis of the major institutions of medical practice in the nineteenth century—the independent practitioner, the medical society, the medical school, and the licensing system. It endeavors to examine changes in these institutions as responses to two major causal forces—the body of medical knowledge used by physicians at any given time and the economic interests of physicians in earning a livelihood.

The nineteenth century is a particularly appropriate period in which to study the independent effects of these causal forces on medical institutions. While the body of medical knowledge changed little in the first half of the nineteenth century, the economic interests of physicians changed considerably. Large numbers of men became professionally trained physicians and sought to earn a livelihood by practicing medicine. Their economic interests in earning a livelihood led them to organize medical societies and medical schools, to seek licensing legislation from state governments, and to standardize their relations with patients. In the second half of the century, the economic interests of physicians stabilized, but the body of medical knowledge increased abruptly. The innovations in medical knowledge caused new and independent changes in the institutions which physicians had established in the first half of the century. Thus the nineteenth century provides

ample material for examining separately the effects of economic interests and the body of medical knowledge on medical institutions.

The measurement of changes in medical institutions and in scientific and economic forces is a matter of major concern in any study of
this kind. One advantage of studying institutions is the ease of measurement of some institutional changes. The number of medical societies, the rate of growth of medical schools, the enactment and repeal
of licensing legislation—all these can be examined quantitatively, at
least to a degree sufficient to establish a demonstrable and objective
basis for analysis. The causal economic and scientific forces are more
difficult to quantify; these must be examined in a more qualitative
manner, using available data to measure the medical knowledge of
physicians, the rate of adoption of new developments in therapeutics,
the popularity of patients' alternatives to physicians, etc. In many
cases, contemporary observers must be relied on, but in some instances,
particularly toward the end of the nineteenth century, more quantita-
tive measures are available.

Establishing a relationship between causal forces and institutional
changes is also a major problem. Although it is possible to establish a
chronological relationship between changes in the postulated forces
and changes in medical institutions, it is impossible to prove a causal
relationship in any historical analysis. This is because it is impossible
to isolate and manipulate the relevant variables while either randomiz-
ing or controlling all the other pertinent variables. Indeed, the word
"proof" has little significance in historical research,[2] and the historical
researcher must perforce be content with the demonstration rather
than the proof of causal relationships.

There are several potential sources for a conceptual and theoretical framework for this analysis. The study of the history of medicine
has itself had a long and productive past. Studies of American medical
history, however, are often inadequate as sources for a theoretical
framework. For one thing, they usually take the form of biographies of
famous American physicians or histories of individual medical societies, medical schools, geographic regions, or some aspect of the development of medical science. This fragmentation hinders systematic analysis
of the effects of economic and scientific forces on medical institutions
or of relations among different medical institutions. Studies of the
development of medical science rarely describe how new advances in

[2] For a discussion of causality in this context, see Hubert M. Blalock, Jr.,
Causal Inferences in Nonexperimental Research (Chapel Hill: University of North
Carolina Press, 1961), p. 12–13.

medicine affect medical societies, and studies of medical societies seldom examine their relations with medical schools.[3]

A second limitation of studies in American medical history is that they tend to examine developments in medical science and changes in medical institutions without reference to the behavior of the individual physicians involved. With respect to developments in medical science, Erwin Ackerknecht has remarked:

... the medical history we read and write today is still based mostly on the *writings* of an *elite* of medical men. We are primarily students of scientific literature. Excellent as this may be, it teaches us relatively little concerning what this elite actually *did*, and even less of what the average physician or surgeon did. ...

I would suggest calling the approach I am here pleading for the "behavorist" approach. . . , [a] more extensive and more critical analysis of what doctors *did* in addition to what they *thought* and *wrote*.[4]

In addition to emphasizing the ideas rather than the behavior of physicians, medical historians have tended to impute motives and ascribe behavior to the medical profession generally, without reference to the needs and interests of individual physicians. Carr's observation that a society cannot be treated as a reified, acting agent applies equally to a profession. A profession does not have economic interests to further or patients to treat; only individual physicians have these, and an adequate explanation must show how changes in economic and scientific forces affect the interests and behavior of individual physicians.[5]

A third limitation of studies of American medical history is the

[3] This, the writer believes, is an observation made by Oscar Handlin in his "Foreword" to Daniel H. Calhoun, *Professional Lives in America* (Cambridge, Mass.: Harvard University Press, 1965), p. vii.

[4] Erwin H. Ackerknecht, "A Plea for a 'Behavorist' Approach in Writing the History of Medicine," *Journal of the History of Medicine and Allied Sciences* 22 (1967): 211, 214. In a somewhat similar vein, a sociologist has written: "Most historians of medicine have been concerned solely with documenting discoveries of those isolated bits of information that we now consider to be scientifically true. . . . the historian is inclined to pass through the centuries picking out the 'valid' elements of medical knowledge and assembling a chronology of truths that add up to become present-day scientific medicine. In such histories, particularly when they are inflamed by undetached conceptions of the dignity and glory of medicine, it is difficult to perceive that in the past (as in the present), the individually discovered truths were often embedded in and undiscriminated from a mass of ineffectual or even harmful procedures. . . . they fail to communicate how inadequate and how radically different from today the everyday work of the practitioner was." Eliot Freidson, *Profession of Medicine* (New York: Dodd, Mead, 1970), p. 13.

[5] This view, known as "methodological individualism" among some philosophers of history, has been examined in some detail in George C. Homans, *The Nature of Social Science* (New York: Harcourt, Brace and World, 1967), pp. 35–75.

opinion of some medical historians that one group of physicians, called "regular physicians," has alone nurtured the seed of medical science when medical science was virtually nonexistent, has alone cultivated its growth until it began to blossom, and therefore alone merits the fruit of praise and honor for its efforts. According to this view, other groups—like the botanics, eclectics, and homeopaths—either retarded the growth of medical science or, at best, watched it skeptically and disapprovingly. Whether a direct lineal progenitor of scientific medicine can be traced exclusively to a single group of medical practitioners is a question to which much of this study will be devoted.

The writings of a number of sociologists provide another source for a theoretical framework for this study.[6] Although different authors stress different aspects of professions, and although there is some disagreement among various authors, one core model appears frequently in the sociological literature. This core model depicts a profession as a community held together by shared norms and values which emphasize self-denying service to others and loyalty of professionals to their professional community. Members of the profession learn these norms and values through the socialization process which is part of their professional education. According to the model, professional institutions serve to strengthen the communal aspects of professions by making professionals dependent on their colleagues, rather than on their clients, for the major rewards of professions, which are considered to be prestige and career advancement. Because professions practice service to others at the expense of self-interest and because they regulate themselves through their own institutions, society gives them a greater degree of autonomy than it gives to other occupations.

It is not possible to undertake a detailed examination of this model here, partly because of the limitations of space and partly because of the difficulty of juxtaposing it into the historical narrative.[7] Nonetheless, several observations can be made about the limitations of this model in the context of this study. First, it fails to provide for the influence of clients and economic forces on professional behavior: as long as physicians derive their incomes from their clients, clients have a great deal to say about the behavior of physicians, independ-

6 Two useful descriptions of a popular model, taken from the large number written, are to be found in William J. Goode, "Community Within a Community: The Professions," *American Sociological Review* 22 (1957): 194–200; and Bernard Barber, "Some Problems in the Sociology of Professions," *Daedalus* 92 (1963): 669–88.

7 The writer has examined the model in greater detail with respect to engineers. See William G. Rothstein, "Engineers and the Functionalist Model of Professions," in *The Engineers and the Social System*, Robert Perrucci and Joel E. Gerstl, eds. (New York: Wiley, 1969), pp. 73–98.

ently of the physicians' colleagues.[8] Second, the model fails to deal with the conflicting interests among the various groups and institutions in a profession: for example, medical societies and medical schools do not have the same interests, and there is frequent conflict between them.[9] Third, the model fails to examine in any detail institutional change in professions—a major aspect of this study.[10] Fourth, like many writings in American medical history, the model tends to reify professions and treat them as historical actors when in fact professions per se cannot undertake the actions attributed to them. These issues, although not discussed explicitly throughout this study, are implicit in it, and the interested reader is invited to evaluate this model in light of the data presented in this study.

To overcome the limitations inherent in the above models, it was necessary to develop a new conceptual framework with which to analyze professional behavior. The remainder of this chapter will present this framework and briefly outline the plan of analysis for the study.

MODEL OF ANALYSIS

The model to be developed in this study consists of a number of definitions, a general axiomatic framework, and several specific hypotheses. The enumeration of hypotheses is not intended to make the data presented here more systematic or scientific than they otherwise would be; rather it is an attempt to make explicit the author's intentions. It is also intended to offer future students of the subject an opportunity to relate their findings to those presented here in terms of these general statements about the behavior of physicians.

A profession can be defined as a manner of earning a livelihood through the application of a body of highly abstract knowledge in some set of institutions. This definition implies that physicians, like all other professionals, are motivated largely by economic needs because they have no significant alternatives for income, that they are constrained in their behavior by competitors and by the body of knowledge available to them, and that the institutions they develop are ways of dealing with these motivations and constraints. Each of these elements will be examined in turn.

8 For a discussion emphasizing the role of clients in contemporary medical practice, see Eliot Freidson, "Client Control and Medical Practice," *American Journal of Sociology* 65 (1960): 374–82.

9 This point has also been made in Rue Bucher and Anselm Strauss, "Professions in Process," *American Journal of Sociology* 66 (1961): 325–34.

10 The argument has been made elsewhere that models of this type, called functionalist models, fail to examine institutional change and institutional development generally. See George C. Homans, "Bringing Men Back In," *American Sociological Review* 29 (1964): 809–18.

THE BODY OF MEDICAL KNOWLEDGE

In order to understand the body of medical knowledge used by physicians, it is necessary to define a number of important dimensions of medical science. Two dimensions have general application to the others: demonstrability and consistency. *Demonstrability* refers to the degree to which medically significant phenomena can be measured objectively. For example, there is a marked difference in demonstrability between a diagnosis of tuberculosis based on a few external symptoms and a diagnosis based on a bacteriological analysis which isolates the tubercle bacillus. *Consistency* refers to the predictability with which an event will recur, given the delineation of the circumstances preceding and surrounding the event. For example, if a drug reduces fever in one patient, increases it in another, and has no effect at all on a third, and if the physician cannot predict which patient will undergo which change, it can be classified as a wholly inconsistent therapy.

Diagnosis refers to the ability of a physician to determine the nature of the pathological condition of a patient. The lack of demonstrable and consistent diagnosis often made it impossible to treat a patient effectively in the nineteenth century. For example, quinine was known to be an excellent palliative for malaria, but because physicians had great difficulty in diagnosing malaria, they were frequently unable to use quinine effectively.

Medical prophylaxis means the prevention of disease through the use of demonstrable and consistent medical treatment, like smallpox vaccination. This can be compared with other forms of prophylaxis, like the use of fresh fruit or vegetables to prevent scurvy. The small number of demonstrable and consistent medical prophylactics that were discovered before the end of the nineteenth century made prophylaxis an unimportant part of the professional activities of physicians during that period. Nonetheless, physicians' acceptance of demonstrable and consistent prophylactics can be used to estimate the nature of their professional knowledge.

Therapy is the treatment of disease by the physician through either palliation or cure. The most important forms of therapy used by physicians in the nineteenth century were drugs and surgery. The medical value of therapies varies along a continuum from a high degree of therapeutic value with practically no side effects to a low degree of therapeutic value with dangerous side effects. In order to minimize any possible misinterpretation of the behavior of physicians, this study will emphasize therapies at the two extremes, which will be called *medically valid* and *medically invalid* therapies respectively.[11] Early in the nineteenth century, there were few medically valid therapies, but after the middle of the century, major discoveries which were made in many areas of medical science augmented the physician's ability to treat his patients effectively.

The body of medical knowledge used by practicing physicians in the nineteenth century was concerned with the diagnosis and individual clinical treatment over a period of time of physiologically pathological states of the human organism.[12] Physicians also used medical knowledge concerning the prevention of disease, but only when it involved individual medical prophylaxis. Thus, for example, many physicians were involved in the promulgation of smallpox vaccination, but only a small number participated in the movement advocating sanitary measures for the prevention of tuberculosis. The theoretical and experimental aspects of medicine rarely concerned nineteenth-century physicians, who emphasized medical knowledge which had immediate significance for clinical medical practice.

While relations between clients and physicians will be examined in this study only in terms of nineteenth-century medical therapeutics, some medical historians have argued that the nineteenth-century physician benefited his patients in non-medical ways. The physician enhanced the likelihood of his patient's recovery by inspiring him with hope and confidence. The therapeutic value of hope and confidence exists solely because of the patient's faith in the physician. Therefore, any practitioner who inspires faith in his patients is the physician's equal in this regard. Indeed, lay healers, faith healers, Indian doctors, nostrum vendors, and the whole range of practitioners who relied largely on their charismatic qualities for their success were probably more successful than most physicians in inspiring hope and confidence in their patients. It must be concluded that the ability to inspire confidence is characteristic to some degree of all medical practitioners sought out by clients, and cannot be used to differentiate physicians from other practitioners.

EARNING A LIVELIHOOD

Medical practice is a profession insofar as it provides the major source of the livelihood of physicians. This study will be limited to an examination of those physicians who earn their livelihood directly from

[11] The concepts of consistency and therapeutic validity used here have been based to some degree on the statistical concepts of reliability and validity, although no exact parallel is intended. Definitions of statistical reliability and validity can be found in any social science statistics textbook.
[12] This study will not examine psychiatric medicine.

clients' fees on a case by case basis, rather than from salaries or other forms of earnings.[13] In seeking to earn a livelihood in this way, a physician must attract clients in competition with other practitioners and patent medicines, and he must do so by means of the existing medical knowledge available to him. Each physician thus has certain economic and scientific constraints which limit his ability to satisfy his economic needs. The economic constraints consist of the competition from other medical practitioners and from self-medication accessible to his clients. The scientific constraints consist of the extent to which a physician's medical knowledge and technical skill enable him to dispense treatments which his clients could neither provide themselves nor obtain from his competitors. These constraints are largely beyond the control of the individual physician. He has virtually no influence over the number and location of other medical practitioners or pharmacists with whom he must compete for clients. Medical knowledge is the result of the cumulative efforts of men all over the world whose contributions are promulgated with extraordinary rapidity wherever numbers of trained physicians are found. The medical knowledge available to any one physician is thus no greater or less than that available to his competitors. Technical skill is the only significant differentiating factor over which an individual physician has some degree of personal control, and it is useful only to the degree that clients are familiar with his work. The independent practitioner, therefore, is placed in a situation where he has very limited control over his ability to earn a living when acting alone.

In earning a livelihood, physicians are brought into regular and routinized relations with both clients and colleagues. Patterned sets of relations in which participants have mutual expectations for each other's behavior are known as "institutions," and the participants in them as "roles." Institutions can consist of roles either related to each other formally, as in a medical society in which each participant has a role defined in the rules of the organization, or related informally, as when each participant has a role defined in terms of relatively vague and poorly defined social norms and values. Informal institutions suffer from a lack of adequate mechanisms to insure conformity of the participants to their roles, sometimes because the roles themselves are not adequately defined and sometimes because few effective sanctions can be imposed on deviants.

Because of the ease with which the participants in informal institu-

---

[13] Different modes of compensation will affect the behavior of physicians in different ways. For a discussion of the effects of different modes of compensation in the twentieth century, see William A. Glaser, *Paying the Doctor* (Baltimore: Johns Hopkins Press, 1970).

tions can violate their roles, physicians would like to formalize institutional relations with both clients and colleagues to regulate their behavior, even though in so doing the individual physician must himself give up some of his independence. Relations between a physician and a client are not readily formalized however, because while a client has considerable influence over a physician through his fees, the physician has no reciprocal influence over his client, who can dispense with the physician's services at will. Thus clients have disproportionate power in the relationship and need not accept restraints imposed by individual physicians. Relations among physicians, on the other hand, can be formalized to the degree that reciprocal dependence exists among the physicians involved, and in those instances medical societies are usually formed. If relations among all or most physicians in a community are formalized in some way, the physicians collectively can exert considerable influence over their clients.

Medical practice as a profession could be successful on a large-scale basis only under two conditions. First, enough clients with enough wealth to support a physician had to reside in a geographic area small enough for the physician to treat all his clients readily. This process of urbanization occurred throughout the nineteenth century and was responsible for much of the growth of the medical profession. Second, professional physicians had to offer services to patients that were demonstrably and consistently superior to those offered by other medical practitioners or to those obtainable by self-medication. Because this did not occur during the first half of the century, other medical practitioners increased proportionately with physicians. The relative importance of physicians in providing medical services increased only after specialization and bacteriology enabled them to offer services to patients that were demonstrably superior to those available elsewhere.

Where institutionalization occurs, it is possible to make predictions about the behavior of the parties to an institutional relationship. Therefore, for each important institution in nineteenth-century medical practice, an effort will be made to identify and describe predictable patterns of behavior and the economic and scientific constraints which affect the behavior. The institutions to be examined are: the independent practitioner, the medical society, the medical school, and the licensing of physicians.

THE INSTITUTION OF THE INDEPENDENT PRACTITIONER

Clients in the nineteenth century tended to employ physicians only when, through self-diagnosis, they perceived the need for medical treatment. They sought out independent practitioners and paid them for individual clinical treatment of their ailments. As a result, medical practice developed as a form of self-employment, in which the physician received his earnings from fees obtained for services rendered on a voluntary case-by-case basis. Physicians in the nineteenth century competed for the patient's dollar not only with other physicians, but also with lay and part-time practitioners, who frequently charged less than physicians and provided serious competition for them during much of the period.

The structuring of practice along these lines made physicians particularly sensitive to the whims and self-diagnosed problems of the patient. A patient wants to be cured of his illness, relieved of his discomfort, and receive proper value for his payments to the physician. If the patient feels he is not receiving adequate treatment from a physician, he can and is likely to seek out other physicians, other practitioners, or patent medicines. It may be hypothesized that *extensive competition from other physicians, other practitioners, and/or other forms of medical treatment (e.g., patent medicines) causes physicians to adopt readily those medically valid therapies which can be administered on a demonstrable and consistent basis.* Physicians who do not adopt medically valid therapies will be at a disadvantage in attracting patients relative to their competitors who do adopt them, because patients will tend to patronize those physicians who offer the best treatment.

In the absence of medically valid therapies, it may be hypothesized that *extensive competition from other physicians, other practitioners, and/or other forms of medical treatment causes physicians to use therapies which produce demonstrable and consistent short-run palliative changes in the patient's condition.* In this way, physicians can show patients that they are doing something to earn their fees even if they cannot cure the patients. It is important to realize that such palliative treatment may not be the most medically valid treatment for the patient. Bed rest and patience may well be the best advice that a physician can give patients with some kinds of illnesses, but competitive pressures induce the physician to provide palliative therapy nonetheless.

An examination of medical therapeutics in the nineteenth century will attempt to demonstrate these hypotheses. It will be shown that, despite their ignorance of the reasons why medically valid therapies were effective, physicians adopted therapies like vaccination and quinine with remarkable rapidity when they could be administered on a demonstrable and consistent basis. Toward the end of the century, despite their opposition to bacteriology generally, physicians adopted its therapeutic by-products with similar rapidity. In those illnesses where medically valid therapies were lacking, physicians tended to pursue a course of active therapy, often dosing the patient with dangerous and toxic palliatives which did more harm than good. For example, throughout the century, physicians endeavored to reduce fever and relieve pain by using treatments which in the short run achieved the desired objective, but in the long run produced serious side effects.

Specialization. The hypotheses advanced above with regard to medically valid therapies must be qualified. Even when medically valid therapies exist, all physicians may not be able to use them. The therapies may be so complex that they require considerable specialized training for proper administration; they may change so rapidly that continuous study is essential: they may, in short, be beyond the capabilities of the general practitioner and require full-time specialization. Under these circumstances, it may be hypothesized that *a significant difference between the ability of specialists and general practitioners to use medically valid therapies and the existence of a sufficiently large demand for the therapies will cause some physicians to specialize on a full-time basis.* The additional training involved in specialization requires considerable expense, time, and ability, and these constraints will tend to limit the supply of specialists. When the supply is restricted in this way, specialists will be able to charge proportionately higher fees and restrict their practice to an upper-class clientele.

Stratification. The differentiation among physicians in terms of clientele is another major characteristic of independent practitioners. *The patronage of a wealthy and influential clientele will cause physicians to amass greater wealth, power, and social position in the profession than their colleagues who lack such patronage.* A wealthy and influential clientele provides a physician with greater income, greater influence in institutions like hospitals and medical schools that are regulated and partly supported by laymen, and greater influence among his colleagues who can benefit from referrals of and consultations concerning his patients. It has been observed that specialists are more likely to have a wealthy clientele than other practitioners, and therefore they will tend to be the leaders of the profession.

These hypotheses will be examined throughout the study. It will be shown that specialization did not develop in medicine until medically valid diagnostic and therapeutic procedures were developed that could not be used by general practitioners. Once specialization did develop, specialists rapidly attained a position of unrivaled wealth and power in the profession. Prior to that time, the highest stratum in the profession was composed of the best educated (often educated in

Europe) physicians, who resided in the largest cities and had the wealthiest clients.

PROFESSIONAL SOCIETIES

Writers on professional societies have often alleged that members of the same profession have some inherent or instinctive fraternal propensity to organize themselves in professional societies. The attribution of professional organizations to collegial affection is inadequate to explain such questions as the rate of growth of professional organizations, the different and varied kinds of professional organizations in the same profession, and any absence of organization in a profession. A more useful approach must look instead to those sets of rewards offered to members of professional organizations that sufficiently offset the basically competitive nature of the relationship among physicians to make professional organizations viable and stable. Two kinds of rewards are especially important—prestige and the regulation of economic competition.

Some associations of physicians can provide their members with a most valuable and commercially desirable commodity—prestige. It is no mean thing to be associated in professional fellowship with a group of illustrious colleagues, and it can be a considerable advantage in soliciting clients, obtaining appointments to hospitals and medical schools, etc. These *exclusive societies* are meaningful in two kinds of situations. Where there are many lay practitioners and the boundary line between them and the professional physicians is poorly defined (as in a situation where no licensing system exists), exclusive societies serve to differentiate the two groups. Where the profession itself is heterogeneous, exclusive societies serve to differentiate some physicians from others. Therefore, it may be hypothesized that *either (1) a high degree of heterogeneity among physicians in terms of the amount and nature of professional training, social class of clientele, or specialization, or (2) the absence of well defined boundaries between professional physicians and other medical practitioners will cause physicians to form exclusive societies.*

The physicians who form and join exclusive societies are those who benefit most from mutual association in terms of appointments to medical schools and hospitals, referrals and consultations with affluent patients, political influence, etc. It may be hypothesized that *the desire of members of exclusive societies to maximize their influence, prestige, and opportunities for additional income will cause them to limit membership to physicians who have high status in the profession in terms of the characteristics necessary to achieve such ends.* Exclusive societies which differentiate physicians from other practitioners will be less restrictive in their membership policies than those which differentiate some physicians from others, but in either case higher-status physicians will constitute the membership of exclusive societies.

Exclusive societies suffer from two major dilemmas. First, an exclusive medical society has no control over non-members, who, if they are envious of the society, will tend to form their own competing societies. Thus individual rivalries are replaced by organized conflict, a phenomenon which often has deleterious consequences. Second, exclusive societies are bound by the very nature of the organization to define every member as worthy and every non-member as less than worthy, even though the society may have some misfits and some eminent men may be excluded because of personal rivalries with members or for other reasons. To concede the exclusion of qualified physicians would cause the public to doubt the organization's ability to select its membership wisely. Interestingly enough, these points were recognized in 1769 by an ex-member of one of America's first medical societies, who attacked the society in these words:

> . . . if any regular practitioner in the county should upon the whole, think it not best to join with the corporation, etc. he must be discountenanced, and all the injury possible done him, so far as the influence of the corporation can extend, but another that has no other qualification to recommend him, but only that he has join'd the medical club, must be carest, and recommended to mankind as an able physician, when he scarcely knows the difference between a Bagpipe and a Glysterpipe [a tube through which enemas were administered]. . . .[14]

Inclusive societies, which are open to virtually all qualified physicians in a community, minimize the problems of factionalism and personal animosities, but they also eliminate the prestige value of membership in the society. In compensation for this loss, they offer their members other benefits. By obtaining the membership of all physicians in a community, inclusive medical societies can regulate, under certain conditions, medical services through "fee bills" (lists of minimum charges for specified services) and codes of ethics and etiquette. They can also maximize the influence of the profession in dealings with governments and other relevant organizations.

The major problem of inclusive societies is the delineation of membership qualifications. Why should an inclusive society exclude graduates of bogus or substandard medical schools, self-educated physicians, midwives, nurses, or pharmacists? This problem can be solved

[14] Byron Stookey, "Found! The Record of the 1767 Medical Society in Litchfield," *Connecticut State Medical Journal* 21 (1957): 347.

only when the state licenses physicians in a manner which effectively limits professional activities to physicians, and therefore establishes a finite and bounded potential membership. Consequently, inclusive medical societies are forced to place the evaluation of candidates for membership in the hands of governmental officials whose judgments are accepted by the society. The society's lack of formal control over its own membership policies is exemplified by the ability of the government licensing agency to change the criteria for obtaining a license without the approval of the society. Historically, effective licensing procedures were established only in the twentieth century, and inclusive medical societies date from that time.

It should not be thought that inclusive societies are always large and exclusive societies always small. In periods without effective licensing systems, exclusive medical societies functioned as informal licensing agencies in the profession and often became quite large. Nonetheless, the difference between the two was that exclusive societies always maintained an examining committee, called a "board of censors," which evaluated applicants for membership on the basis of rather subjective criteria. Inclusive societies, on the other hand, accepted practically all qualified candidates on the basis of outside evaluation by the licensing agency, and opponents of a candidate were forced to demonstrate that he was unworthy of membership.

Both types of medical societies share similar concerns in some areas. Neither wishes to see desirable members remain outside the organization, and both wish to regulate the behavior of their members in certain areas. The success of the societies in achieving these goals can be hypothesized as follows: *high dependence of physicians on the economic rewards of membership in professional societies and/or high susceptibility of non-members to economic deprivations will cause physicians to accept membership in and conform to the regulations imposed on members by the medical societies.*

Exclusive societies depend primarily on the rewards of membership to control the behavior of members; inclusive societies induce conformity primarily by depriving non-members of participation in essential activities. The difference can be illustrated by several common activities of mutual benefit to physicians. Serving on the faculty of a medical school brings a physician much business and income he would otherwise forgo. However, medical-school faculties in the nineteenth century were small, which permitted only a few physicians to serve on a faculty. Thus, this highly desirable reward was useful in controlling the behavior of very few physicians. Opportunities for consultations and referrals were also limited in an era without much specialization. Furthermore, these activities were not absolutely essential to a physician's ability to practice. Therefore, they were useful sanctions only in small exclusive societies. On the other hand, support from one's colleagues in malpractice suits, malpractice insurance, and access to hospital beds for one's patients are essential to a physician's survival, and denial of them would seriously endanger any physician's ability to practice. These are therefore useful sanctions for inclusive societies. Malpractice suits and hospitalization of patients became common only in the twentieth century, which was another reason for the establishment of inclusive societies at that time.

Another consequence of the sanctions associated with society membership can be hypothesized as follows: *The local nature of the market for medical services causes general local societies to be more stable and successful than general societies drawing members from larger geographic areas.* Because physicians compete with each other in a local area, they are most affected by local colleagues. State and national organizations developed later in the nineteenth century than did local societies and usually had more difficulty in establishing themselves. Specialty societies, which have few potential members in any one locality, are not necessarily more successful at the local than at the national level.

MEDICAL SCHOOLS

Education can be considered a product dispensed like other services, and in this study it can best be analyzed in those terms. Medical colleges in the nineteenth century rarely received significant public support and were generally financed wholly out of tuition fees, which was then economically feasible. The physicians who operated medical colleges expected to earn a profit from their ventures, or at least not to support the schools as a financial burden. Furthermore, physicians also expected to derive some prestige in the community from their role as educators, as well as to profit from referrals and consultations from their former students and fellow teachers. In short, physicians who operated medical colleges did so in order to realize certain economic objectives.

Because medical knowledge was limited and unscientific during much of the nineteenth century, most instruction was provided in lecture courses with very little, if any, clinical or laboratory instruction. Consequently, the only essential prerequisites for founding a medical school were a faculty, which was easily obtained from among local practitioners, a lecture hall, and a room for dissections. Furthermore, the only additional cost of expanding the institution was for the additional chairs in the lecture hall. Thus the rate of growth of medical colleges was a useful index of the popularity and rate of growth of the profession, because a school's survival depended solely on its ability to attract students.

When medical knowledge became scientific, it was necessary to incorporate laboratory and clinical work into the curriculum if students were to obtain a practical and useful education. When this occurred, schools were no longer profitable and had to depend on some form of subsidization. This led to the demise of many medical schools, and made the remainder more susceptible to regulation by medical societies and the state.

The relationship between medical colleges and physicians was a hostile one throughout the nineteenth century, a situation brought about by the strikingly different economic interests of the two groups. Physicians were concerned with keeping the profession from being overcrowded, and wanted to keep the number of graduates small. Educators wanted to increase the number of students and graduates as much as possible to augment their incomes. Physicians wanted to use medical students as sources of income and of cheap labor. Under the old apprenticeship system, apprentices paid physicians for their education and also performed many of the tasks now delegated to nurses and pharmacists, but which then were performed by physicians. The schools did not consider bandaging wounds and mixing drugs for physicians to be of primary educational value, and abandoned these elements of medical education.

As a result of these differences, two major issues developed between physicians and medical educators: (1) who shall educate the medical students and how; and (2) who shall decide whether or not a student is competent to enter medical practice by receiving a degree or a license. The resolution of the first issue depended on the relative strength of the medical colleges and physicians. When the colleges had few students and apprenticeship was common, they depended on physicians to send their apprentices to the medical schools for their academic training, and therefore were willing to let physicians exert considerable control over the educational process. When the schools became large and powerful in their own right, they abandoned their relationship with physicians and disregarded them. The second issue between medical educators and physicians concerned the determination of who was competent to practice medicine. This issue can best be understood by examining the role of licensing in the profession.

LICENSING

Licensing can be defined as certification by the state of a member of a profession (or an occupation) who meets certain criteria pertaining to competence to practice that profession. Customarily, but not always, a license provides the practitioner with some legal rights and privileges (in addition to the display of his license) that are denied to unlicensed practitioners. Members of almost all professions are motivated to seek licensing legislation as a means of regulating the supply of labor in their professions. Two major factors affect the ability of the members of a profession to have a licensing system enacted into law. The first concerns whether or not the practice of the profession is amenable to regulation by licensure, and the second concerns whether or not the members of the profession have sufficient political influence relative to other interested groups to have the legislation enacted and enforced.

The effectiveness of licensing laws depends on the nature of medical practice in any period. It can be hypothesized that *the existence of easily identifiable and regulable goods or services restricted by law to licentiates causes licensing to be effective in limiting the supply of those specific goods or services.* For example, dispensing drugs or granting permission to obtain drugs is a major part of the professional activities of the physician. During much of the nineteenth century, the drugs used by physicians were common minerals and local herbs, and the latter often grew wild throughout the regions where they were used. Obviously, it was impossible to enforce legislation permitting only licensed physicians to dispense them. The great drug discoveries in the twentieth century were manufactured by pharmaceutical firms, and it became possible to regulate their sale effectively. Another illustration is the hospital, which was an insignificant part of medical practice during the nineteenth century. Restricting hospital privileges to licensed physicians at that time did not deprive unlicensed physicians of anything they needed to practice medicine. During the twentieth century, when hospitals became an indispensable part of medical care, access to hospitals became vital for physicians and hence strengthened the licensing system.

The ability of physicians to have licensing legislation enacted and enforced depends on the amount of their influence relative to that of groups opposing licensing. During the nineteenth century, groups opposing all licensing legislation or opposing the specific licensing legislation sought by the regular physicians were sufficiently powerful to prevent legislation from being enacted, to dilute the legislation if it was enacted, or to render enforcement almost impossible. By the turn of the century, changes in the relative balance of power of the groups involved and in the type of legislation acceptable to regular physicians made effective licensing legislation possible.

MEDICAL SECTS

One area where medical societies were effective in regulating the behavior of their members was the standardization of therapies. In a period when few medically valid therapies are available, standardization of medically invalid therapies is useful because it reduces therapeutic conflicts among physicians, presents a united front to the physicians' clients, and offers a means of professional validation of therapies through social norms when no objective validation is possible. In this way physicians can attribute their use of particular medically invalid therapies to the carefully considered professional judgment of their colleagues. Standardization is equally useful in both exclusive and inclusive societies; thus a distinctive set of medically invalid therapies, known as "heroic" therapy, was shared by most regular (i.e., regularly educated) physicians of the first half of the century.

Because the standardized system was medically invalid, dissatisfied physicians periodically devised other medically invalid systems which differed from the standardized one. The advocates of the standardized system, including the leaders of the profession, responded to these novel systems in ways varying from receptiveness to ostracism of their proponents, depending on the system proposed. Why such differences in responses should have occurred has always constituted a problem for medical historians. Many historians have argued that the ostracized systems were dogmatic and based on "monistic pathologies" which traced all diseases to single ultimate causes. These historians state that the regular system and other systems accepted by regular physicians were empirical and based on observation and experiment.

This explanation suffers from several weaknesses. All medically invalid systems are dogmatic in their arbitrary selection of pathological symptoms on which to base the system. All are empirical in their concern with producing demonstrable and consistent effects on the patient. A more fundamental criticism of this explanation is that physicians were rarely concerned with the theoretical explanations advanced by the originators of systems. Physicians then as now earned their livelihood by administering therapies to clients, and the most probable source of conflict among them was the therapeutic differences between systems, not the causes of diseases advanced by them.

The question one physician asked of another was not what system of pathology he used, but rather the more practical question—what kind of treatment did he apply in a given situation. Nowhere was this better illustrated than in a popular *vade mecum* of medical practice, written around 1880 by a regular physician, D. W. Cathell. In one section the author discussed consultations between regular physicians and homeopaths, a group of non-regular physicians who advocated the use of very small doses of highly diluted drugs instead of the more drastic palliative treatment of the regular physicians. Cathell stated:

> Imagine an attempt to consult, say, with a Homeopath—patient has, for example, convulsions, the result of teething. You examine the case to- gether and retire for consultation; the subject of treatment is finally reached. You, true to humanity, survey the whole field of rational therapeutics and conclude: first, that the cause should be removed as far as possible by incising the gums for purpose of severing their irritated nerves; second, that sedatives and antispasmodics are indicated. He, true to his creed, puts on his homeopathic spectacles, surveys the totality of symptoms by the square and compass of [his therapeutics] and arrives [at an infinitesimal dose of some highly diluted drug]. . . . Result, emphatically a therapeutic deadlock, unless—false to your profession, and false to the needs of humanity—you agree to give up your sense for [his] nonsense.[15]

Other physicians emphasized that even the fundamental theories of systems were based on inductions from the effects of therapies. One regular physician wrote in 1852:

> The entire profession of medicine may . . . be in accord as to certain facts, but may differ as to the general law influencing these facts. The facts alone are part of the profession. . . . Difference of theory does not necessarily imply difference of treatment; indeed, the treatment of a disease upon which all are agreed, may be one of the facts upon which is founded different theories as to the nature of the disease.[16]

Thus, for all physicians of the period, the theoretical differences among systems were less significant than the therapeutic ones which constituted the major source of conflict among advocates of different systems.

With these observations in mind, it is possible to develop a hypothesis to explain the varying reactions of regular physicians to novel systems. It may be hypothesized that *the espousal in different systems*

---

[15] D. W. Cathell and William T. Cathell, *Book on The Physician Himself* (Philadelphia: Davis, 1902), 11th ed., p. 303.

[16] William Maxwell Wood, *Hints to the People upon the Profession of Medicine* (Buffalo: Derby, 1852), pp. 20–21.

of mutually incompatible, medically invalid therapies which cannot be evaluated objectively, and the existence of a popular demand for the systems' therapies, causes adherents of the conflicting systems to form separate medical societies, medical schools, and other institutions. Only when mutually incompatible therapeutic differences exist between systems do relations among their advocates reach the breaking point. Differences in etiology, pathology, or other aspects of medicine are insufficient to create open conflict among advocates of different systems.

Physicians who adopt different systems and form the related institutions have been called sects, a term which can be defined as follows: *A sect consists of a number of physicians, together with their professional institutions, who utilize medically valid therapies when they exist, but otherwise utilize a distinctive set of medically invalid therapies rejected by other sects.* Sects cannot consist of a few isolated practitioners, because such a definition would be too inclusive to be useful. The definition of a sect also stated that medically valid therapies cannot be used to differentiate sects. The reason for this was hypothesized above. Sectarian physicians depend for their existence on a clientele that is willing to pay for services received, and if members of other sects offer superior services by dispensing medically valid therapies, the sects which refuse to accept them will tend to lose their clientele. This is not to say that members of sects adopt medically valid therapies willingly, or that medically valid therapies are compatible with all of the doctrines of the sects, but rather that physicians are forced by competitive pressures to accept them. Consequently, medically valid therapies tend to be adopted with surprising rapidity, especially considering the accumulated traditions and dogmas which they must overcome. Sects could survive in medicine only so long as medically valid therapies constituted a small part of the therapies used by physicians. Once medically valid therapies became the dominant part of medical practice, medical sectarianism declined markedly.

A major part of this study will be devoted to the rise and fall of sectarianism in medicine. It will be shown that regular physicians adopted sectarian dogmas, that public opposition to their practices enabled several other sects to develop, and that the institutions of the regular sect and two competing sects dominated American medical practice during the second half of the nineteenth century. The regular sect ostracized its competitors in most professional matters involving therapeutics, but in scientific matters like specialization and public health, physicians of all three sects adopted similar practices and cooperated. Ultimately, the additional impact of bacteriology nullified the rationale for sectarianism and the regular physicians abandoned their policy of ostracism at the end of the century.

One other group of practitioners must be defined. These practitioners, called quacks, either rejected medically valid therapies outright or else dispensed fraudulent drugs or medical services. Quacks have usually been nostrum vendors, patent medicine manufacturers, perpetrators of mail fraud through advertising, etc. Quacks rarely organized themselves, probably because each was marketing a unique product. They therefore were clearly distinguished from physicians, and will not be dealt with in this study in any detail.

OTHER CONSIDERATIONS

This study does not attempt to describe the historical role of all medical institutions and the nature of all medical practice in the nineteenth century. Hospitals, for example, played a minor role in nineteenth-century medical practice and will not be discussed here. Regional differences among physicians were important in the nineteenth century (primarily in the rapidity of adoption of innovations), but these will not be discussed either. This study will not discuss the many physicians who never joined medical societies and who were in many respects marginal members of the profession. Because these physicians were influenced by the actions of medical societies and medical colleges in the same way and often to the same degree as their colleagues, this omission is not believed to be a serious one.

Physicians, unlike carpenters or longshoremen, have left behind an extraordinarily large mass of detailed information about themselves in their books and their journals, the latter being the more important source. The use of such information, which constitutes the major source of original data for this study, has certain dangers. Contemporary writers are often so bound up with the issues of the moment that they cannot clearly see the forces behind the issues or the merits of the different positions taken by different groups on the same issue. Nathan Smith Davis, one of the founders of the AMA and one of the most important figures in the American medical profession during the second half of the nineteenth century, stated in 1883: "our minds are so liable to be influenced by such part of the events transpiring in the present as are most nearly related to our own interests, that we find great difficulty in comprehending with equal clearness all the influences at work around us. . . ."[17] It behooves those of us who write

17 N. S. Davis, "Address on the Present Status and Future Tendencies of the Medical Profession in the United States . . . ," *Journal of the American Medical Association* 1 (1883): 33.

history to recognize these human failings of past writers and to analyze their writings in terms of their own interests. We are also obliged to examine the writings of as many different and varied participants as possible in order to obtain their different perspectives. At the same time, we must recall that the writings of these men reflected rather than caused the situations in which they found themselves, and we must endeavor to look beyond the words to the situations which brought the words forth. In this way we can gain a deeper and more lasting insight into the behavior of nineteenth-century physicians and utilize those insights to understand not only nineteenth-century physicians, but physicians of our own time and of other times as well.

CHAPTER 2 PROLOGUE:
THE COLONIAL PERIOD

THIS CHAPTER will examine several aspects of colonial medicine that are particularly important for this study. The first of these is developments in medically valid therapeutics. During the colonial period two important medically valid therapies were discovered: the use of the bark of the cinchona tree in malaria, and inoculation and later cowpox vaccination for smallpox. Another relevant aspect of colonial medical practice was the small number of full-time professionally trained physicians, who practiced almost exclusively in the urban areas. Finally, the colonial American public maintained a skeptical attitude toward the medical profession. This was exemplified by popular reliance on self-medication, especially botanical medicines, by frequent use of other kinds of medical practitioners, and by the lack of any medical licensing legislation which would give physicians control over admission to the profession.

MEDICAL PRACTICE IN THE COLONIAL PERIOD

The great contributions to science made during and after the Renaissance had little impact on colonial medical practice, which changed little from the practices of physicians for centuries before that time. Vesalius's anatomical dissections were a major scientific innovation of the sixteenth century, but their impact on medical practice was negligible, and their impact on surgery was limited by the nonexistence of anesthesia and a means of preventing post-operative sepsis. William Harvey discovered the circulation of the blood in the early seventeenth century, but, according to a well-known late nineteenth-century physician, this discovery failed "to influence medical practice immediately or largely." Harvey himself did not realize the significance of the pulse rate, and only mentioned that it varied from one to four thousand beats per half hour. Furthermore, he did not know why the blood circulated. He surmised that the blood became "thick or congealed by the cold of the extreme and outward parts," and circulated to the heart in order to "receive heat and spirits, and all else requisite to its preservation." He suggested that the blood circulated to the lungs in order to be "prevented from boiling up" because of the heat it received in the heart. Nor did Harvey discover how the blood circulated from the arteries to the veins. Throughout his life he denied the existence of the capillaries which in fact connected them. Thus, although both discoveries contributed to the development of medical science, they required centuries of additional research before they could benefit the physician's daily work.[1]

American colonial medical practice, like European practice of the period, was characterized by the lack of any substantial body of usable scientific medical knowledge. Physicians knew nothing of the role of bacteria or viruses in disease, and therefore lacked even the most rudimentary understanding of infection. They had no valid knowledge of contagion or its vectors. They were unable to diagnose diseases except by observable pathological symptoms like fever or skin eruptions, and therefore grouped completely different diseases under the same name because of some superficially similar symptoms. Their inability to make an accurate diagnosis of a patient's illness also prevented them from testing the effects of therapies scientifically. Physicians used therapies which produced gross physiological changes in the body, like the reduction of fever, without any real knowledge of how that change affected the patient's actual illness.

Nevertheless, by the end of the colonial period, three major medically valid therapies had been developed. The first in order of chronology, surgery, antedated the colonial period by many centuries. While surgeons in the colonial period knew nothing of infection or anesthesia and little of anatomy, they were able to amputate limbs, set dislocations and fractures, remove foreign bodies near the surface of the skin, treat skin diseases like ulcers and inflammations, and cure some diseases of the eye and ear.[2] Many of these procedures were use-

[1] S. Weir Mitchell, "The History of Instrumental Precision in Medicine," *University Medical Magazine* 4 (1891): 7, 13; William Harvey, "An Anatomical Disquisition on the Motion of the Heart and Blood in Animals," in C. N. B. Camac, ed., *Classics of Medicine and Surgery* (New York: Dover, 1959), pp. 94, 64; Walter Pagel, "William Harvey and the Purpose of Circulation," *Isis* 42 (1951): 22–38; Yehuda Elkana and June Goodfield, "Harvey and the Problem of the 'Capillaries'," *Isis* 59 (1968): 61–73.

[2] Owsei Temkin, "The Role of Surgery in the Rise of Modern Medical Thought," *Bulletin of the History of Medicine* 25 (1951): 252. Other developments in the eighteenth century had major implications for disease without involving medical therapeutics. One of the most important was the discovery that scurvy was caused by a deficiency of certain foods, and the consequent use of prophylactic and curative dietary measures.

ful and beneficial; others, like amputations, although dangerous, consistently and demonstrably lowered the probability of death.

CINCHONA BARK

The discovery of the therapeutic value of the bark of the cinchona tree (the source of quinine) in the treatment of malaria was the second major contribution to medical therapeutics. Seventeenth-century European explorers learned of the therapeutic value of the bark in South America, where the tree grew wild. This discovery was significant for American life because malaria was one of the two leading colonial infections (dysentery was the other). Periodic spring and fall outbreaks of malaria occurred in most inhabited areas in the north and south, and sickened large segments of the population. While the death rate from malaria was not high, the recurring attacks debilitated their victims and rendered them more susceptible to other more fatal diseases.[3]

Given the prevalence of the disease, it might be expected that the discovery of the therapeutic value of cinchona bark would be rapidly accepted by colonial physicians and patients alike. This did not occur for two major reasons. First, the drug did not produce consistently useful results because the therapeutic value of the bark varied significantly among the four species of the tree, and exporters did not distinguish among species. A second reason also lay with the problem of consistency, but in this case it was a diagnostic problem. The symptoms of malaria are chills, shaking, and then a high fever which comes and goes in cycles of twenty-four, forty-eight, seventy-two, etc., hours, and leaves the patient bathed in sweat and exhausted each time, although the fever need not abate totally after each paroxysm. Because of the cyclic nature of the fever, malaria was frequently called intermittent fever. While these symptoms may be easily observed, they are not clearly distinguishable from the symptoms of many other fevers. Malaria has no distinctive stigmata, no eruptions, no unique physiological manifestations. Consequently, malaria was not readily distinguished from many other very common fevers of the time, such as typhoid fever. This was true as late as the twentieth century. An 1897 study in Baltimore, Maryland, found that the death rate from typhoid was sixteen times as great as that from malaria in the hospital of The Johns Hopkins University medical school, but that the two were

---

[3] A history of quinine is found in M. L. Duran-Reynals, *The Fever-Bark Tree* (Garden City, N. Y.: Doubleday, 1946); John Duffy, *Epidemics in Colonial America* (Baton Rouge: Louisiana State University Press, 1953), p. 214; and Erwin H. Ackerknecht, *Malaria in the Upper Mississippi Valley 1760–1900* (Baltimore: Johns Hopkins Press, 1945), pp. 54–55.

equally common causes of death in the remainder of the city. This difference can be explained only by faulty diagnosis in the city. These problems were augmented by the peculiar therapeutic properties of cinchona. Cinchona did not cure malaria, but it suppressed the symptoms of the disease and averted the paroxysms (as long as it was not administered during the paroxysms, when it was useless). In other fevers, its effects were very different, and in large doses it was more harmful than beneficial. The colonial physician using cinchona, therefore, found that the bark produced rather mysterious and inconsistent results. When administered during a remission of one case of fever, it would prove miraculous; when administered during a remission of another case of fever, it would prove useless. Furthermore, cinchona bark was usually administered as a powder ground from the crude bark. Its bitter taste and great bulk were so unpalatable that patients were unable to consume a sufficient quantity of the bark without emesis to prevent the approaching paroxysm. Quinine, the more concentrated alkaloid of cinchona, was discovered in 1819, but became available in large quantities at low cost only around the middle of the century. Until these diagnostic and pharmacological problems were solved, the use of both cinchona bark and quinine was not widespread.[4]

This analysis of the use of cinchona illustrates the immense problems which had to be overcome to develop a truly useful medical practice. Not only was it necessary to discover medically valid therapies; it was necessary to develop some knowledge of etiology, diagnosis, and pharmacology in order to apply those therapies demonstrably and consistently.

INOCULATION AND VACCINATION

The eighteenth century also witnessed the third great contribution to medical therapeutics—the discovery of inoculation and vaccination for smallpox. Knowledge was brought to Europe from the

[4] Duran-Reynals, *Fever-Bark Tree*, pp. 94–95, 99, 105; M. A. Barber, "The History of Malaria in the United States," *Public Health Reports* 44 (1929): 2575; G. S. B. Hempstead, "Reminiscences of the Physicians of the First Quarter of the Present Century . . . ," *Cincinnati Lancet and Clinic* 40 (1878): 55; Erwin H. Ackerknecht, "Aspects of the History of Therapeutics," *Bulletin of the History of Medicine* 36 (1962): 410. By the 1840's, quinine was so widely used in the Midwest, where malaria was far more widespread than in the East, that severe epidemics would cause its price to increase as much as ten times the normal price. It was sold in quantities which, according to one physician, "would astonish an eastern dealer in drugs." Although quinine was five times as expensive as cinchona, much larger amounts of it were sold than the crude bark; A. B. Shipman, "Professional Matters at the West—Malarious Fever," *Boston Medical and Surgical Journal* 40 (1849): 69–71, 239.

near east around 1720 that transfering a small amount of pus from the pustule of a smallpox victim into the arm of a healthy person would give that person a mild case of smallpox which would render him relatively immune to severe attacks of the fully virulent disease. Even if the induced case were not so mild, the chances were very good that it would be considerably milder than a case contracted through infection. This process was called "inoculation." The discovery was of major importance because of the recurrence of smallpox throughout the colonial period, the high mortality, the possibility of lifelong disfigurement, and the particular prevalence of smallpox among children. Furthermore, smallpox, unlike malaria, was readily diagnosed by the distinctive pustules, or pox, which developed on the face of the infected person, and it was the first specific disease in which mortality statistics were used. The accuracy of diagnosis of smallpox meant that any treatment could be evaluated carefully and scientifically. Consequently, the therapeutic validity of inoculation was easily proven by analyzing the incidence of smallpox among inoculated and uninoculated persons.[5]

However, a number of difficulties associated with inoculation limited its acceptance. First of all, many physicians thought it a very illogical procedure. One contemporary physician stated: "The Novelty of seeking Security from a Distemper [i.e., smallpox], by rushing into the Embraces of it . . . could naturally have very little Tendency to procure it a good Reception on its first Appearance." A second reason was that inoculation could cause a severe case of smallpox, although this was not common. The most important criticism of the use of inoculation was that a person suffering from smallpox via inoculation, although unlikely to receive a virulent case himself, could easily pass on the disease in its virulent form to others around him. A number of epidemics, such as the 1752 epidemic in Boston which caused over five hundred deaths, have been traced to inoculation. The danger of contagion from inoculated cases of smallpox led public authorities to regulate its use in the city of Boston and the states of Virginia, New Hampshire, Connecticut, and New York during much of the eighteenth century.[6]

Despite these problems, the use of inoculation increased through-

[5] Duffy, *Epidemics in Colonial America*, pp. 16, 105, 22; John B. Blake, *Public Health in the Town of Boston 1630–1822* (Cambridge, Mass.: Harvard University Press, 1959), pp. 105–7.

[6] Daniel J. Boorstin, *The Americans: The Colonial Experience* (New York: Random House, 1958), p. 226; Blake, *Public Health in Boston*, pp. 82, 86, 111–12; Solon S. Bernstein, "Smallpox and Variolation: Their Historical Significance in the American Colonies," *Journal of the Mount Sinai Hospital* 18 (1951): 237.

out the century. In Boston, for example, only two percent of the cases of smallpox recorded in 1721 were caused by inoculation, but this increased to 28 percent in 1752 and 87 percent in 1764. Inoculation was not practiced in rural areas where smallpox rarely occurred, which created a major problem for Revolutionary War soldiers recruited from these areas. George Washington called smallpox "more destructive to an army in the natural way than the sword," and after 1777 he ordered the entire army to be inoculated. After the Revolution, inoculation was rendered safer by the establishment of hospitals and farms where inoculated persons could be isolated from the remainder of the community and therefore were not potential carriers of the disease. In this way, the practice became reasonably widespread.[7]

In the 1790's Edward Jenner, a British physician, began to experiment with the relationship between smallpox and cowpox, a much milder and less dangerous form of the same disease. Jenner confirmed the fact that persons who contracted cowpox were immune to smallpox, and demonstrated that cowpox could be inoculated in the same way as smallpox. He called this form of inoculation "vaccination," from the Latin word for cow, *vacca*.[8]

Jenner first published an account of his findings in 1798; in that year and the following year, several American physicians, notably Benjamin Waterhouse of Boston, obtained a supply of cowpox lymphatic matter from England (cowpox was unknown in America at the time). The news of the new vaccine aroused considerable public interest, and Waterhouse wrote early in 1799 that it excited "the public curiosity as much as anything that has occurred in the medical line since my remembrance." By 1802, the vaccine was being used in all the major seaports and in such inland places as Mississippi, Kentucky, and Ohio. The editors of an American medical journal wrote: "we believe no improvement in the practice of physic, of any great importance, was ever adopted by the community with so much readiness as the vaccine inoculation." Furthermore, its use was soon publicly supported. In New York City, a voluntary association was founded in 1802 to provide free vaccination for the poor and to maintain a supply of the vaccine, and about the same time the city appropriated $200 annually for vaccination of the indigent. In Massachusetts, the state legislature authorized towns in 1810 to raise money to cover the expenses of vaccination. In Maryland, James Smith, one of the first

---

[7] Blake, *Public Health in Boston*, p. 244; Bernstein, "Smallpox and Variolation," pp. 239–44.

[8] H. J. Parish, *A History of Immunization* (Edinburgh: Livingstone, 1965), pp. 25–26.

American users of the vaccine, was appointed state vaccine agent for both Maryland and Virginia, and national vaccine agent, in which capacity Congress authorized him to send vaccine anywhere in the country, postage free. In 1818 Smith endeavored to establish a national institute for the dissemination of vaccine and raised $26,000 in two years from public contributions.[9]

Thus, within a few years after its discovery, vaccination became widely used in the United States, despite several serious problems. First, the exact manner of using the vaccine had to be developed experimentally, and considerable harm was done on some occasions through ignorance of its proper use. Second, pure vaccine was not always used, and vaccinated individuals were not always protected and sometimes made ill by the spurious products. Third, no one knew how or why vaccination worked. Jenner himself surmised that "the small-pox and the cow-pox were the same diseases under different modifications" and suggested that the reason for the vaccine's effectiveness was that "two diseased actions cannot take place at the same time in one and the same part."[10]

The success of the vaccine therefore cannot be attributed to the development of medical science. Rather, there seem to be two reasons for its immediate acceptance. First, it was very similar in its use and effects to inoculation, and therefore lacked striking novelty. Second, it could be demonstrably and consistently shown that cowpox vaccination worked, and indeed on several occasions physicians in New England, for example, demonstrated its effectiveness experimentally.[11] For the average physician and patient, this criterion rather than any theoretical one was adequate justification for its use.

BOTANICAL MEDICINE

The earliest Spanish explorers of central and South America recognized the value of drugs used by the natives and soon began to export American medicinal plants to Europe through Spain. By the seventeenth century, quantities of cinchona bark, sarsaparilla, coca

9 John B. Blake, *Benjamin Waterhouse and the Introduction of Vaccination* (Philadelphia: University of Pennsylvania Press, 1957), pp. 77, 61–64; John Duffy, *A History of Public Health in New York City 1625–1866* (New York: Russell Sage Foundation, 1968), p. 246; Josiah Bartlett, *A Dissertation on the Progress of Medical Science in the Commonwealth of Massachusetts* (Boston: 1810), p. 31; Whitfield J. Bell, Jr., "Dr. James Smith and the Public Encouragement for Vaccination for Smallpox," *Annals of Medical History*, Ser. 3, vol. 2 (1940): 505, 508–9.

10 Blake, *Waterhouse*, pp. 23–28; Edward Jenner, "A Continuation of Facts and Observations Relative to the Variolae Vaccinae, or Cow-Pox," in Camac, *Classics of Medicine*, p. 281n.

11 Blake, *Waterhouse*, pp. 31, 46–47.

leaves (the source of cocaine), and other drugs were being brought to Europe from South America. These drugs had a major impact on sixteenth- and seventeenth-century European therapeutics.[12]

The profitability of this trade encouraged the Europeans who colonized North America to instruct their representatives to search out plants which might have medicinal value. In Virginia, trade in botanicals between Great Britain and the colonists occurred throughout the seventeenth and well into the eighteenth century. A similar situation prevailed in French-occupied Louisiana, where French officials, travelers, and colonists displayed considerable interest in local medicinal botany. Expectations about the medicinal properties of North American flora were overly optimistic, and the colonists were soon forced to import large quantities of medicine from Europe. The high cost of imported botanical and non-botanical medicines encouraged colonists to import the seeds of European medicinal plants and grow their own botanicals. Plants first cultivated in America in this way include dandelion, wormwood, burdock, mint, plantain, and catnip.[13]

Most American families in the colonial period used these botanical medicines when illness occurred. Each fall, housewives gathered domesticated and wild herbs like sarsaparilla, horehound, sassafras, and dandelion, dried them, and hung them up in bundles for future use like articles of food. When illness came, housewives turned to notebooks of recipes compiled from newspapers, almanacs, neighbors, and relatives, and concocted some remedy to meet the need. As can be seen from the kinds of herbs used, most remedies could neither help nor hurt the patient. Early in the nineteenth century, books on domestic medicine replaced the old recipe notebooks and provided housewives with more professional, if not more valid, advice on the treatment of disease. About the same time, the patent medicine industry, which also used many botanicals, began to assist the American family in its self-medication.[14]

[12] Duran-Reynals, *Fever-Bark Tree*, pp. 25–26; Ackerknecht, "Aspects of the History of Therapeutics," p. 394.

[13] Wyndham B. Blanton, *Medicine in Virginia in the Seventeenth Century* (Richmond: William Byrd Press, 1930), pp. 99–108; John Duffy, ed., *The Rudolph Matas History of Medicine in Louisiana* (n.p.: Louisiana State University Press, 1958), I: 112–13; Wyndham B. Blanton, *Medicine in Virginia in the Eighteenth Century* (Richmond: Garrett and Massie, 1931), p. 33; Samuel Abbott Green, "A Centennial Address," *Medical Communications of the Massachusetts Medical Society* 12 (1881): 563–64.

[14] Barnes Riznik, "The Professional Lives of Early Nineteenth-Century New England Doctors," *Journal of the History of Medicine and Allied Sciences* 19 (1964): 2; Malcolm Sydney Beinfield, "The Early New England Doctor: An Adaptation to a Provincial Environment," *Yale Journal of Biology and Medicine* 15 (1942): 277–78; Green, "Centennial Address," pp. 564–65.

If the patient did not respond to the ministerings of his family, more professional assistance would be called for. Professional physicians, however, constituted only a small part of the personnel who performed medical services.

THE OCCUPATIONAL ROLE OF THE PHYSICIAN

The practice of medicine as a full-time vocation was rare in the American colonies during the seventeenth and early eighteenth centuries. The population of most communities was too small and too poor to support a full-time physician. Most colonial physicians earned their livelihood as clergymen, teachers, government officials, or at other vocations, and practiced medicine only part-time. As late as 1789, Benjamin Rush, an eminent physician of the period, advised medical students planning to practice in rural areas to purchase and operate small farms partly in order to furnish occupation during the lax season.[15]

Gradually, the practice of medicine became a vocation. As it did, it became stratified, primarily by the amount and nature of the education of medical practitioners, which affected the kind of clientele they attracted. Because colonial America had no medical schools before the second half of the eighteenth century, and only a few small ones until the nineteenth century, the wealthiest medical students went to Europe to obtain a formal medical education. Between 1749 and 1812, 139 Americans attended the medical school at Edinburgh, which was the most popular of the European medical schools among American students. This elite of European-educated physicians constituted only a small minority of all practitioners. Blanton has estimated that about 55 of the approximately five hundred physicians in Virginia at the end of the eighteenth century held medical degrees (some of the degrees were obtained from the recently established American medical schools).[16]

The great majority of American practitioners at the time of the American Revolution were products of the apprenticeship system, which will be described thoroughly in Chapter 5. The extent and nature of apprenticeship training depended on the quality of the tutor, the length of the apprenticeship, and the ability and motivation

[15] Beinfield, "Early New England Doctor," p. 101; Joseph M. Toner, *Contributions to the Annals of Medical Progress and Medical Education in the United States before and during the War of Independence* (Washington: U. S. Government Printing Office, 1874), pp. 58–59; Henry Burnell Shafer, *The American Medical Profession 1783 to 1850* (New York: Columbia University Press, 1936), p. 76.

[16] Blanton, *Medicine in the Eighteenth Century*, pp. 86, 207–8.

of the student. Apprentice-trained physicians varied greatly in their medical knowledge.

At the bottom of the hierarchy were the so-called "empirics," who lacked any professional training, but were often quite knowledgeable in the therapeutic properties of botanical drugs, often learned through an informal system of apprenticeship with botanical practitioners. A Maryland physician named Alexander Hamilton wrote about his tour of the colonies in 1744:

The doctors in Albany [New York] are mostly Dutch, all empirics, having no knowledge or learning but what they have acquired by bare experience. They study chiefly the virtues of herbs, and the woods there furnish their shops with all the pharmacy they use. A great many of them take the care of a family for the value of a Dutch dollar a year, which makes the practice of physick a mean thing, and unworthy of the application of a gentleman. The doctors here are all barbers. . . .

Among the rest [elsewhere in his travels] was a fellow with a worsted cap and great black fists. They styled him doctor. Flat told me he had been a shoemaker in town, and was a notable fellow at his trade, but happening two years ago to cure an old woman of a pestilent mortal disease, he thereby acquired the character of a physician, was applied to from all quarters and finding the practice of physic a more profitable business than cobbling, he laid aside his awls and leather, got himself some gallipots, and instead of cobbling of soales fell to cobbling of human bodies.[17]

Many of these empirics were called "root and herb" or "Indian" doctors; they limited their entire practice to roots and herbs, which they sometimes claimed they learned from the Indians. Other colonial practitioners who lacked professional training included the midwives, who took care of most obstetrical practice, and bonesetters, who corrected dislocations.[18]

The educated physicians congregated in the larger cities and towns almost exclusively. In Virginia, the eleven largest towns and cities had only three percent of the state's 880,000 persons in 1800, yet 25 percent of the approximately 700 physicians known to have practiced in Virginia during the eighteenth century lived in them. In Massachusetts around 1780, the few well-educated practitioners resided in the larger cities and towns. In colonial Louisiana, physicians congregated in New Orleans to the exclusion of other areas until other towns

[17] Alexander Hamilton, *Hamilton's Itinerarium* (St. Louis, Mo.: 1908), pp. 79, 110.

[18] Blanton, *Medicine in the Eighteenth Century*, p. 22; John B. Beck, *Medicine in the American Colonies* (Albuquerque, N. M.: Horn and Wallace, 1966; originally published in 1850), p. 23; Robert T. Joy, "The Natural Bonesetters with Special Reference to the Sweet Family of Rhode Island," *Bulletin of the History of Medicine* 28 (1954): 416–41.

and cities developed. This occurred because physicians found enough clients able to support them only in the urban areas. In the rural areas, physicians were often paid in farm produce rather than cash, which was hardly likely to attract the better-educated members of the profession to those areas.[19]

The empirics practiced in communities of all sizes. They were the only practitioners in most rural areas, as Hamilton found in Albany in 1744. They were also numerous and popular in the cities, to the consternation of the better-trained physicians. A New York City historian wrote in the middle of the eighteenth century that "quacks abound like Locusts in Egypt, and too many have recommended themselves to a full Practice and profitable Subsistence." Many of the better-trained physicians felt that the empirics overshadowed and degraded the entire profession. One Virginia doctor suggested a coat of arms for the profession ornamented with three duck heads and containing the motto, "Quack, Quack, Quack."[20]

The differences in therapeutics among the three groups of practitioners, although significant, rarely benefited the patient in proportion to the amount of training of the physician. Medical schools of the period were characterized by a dogmatic pedagogy based on doctrinaire and unscientific systems of therapeutics. An apprentice-trained Virginia physician complained about

those selfswolen sons of pedantic absurdity, fresh & raw from that universal asylum of medical perfection, Edinburgh, . . . [who] enter with obstinate assurance upon the old round of obsolete prescription, which their infallible masters taught them, &, like the mule that turns aside for no man, push on in their bloody career till the surrounding mortality, but more especially the danger of their own thick skulls, brings them to a pause, & works in them a new conviction.[21]

Far more important than the nature of medical education was the kind of medical knowledge available to all physicians of the period. Well-educated physicians were unable to offer their patients therapies superior to those of the empirics. For example, because of the absence of any knowledge of infection, even the best trained physicians could unknowingly transmit puerperal fever to their obstetrical cases. Because a midwife had fewer patients than a full-time physician

[19] Blanton, *Medicine in the Eighteenth Century*, p. 313; Reginald H. Fitz, "The Rise and Fall of the Licensed Physician in Massachusetts, 1781–1860," *Transactions of the Association of American Physicians* 9 (1894): 2; Duffy, *Medicine in Louisiana* I: 159–60.

[20] William Smith, *The History of the Province of New-York . . . to the Year M.DCC.XXXII* (London: 1757), quoted in Whitfield J. Bell, Jr., "Medical Practice in Colonial America," *Bulletin of the History of Medicine* 31 (1957): pp. 442–43; Blanton, *Medicine in the Eighteenth Century*, p. 209.

[21] Bell, "Medical Practice in Colonial America," p. 444.

and usually did not examine her patients before delivery, she was less likely than a physician to be a carrier of puerperal fever. Few physicians practiced surgery during the colonial period, and those who did were rarely capable.[22] Even the general therapeutic philosophy of educated physicians was not such as to make them preferable to their lesser trained competitors. An outstanding Boston physician of the period wrote:

In general the physical practice in our colonies is so perniciously bad that, excepting in surgery and some very acute cases, it is better to let nature, under a proper regimen, take her course than to trust to the honesty and sagacity of the practitioner; our American practitioners are so rash and officious. . . . Frequently there is more danger from the physician than from the distemper. Our practitioners deal much in quackery and quackish medicines . . . In the most trifling cases they use a routine of practice. When I first arrived in New England . . . a most noted facetious practitioner . . . told me their practice was very uniform: bleeding, vomiting, blistering, purging, anodynes, etc., if the illness continued, there was *repetendi*, and finally *murderandi*; nature was never to be consulted or allowed to have any concern in the affair.[23]

MEDICAL LICENSING

The limited nature of medical knowledge and the lack of skill of American physicians were reflected in colonial medical licensing laws. Throughout the colonial period, physicians attempted to obtain licensing legislation limiting the practice of medicine to qualified practitioners. Most legislatures, however, would enact only honorific licensing measures which recognized merit and service to the community. In Connecticut, for example, in 1652 the General Assembly granted a license and an annual retainer to a physician "for setting of bones and otherwise, as at all times, occasions and necessities may require."[24] It was apparently the opinion of the legislators that the primary medical contribution of physicians involved setting fractures

[22] Blanton, *Medicine in the Seventeenth Century*, p. 164; Courtney R. Hall, "The Rise of Professional Surgery in the United States: 1800–1865," *Bulletin of the History of Medicine* 26 (1952): 231, 236.

[23] William Douglass, quoted in James J. Walsh, *History of the Medical Society of the State of New York* (n.p., 1907), pp. 31–32. Alexander Hamilton met Douglass when he visited Boston in 1744 and referred to him in the following words: "Douglass, the physician here, is a man of good learning, but mischievously given to criticism, and the most compleat snarler ever I knew. He is loath to allow learning, merit, or a character to anybody. He is of the clinical class of physicians, and laughs at all theory and practice founded upon it, looking upon empiricism or bare experience as the only firm basis upon which practice ought to be founded." Hamilton, *Itinerarium*, p. 142. Although Hamilton stated that Douglass had a number of disciples in Boston, there is much evidence that his opinions were as deviant as Hamilton felt they were.

[24] George O. Sumner, "Early Physicians in Connecticut," *Connecticut State Medical Journal* 6 (1942): 459. (Article originally published in 1851.)

and dislocations. Midwives assisted in obstetrical cases, and most families prepared, prescribed, and administered their own botanical drugs.

In the middle of the seventeenth century, Massachusetts, New Jersey, and New York enacted legislation regulating the practice of medicine in the following language:

. . . no person or persons whatsoever that are employed about the bodies of men, women, and children for preservation of life or health, as physicians, surgeons, midwives, or others, shall presume to exercise or put forth any act contrary to the known rules of art, nor exercise any force, violence, or cruelty upon or toward the bodies of any, whether young or old— no, not in the most difficult and desperate cases—without the advice and consent of such as are skillful in the same art, if such may be had, or at least of the wisest and gravest then present, and consent of the patient or patients (if they be mentis compotes), much less contrary to such advice and consent. . . .[25]

The obvious implications of this legislation are that (1) the "rules of art" of medicine were known to most people; and (2) in case the physician departed from such known rules, the "wisest and gravest then present," even though they were laymen, were competent to overrule the physician. The legislators, therefore, did not consider the physician's knowledge to be so specialized and advanced that it was beyond the comprehension of laymen.

The two most important regulatory licensing laws enacted in the eighteenth century before the Revolution gave laymen a similar role, even though the professionalization of medicine had developed greatly in the succeeding century. These laws were passed in New York State in 1760 (but applied only to New York City), and in New Jersey in 1772. Both laws placed responsibility for granting licenses exclusively in the hands of laymen (political and judicial office-holders) who were empowered to solicit the advice of physicians.[26] Here, too, it was believed that intelligent laymen were quite competent to evaluate the ability of physicians.

With this background, it is now possible to turn to the main focus of this study—the nineteenth-century physician. The next several chapters will examine the development of medicine as a profession in the first half of the nineteenth century.

[25] The spelling of the law has been modernized. Fitz, "Licensed Physician," p. 2; Fred B. Rogers and A. Reasoner Sayre, *The Healing Art: A History of the Medical Society of New Jersey* (Trenton, N. J.: 1966), p. 5; Duffy, *Public Health in New York*, p. 33.

[26] Louis G. Caldwell, "Early Legislation Regulating the Practice of Medicine," *Illinois Law Review* 18 (1923): 234.

PART II THE REGULAR MEDICAL PROFESSION IN THE FIRST HALF OF THE NINETEENTH CENTURY

IF . . . WE LOOK into the profession of physic, we shall find a most formidable body of men; the sight of them is enough to make a man serious, for we may lay it down as a maxim that when a nation abounds in physicians it grows thin in people. This body of men in our own country may be described like the British army in Caesar's time—some of them slay in chariots and some on foot.

JOSEPH ADDISON, *The Spectator*

CHAPTER 3 MEDICAL PRACTICE AMONG PHYSICIANS

THE FIRST HALF of the nineteenth century was the period in which the American medical profession became firmly established. Thousands of men became professionally trained, full-time physicians; they organized medical societies and medical schools, obtained licensing legislation, and established institutional relations with clients. The last of these activities will be the subject of this chapter; the other three will be analyzed in subsequent chapters.

The model presented in Chapter 1 analyzed the relationship between physicians and clients in terms of the therapeutics used by the physician to treat patients. It will be shown in this chapter that standard therapeutics in the early nineteenth century consisted of a small number of treatments distinguished by their immediate and drastic impact on the organism. Active therapy was the hallmark of medical practice of the period; the patient was dosed, bled, and blistered by physicians who adhered tenaciously to the belief that the best therapy produced the most rapid and observable symptomatic changes in the patient.

The state of health of the American population influenced the physician's determination to make an impression on the patient. Diseases like malaria and dysentery were so widespread that they afflicted a large proportion of the population. Cholera and yellow fever attacked occasionally, but with such severity that they could paralyze most productive activities in a community. The physicians who confronted these harsh diseases often responded by using the most active therapies available.

THE BASIS OF MEDICAL THERAPEUTICS

Inasmuch as early nineteenth-century physicians were ignorant of the etiology and means of contagion of diseases, the relationship between their theories of medicine, their therapies, and the actual disease states had no scientific basis. Contemporary medical theorists constructed nosologies, in which they categorized diseases into families based on some assumed or symptomatic similarity, e.g., eruptive diseases. They thereupon deduced that the same therapies would be suitable for all diseases within each family. In this way, physicians established a relationship among diseases, theories, and therapies.

Theory-building was a popular pastime of the period, and Thomas Jefferson, who distinguished himself in many areas, spoke critically of them in this way:

> . . . the adventurous physician . . . substitutes presumption for knolege. From the scanty field of what is known, he launches into the boundless region of what is unknown. He establishes for his guide some fanciful theory of corpuscular attraction, of chemical agency, of mechanical powers, of stimuli, of irritability accumulated or exhausted, of depletion by the lancet & repletion by mercury, or some other ingenious dream, which lets him into all nature's secrets at short hand. On the principle which he thus assumes, he forms his table of nosology, arrays his diseases into families, and extends his curative treatment, by analogy, to all the cases he has thus arbitrarily marshalled together. I have lived myself to see the disciples of [a number of theorists] succeed one another like the shifting figures of a magic lantern, & their fancies, like the dresses of the annual doll-babies from Paris, becoming, from their novelty, the vogue of the day, and yeilding to the next novelty their ephemeral favor.[1]

While theory-building was popular, it was of only marginal importance for the medical practice of the period. Actual medical therapeutics was based on a system of superficial observation and analysis guided by two major principles. One was that the pathological state of the organism could be understood by reliance on external symptoms exclusively. Under this principle, for example, fever constituted a disease state which could be treated by itself. Because thermometers were not yet used to determine the temperature of the patient, a number of symptoms were considered necessary for a diagnosis of fever. William Buchan wrote in his *Domestic Medicine*, an extremely popular medical guide for laymen early in the nineteenth century, that the symptoms of fever were "increased heat, frequency of pulse, loss of appetite, general disability, pain in the head and a difficulty in per-

---

[1] Wyndham B. Blanton, *Medicine in Virginia in the Eighteenth Century* (Richmond: Garrett and Massie, 1931), p. 199. Mention of the major etiological theories popular in the first half of the nineteenth century may be found in Phyllis Allen, "Etiological Theory in America Prior to the Civil War," *Journal of the History of Medicine and Allied Sciences* 2 (1947): 489–520.

The epigraph for this Part is quoted in A. Y. P. Garnett, "The Mission of the American Medical Association," *Journal of the American Medical Association* 10 (1888): 577.

forming some of the vital or animal functions." Buchan classed fevers
into four groups: continual, remittent (up and down but never wholly
absent), intermittent (comes and goes periodically), and attended with
eruptions (e.g., smallpox).[2] Jefferson was quite correct in his criticism
of such nosologies; these categories were wholly arbitrary and confused
many different diseases.

The second major principle was that anything which produced
desired changes in the gross pathological symptoms of the patient was
acting on the disease and was therefore a useful therapy. For example,
virtually anything which reduced fever in a patient was considered a
desirable therapy, even though the reduction in fever might be wholly
unrelated to any change in the patient's illness and even might be
injurious in the long run. Consequently, physicians adopted therapies
largely because they produced desirable short-run symptomatic changes
in the patient. Indeed, many physicians went so far as to argue that a
therapy which had a profound physiological effect of any kind on the
patient must be a source of benefit. In a paper about the effects on
children of blisters induced by plasters, a common treatment for many
diseases, a physician observed that blisters affected children far more
severely than adults, sometimes producing convulsions, gangrene, and
even death in children. He concluded from this that blisters "ought to
hold a high rank" as remedial agents in the diseases of children, although he also criticized their "indiscriminate application" by many
physicians.[3] While some physicians would have agreed with the criticism, most others would have agreed more readily with the conclusion
that powerful agents were powerful remedies.

While these views were held by the overwhelming majority of
physicians, they were opposed by a few physicians and laymen who
argued that the physician should wait on the therapeutic effects of
nature whenever he was not confident of his therapies. Thomas Jefferson, for example, stated:

Where . . . we have seen a disease, characterized by specific signs or phenomena, and relieved by a certain natural evacuation or process, whenever
that disease recurs under the same appearances, we may reasonably count on
producing a solution of it, by the use of such substances as we have found
produce the same evacuation or movement. Thus, fulness of the stomach we
can relieve by emetics; diseases of the bowels, by purgatives; inflammatory
cases, by bleeding; intermittents, by the Peruvian bark; syphilis, by mercury;

[2] William Buchan, *Domestic Medicine*, Revised and adapted to the Diseases
and Climate of the United States of America by Samuel Powell Griffitts (Philadelphia: Dobson, 1809), p. 145.

[3] John B. Beck, "On the Effects of Blisters on the Young Subject," *New York
Journal of Medicine* 9 (1847): 9–10.

watchfulness, by opium; etc. So far, I bow to the utility of medicine. It goes
to the well-defined forms of disease, & happily, to those the most frequent.
But the disorders of the animal body, & the symptoms indicating them, are
as various as the elements of which the body is composed. The combinations,
too, of these symptoms are so infinitely diversified, that many associations of
them appear too rarely to establish a definite disease; and to an unknown
disease, there cannot be a known remedy. Here then, the judicious, the
moral, the humane physician should stop. Having been so often a witness
to the salutary efforts which nature makes to re-establish the disordered
functions, he should rather trust to their action, than hazard the interrup-
tion of that, and a greater derangement of the system, by conjectural experiments on a machine so complicated & so unknown as the human body, & a
subject so sacred as human life. . . . I would wish the young practitioner,
especially, to have deeply impressed on his mind, the real limits of his art, &
that when the state of the patient gets beyond these, his office is to be a
watchful, but quiet spectator of the operations of nature, giving them fair
play by a well-regulated regimen, & by all the aid they can derive from the
excitement of good spirits & hope in the patient.[4]

Most physicians did not take Jefferson's advice. They were earning
a livelihood at the practice of medicine, and knew the patient expected more than "a watchful, but quiet spectator of the operations of
nature" from a physician. Jefferson, who was a wise man, recognized
this:

. . . if the appearance of doing something be necessary to keep alive the
hope & spirits of the patient, it should be of the most innocent character.
One of the most successful physicians I have ever known, has assured me,
that he used more bread pills, drops of colored water, & powders of hickory
ashes, than of all other medicines put together. It was certainly a pious
fraud.[5]

The problem, however, was that patients expected more than this from
their physicians. One contemporary physician, G. S. B. Hempstead,
recalled that, "When dispensing medicine to a patient it was quite
common for him to say, 'now doctor, if you give me a dose, give me a
big one.'" Physicians were quite willing to outdo one another in
soliciting the favors of their patients, and rapidly developed a vigorous
therapy which demonstrated to the patient and his friends that the
physician was earning his fee not by idle looking on, but by actively
attacking the source of the patient's troubles. The effect on the patient,
however, was so violent that, according to Jefferson, "the inexperienced & presumptuous band of medical tyros let loose upon the world,

[4] Blanton, *Medicine in the Eighteenth Century*, pp. 198–99.
[5] *Ibid.*, p. 199.

destroys more of human life in one year, than all the Robinhoods, Cartouches, & Macheaths do in a century."[6] The primary agents of destruction in this onslaught were bloodletting and calomel.

BLOODLETTING

The use of bloodletting, which had a long history of medicinal use, was based on the symptomatic treatment of the period. If a patient had a fever, the physician endeavored to reduce it. This treatment was called "antiphlogistic," and bleeding was the chief antiphlogistic therapy. When a patient was bled, the effects were demonstrable, consistent, and rapid, according to a contemporary physician: "Often within ten to twenty minutes after faintness or sickness occurred the subject of [bloodletting] would become bathed in a copious perspiration, and the violent fever and delerium existing a short time before would have entirely passed away." These physicians apparently did not recognize that the changes were merely symptomatic and were in no way evidence of any cure or actual improvement in the patient's condition. When bloodletting was administered to excess, the effects were somewhat different. One physician stated they were "a frequent and forcible pulse, beating in the temples, throbbing pain in the head, intolerance of light and sound, and delirium." As a remedy for these effects, he recommended rest and quiet, mild sedatives and nutrients, and "lastly and above all, time."[7] Time, of course, was the best treatment.

Bleeding rapidly became a panacea and was used for every conceivable illness. Buchan recommended its use not only in fevers, but also in wounds, burns, bruises, and fractures. In his history of the New York Medical and Surgical Society, Van Ingen cited the following illnesses in which the use of bleeding was reported: convulsions, concussion, subdural hemorrhages, puerperal convulsions, irreducible hernia, asthenia, enteritis, croup, smallpox, "and of course always pneumonia." The variety of places in which individuals were bled, and the relative difficulty of each, was indicated by a 1798 fee bill of the Medical Society of New York (city). Bleeding from the arm cost $1, from

[6] G. S. B. Hempstead, "Reminiscences of the Physicians of the First Quarter of the Present Century . . . ," *Cincinnati Lancet and Clinic* 40 (1878): 34; Blanton, *Medicine in the Eighteenth Century*, p. 199.

[7] B. M. Randolph, "The Blood Letting Controversy in the Nineteenth Century," *Annals of Medical History* n.s. 7 (1935): 178; Joel Pennington, "Early History of Eastern Indiana," in G. W. H. Kemper, ed., *A Medical History of the State of Indiana* (Chicago: American Medical Association Press, 1911), p. 35; "Reaction after Bloodletting," *Boston Medical and Surgical Journal* 3 (1831): 134.

the foot $2, from the jugular vein $2 (used in young children), and opening an artery $5.[8]

There were two major positions concerning the quantity of blood to be taken. The dominant school of thought advocated bleeding until syncope, or unconsciousness, arguing that the effect produced was more important than the quantity of blood extracted, the "object being to produce a decided impression upon the heart's action." The other school felt this was too extreme. Buchan said that bleeding until unconsciousness was "ridiculous," and that "one person will faint at the sight of a lancet, while another will lose almost the whole blood of his body before he faints. Swooning often depends more upon the state of the mind, than of the body."[9]

Bloodletting enjoyed popularity throughout the colonial period,[10] but the statements of contemporary observers all agree that its extent and use increased considerably in the first half of the nineteenth century. Hempstead stated with reference to the first quarter of the century:

I was acquainted with a neighboring physician who proposed to cure and did cure common intermittent [malaria] by blood-letting alone; he bled the patient till he was too weak to shake, and then the disease and the patient went off together. I mention [this] to show the recklessness of doctors in the use of the lancet, and of patients in submitting to it. You can have no conception of the extent of this devotion to the use of the lancet, scarce a case of any disease was permitted to pass through the hands of a physician without its use; even the non-professionals, many of them carried a lancet, . . . and upon the occurrence of any indisposition, no matter what, would tie up an arm and let the blood flow. Many there were who upon the slightest feeling of malaise would tie up their own arms and use the lancet on themselves.

It was fortunate in that day that we had a hardy, well developed race of men and women, possessing sufficient tenacity of life to not only resist the disease, but the remedies used to combat it. Should this practice again prevail with the badly developed race we now have, the percentage of deaths would be largely increased, and few would come safely out of the hands of the doctors.[11]

[8] Buchan, *Domestic Medicine*, pp. 581–82, 584, 596; Philip Van Ingen, *A Brief Account of the First One Hundred Years of the New York Medical and Surgical Society* (n.p., 1946), pp. 29–30; James J. Walsh, *History of Medicine in New York* (New York: National Americana Society, 1919), 1: 71–72.

[9] Pennington, "Early History of Eastern Indiana," p. 35; Buchan, *Domestic Medicine*, p. 573.

[10] Wyndham B. Blanton, *Medicine in Virginia in the Seventeenth Century* (Richmond, Va.: William Byrd Press, 1930), p. 137; Blanton, *Medicine in the Eighteenth Century*, pp. 5–6; John Duffy, *Epidemics in Colonial America* (Baton Rouge: Louisiana State University Press, 1953), p. 9.

[11] Hempstead, "Reminiscences," pp. 54–55.

The most extraordinary fact was not that bloodletting was used so widely, but that blood was drawn in such large quantities and repeated over such a length of time. One physician wrote in 1851 that he administered the following treatment to a woman who had just been delivered of a child and was suffering from puerperal convulsions (childbed fever):

I opened a large orifice in each arm and cut both temporal arteries and had blood flowing freely from all at the same time, determined to bleed her until the convulsions ceased, or as long as the blood would flow. How much she bled, I have no means of judging, for I designedly prevented any attempt to catch the blood and the convulsions were so violent and so frequent it could not have been caught if attempted. I suffered her to bleed until the pulse could not be felt at the wrist, and beat but feebly in the carotid arteries by which time the convulsions ceased. . . . The woman recovered rapidly without subsequent inconvenience. . . . My practice has been to bleed as long as I thought the bleeding itself would not endanger life. I prefer to cut the temporal arteries in bad cases.[12]

Physicians had no hesitation about continuing bloodletting for extended periods. During an epidemic of bilious fever in Pennsylvania in 1804, a man was bled an average of fourteen ounces of blood a day for ten of eleven successive days; he recovered—"rapidly," according to the report. What Hempstead said about another patient must have been true of this man: "He was a burly, sanguine [man], or probably he never could have lived to thank the doctor for taking so much bad blood out of him."[13]

These heroic efforts frequently had tragic consequences. Salmon P. Chase, Abraham Lincoln's Secretary of the Treasury and later Chief Justice of the United States, described the death of his first wife, two weeks after childbirth, in Cincinnati in about 1837. It was believed that she had puerperal fever, and the family physician, Dr. Colby, was sent for. He in turn requested a consultation with Dr. Daniel Drake. Chase's diary went on to say:

. . . before he arrived Dr. Colby had made preparations for bleeding her, thinking prompt blood-letting necessary, and that a high peritoneal inflammation existed. Dr. Drake concurred, and they proceeded to bleed. When six or eight ounces were abstracted, Dr. Colby, thinking she had been bled as much as her constitution would bear, and becoming satisfied from the effect of the bleeding that the high state of inflammation supposed did not really exist, arrested the flow of blood. Dr. Drake was much dissatisfied, and insisted

12 W. H. Witt, "The Progress of Internal Medicine since 1830," in *The Centennial History of the Tennessee State Medical Association 1830–1930*, Philip M. Hamer, ed., (Nashville: Tennessee State Medical Association, 1930), p. 265.

13 Robert M. Cunningham, *An Inaugural Essay on the Inflammatory Bilious Fever* (Philadelphia: 1806), p. 11; Hempstead, "Reminiscences," p. 54.

on a more copious bleeding. The bandage was accordingly removed, and more blood taken. It was then replaced. Dr. Drake still remained unsatisfied, urging that it was necessary to bleed to fainting. [The difference of opinion was presented to the family, and Dr. Richards was brought in. Drs. Richards and Drake] both soon agreed as to the necessity of bleeding, and she was again bled. . . . Forty grains of calomel were then administered. Thirty ounces of blood had been taken. Still Drs. Drake and Richards were not satisfied—they thought further bleeding was necessary, yet postponed it till morning. . . .

[The next morning.] Such was her condition on the morning of this unhappy day, there was a fair prospect of her recovery. All the symptoms boded well. But Drs. Drake and Richards were of the opinion that she had not been bled sufficiently, and that the disease had not been subdued. They accordingly recommended further bleeding; Dr. Colby opposed it, saying that all her symptoms were improved, and they ought to watch the result. The other physicians insisted, however. [A fourth physician, Dr. Eberle, was sent for.] He concurred with the majority, and further bleeding was consequently resolved upon. It was anticipated that the effect would be to reduce the frequency of the pulse, and augment its volume! Kitty was told that the doctors thought of bleeding her again, and was asked if she was willing. She said "Yes, anything." She was then raised up in bed, and twenty ounces of blood were taken from her. *The effect on the pulse was the exact contrary of what was anticipated.* It became more frequent and more feeble, but in other respects she seemed somewhat easier. The physicians seemed to entertain some hopes of her recovery, and agreed upon a course of treatment to be adopted. The [patient's] father came into [her] room exclaiming, "Thank God, my child, the doctors say there is hope." She said nothing. All hope had vanished. . . . Dr. Drake felt her pulse, and said she was dead.[14]

These physicians were not exceptional in their reliance on the lancet. Drake and Eberle were two of the most eminent American physicians of the first half of the century, and Eberle was the author of a widely used textbook on therapeutics.

Several advantages rendered bloodletting highly desirable as a therapy. Its effects were demonstrable and consistent, and certainly made the patient aware that the physician was not indifferent to his plight. From the physician's viewpoint, it seemed particularly well suited to the many kinds of fevers—malaria, typhoid, yellow fever, pneumonia, etc.—so common in the country at this time. Last, it was a genteel and elegant therapy, well suited to all social classes, as one physician reminisced:

Set the patient up in a chair, cord his arm, have the bowl ready, a folded piece of cotton cloth to apply to the wound, and a bandage. Click goes the lance, and the warm, red current spins from the wound, a little upward so as to describe a curve, and is caught in the wide-topped bleeding bowl. For

[14] [A. J. Howe], "Phlebotomy Forty Years Ago," *Eclectic Medical Journal* 47 (1887): 402–3.

two or three minutes all goes well, the vessel is filling up, when the patient growing a little pale, he is told to look away from the blood; but sharp, the doctor says—"catch his head," and quick as thought he claps his compress on the orifice, passes the bandage deftly around so as to secure it, pins it, and—we *carry* the patient to bed. The operation is well done, is nice and cleanly, no bad smell, and no recurrence, unless the physician chooses.[15]

Indeed, bloodletting had a remarkable virtue in its cleanliness and limited aftereffects (when blood was drawn in small quantities) over other therapies.

Some patients resisted the use of the lancet. One physician related this anecdote about his own childhood:

Old Dr. Colby was in the habit of getting his lancet out and laying it upon the table before even removing his hat, or before ascertaining what the disease might be that he was called to see. Bleeding was done in any event. It was all part of the routine of practice. . . . Bleeding was primary, first and foremost in all cases and conditions. I remember that a horse kicked me once as Dr. Colby was passing the house. I was not injured much, yet mother called in the doctor, and he at once proceeded to bleed me—I presume on general principles. I had seen my mother bled a great many times. The doctor would always bleed her sitting up in the bed, and when she would faint and fall over in the bed he loosened the bandages. The doctor had me sitting upon the bed, and when a small quantity of blood escaped, I shut my eyes and fell over on the bed. I remember he told mother that he never saw any one so speedily affected by bleeding. This was the only time I ever was bled.[16]

PURGATIVES AND EMETICS

In his concern for symptomatically demonstrative therapies, the early nineteenth century physician turned to medicines to "cleanse the stomach and bowels," as Buchan phrased it. Two kinds of drugs were used: emetics which produced emesis or vomiting, and cathartics or purgatives which acted as extremely powerful laxatives. These drugs should not be confused with twentieth-century medicines; their effect was much more drastic and immediate. One country physician recalled: "If vomited, they did not come up in gentle puffs and gusts, but the action was cyclonic. If, perchance, the stomach was passed the expulsion would be by the rectum and anus, and this would be equal to a regular oil-well gusher."[17]

Cathartics were by far the more important of the two and were

15 [John M. Scudder], "Bloodletting," *Eclectic Medical Journal* 36 (1876): 186.
16 George J. Monroe, "Old-Time Practice," *Cincinnati Lancet-Clinic* n.s. 46 (1901): 363.
17 Buchan, *Domestic Medicine*, p. 154; Monroe, "Old-Time Practice," p. 362.

used in America as early as the seventeenth century. In the eighteenth century, calomel was introduced as a cathartic.[18] Calomel is a chloride of mercury which is therapeutically useless, but in the intestine it breaks down into highly poisonous components, which irritate and purge. Continued use of calomel over a long period induces salivation, which was considered to be evidence of the drug's effectiveness. (Mercury itself had become important as a therapy for venereal diseases, where it had some therapeutic value, although the side effects were very dangerous.) Late in the eighteenth century, calomel gained great popularity when Benjamin Rush used doses of ten grains of calomel and ten of jalap (another powerful purgative) in treating patients during the 1793 Philadelphia yellow fever epidemic. According to one of Rush's students, this dose was considered at the time to be "perfectly enormous," two or three times the dose previously considered "ample." Rush was criticized extensively by his colleagues in Philadelphia, including members of the College of Physicians, an exclusive local medical society.[19]

Nonetheless, Rush's prescription soon became widely known and, according to Hempstead, was the "standing cathartic" during the first quarter of the century, not only in the minds of many physicians, but self-administered by patients as well. Calomel alone was probably even more widely used in many circumstances, and like bloodletting it became a panacea for all ills. One physician reminisced that in the early decades of the century, "when a practitioner was puzzled about the administration of any medicine in a disease, it was deemed perfectly proper for him to prescribe a dose of calomel; which he did conscientiously, with well satisfied assurance, that if he did not give the exact medicine adapted to the case, he could not be far wrong!" Many physicians believed that the omission of calomel in desperate cases was tantamount to abandoning the patient without a final saving effort.[20]

Unfortunately, calomel had side effects that were detrimental to health. One physician distinguished three gradations of the action of

18 Blanton, *Medicine in the Seventeenth Century*, p. 136. The therapeutic properties of calomel were well known as early as the sixteenth century. *Encyclopedia Britannica* (Cambridge, Eng.: Cambridge University Press, 1910), 11th ed., s.v. "Calomel."

19 Charles Caldwell, *Autobiography* (Philadelphia: Lippincott, Grambo, 1855), pp. 183–84.

20 Hempstead, "Reminiscences," p. 55; Edward H. Barton, quoted in *The Rudolph Matas History of Medicine in Louisiana*, John Duffy, ed., (n.p.: Louisiana State University Press, 1962), II: 5–6; George T. MacCoy, "Pioneer Physicians of Bartholomew County," in Kemper, *Medical History of Indiana*, p. 111.

the drug. In the first stage, purging and salivation occurred. In the second stage, the gums, tongue, and salivary glands became sore, inflamed, and painful.[21] Soon, according to another writer, if the dosing were continued:

The mouth feels unusually hot, and is sometimes sensible of a coppery or metallic taste; the gums are swollen, red, and tender; ulcers make their appearance and spread in all directions; the saliva is thick and stringy, and has that peculiar, offensive odor characteristic of mercurial disease; the tongue is swollen and stiff, and there is some fever, with derangement of the secretions. The disease progressing, it destroys every part that it touches, until the lips, the cheeks, and even the bones have been eaten away before death comes to the sufferer's relief.[22]

The most common and noticeable effect appears to have been on the teeth and mouth:

The teeth, those valuable instruments of our most substantial enjoyments, become loose and rot, perhaps fall out; or worse still, the upper and lower jaw-bones exfoliate and rot out sometimes, as I have witnessed in the form of horse shoes; parts of the tongue and palate are frequently lost, and the poor object lingers out a doleful existence during life. . . . This happens when mercury performs *a cure!* [23]

These effects were not due to single large doses of calomel alone. Because most minerals tend to remain in the body, the effect of the drug was cumulative. One patient took three-fourths of a grain per day—a very small dose, often recommended for children and infants—for six months. When examined by a physician at that time, his mouth was sore, his gums were soft and spongy, and he could not bite bread comfortably. Shortly afterward, three of his molars fell out.[24]

Perhaps the most extraordinary aspect of the use of calomel was that physicians recognized its side effects, and yet continued to give it in large doses. When a cholera epidemic came to St. Louis, physicians went around with calomel loose in their coat pockets, and dosed it out in teaspoonfuls. The author of a well-known volume on domestic medicine said calomel was a valuable medicine for children, "and per-

21 Nathan Knepfler, "Report on the Uses and Abuses of Mercury," *Transactions of the Indiana State Medical Society* 9 (1858): 37.

22 John M. Scudder, *The Eclectic Practice of Medicine* (Cincinnati: Medical Publishing Co., 1870), revised ed., p. 338. See also T. H. Phillips, "Mercurial Fever and Medical Progress," *Eclectic Medical Journal* 39 (1879): 260.

23 A. Hunn, "Essay on Bilious Fever and the Use of Calomel," *Thomsonian Recorder* 1 (1832): 53–54.

24 [A. J. Howe], "Mercurial Necrosis," *Eclectic Medical Journal* 47 (1887): 454.

fectly safe, provided we do not continue it long."[25] Most physicians had few qualms about its use in virtually any situation.

A number of other emetics and purgatives supplemented or replaced calomel in many situations. Some were minerals and deadly poisons, others were powerful botanical drugs; all produced consistent and demonstrable changes in the patient's condition. One of the most popular was "tartar emetic," which was tartrate of antimony. In small doses, it produced vomiting. In large doses, it reduced the force and frequency of the heart beat, lowered the body temperature, and thus was an antiphlogistic. It was also a lethal poison. Another popular every-day purgative was nitre, or salt-peter, which also depressed the heart beat. Nitre was a mineral and a lethal poison, and undoubtedly made its contribution to the mortality of the period. One last common purgative was jalap, which Benjamin Rush made so famous. Because its action was so harsh, it was often mixed with other drugs to reduce its dangers. Its harshness can best be judged by recognizing that it was mixed with calomel to make it more palatable.[26]

The effect of these purgatives on the patient's system was debilitating and dehydrating in the extreme. One physician condemned his colleagues' callousness in their frequent resort to purgatives and urged them to take some of their own medicine so as to cause five or six evacuations a day for a week. He said, "It will take all your strength, your flesh, your blood, your appetite, your functions of all kinds, just as certainly as a bloodletting, and you will be able to realize the influence of similar catharsis on the sick."[27]

OTHER THERAPIES

Once the patient's system was properly cleaned out and his fever reduced by bloodletting, he was ready to be restored to health by the use of tonics. Tonics were supposed to build up the system through improved appetite, digestion, etc. One of the most popular tonics was arsenic, used in Fowler's solution or other compounds. Arsenic is a

[25] J. W. Pruitt, "The Olden Time," *Eclectic Medical Journal* 38 (1878): 532–33; Horatio Gates Jameson, *The American Domestick Medicine* (Baltimore: 1817), p. 592. See also Alex Berman, "The Heroic Approach in 19th Century Therapeutics," *Bulletin American Society of Hospital Pharmacists* 11 (1954): 322. Medicines were not administered in the form of pills during most of the nineteenth century, but rather directly as a powder or in solutions with alcohol or water.

[26] *American Cyclopedia* (New York: Appleton, 1881), s.v. "Antimony"; *Encyclopedia Britannica*, 11th ed., s.v. "Salt-peter"; *Johnson's Universal Cyclopedia* (New York: Johnson, 1894), s.v. "Jalap."

[27] [Scudder], "Bloodletting," p. 187.

deadly poison, and in overdose or excessive use it produces dangerous and toxic side effects.[28]

Cinchona bark and quinine were beginning to assume an important role in therapy during this period, especially in the treatment of malaria. But for the reasons discussed in Chapter 2, they were to become more important in the second half of the century. Crude opium was also used at this time, but its deficiencies were similar to those of cinchona. Like cinchona also, opium was largely replaced in the second half of the century by its alkaloid, morphine.

In addition to bloodletting and drugging, cantharides, or skin irritants, were very popular remedies. The most common of these was blistering. A blister was raised on the affected part of the anatomy with a plaster and then broken; the pus flowing from the blister was believed to be a desirable emission of harmful matter. The sores made by the blisters were often irritated to make the effect more intense, which delayed healing and sometimes produced gangrene or ulcers. One physician, describing how he saved the population of Middletown, Connecticut from the ravages of an obviously mild epidemic (judging from the low mortality) of sinking typhus, or spotted fever, considered blistering a vital part of the treatment: "In every case (the very mildest are not with safety excepted,) the forehead, and in the severe, the vertex should be immediately blistered. Shaving the head and blistering it *early*, is more serviceable than any other external application." He stated that he gave one patient over thirty blisters to save him. Probably the most disturbing aspect of blistering was that, like calomel, it was considered to do little harm, even if it did no good. Therefore it was used very frequently on children. Another less prevalent cantharide was the seton, a thread placed under the skin and kept there to irritate and inflame: the pus emitted was considered beneficial.[29]

Infants were afflicted with a disease not existent among the adult population—teething. Many physicians attributed almost all children's diseases to the irritation caused by cutting of the teeth. Buchan, for example, apparently believed that one-tenth of teething infants died from it. Although many treatments were recommended to save infants from the horrors of this disease, including purgatives, many physicians

[28] *American Cyclopedia*, s.v. "Arsenic."
[29] Thomas Miner, *Typhus Syncopalis, Sinking Typhus, or the Spotted-Fever of New England, as it Appeared in the Epidemic of 1823, in Middletown, Connecticut* (Middletown: 1825), pp. 17–18; Beck, "Effects of Blisters," p. 14; Madge E. Pickard and R. Carlyle Buley, *The Midwest Pioneer* (New York: Schuman, 1946), p. 112.

agreed with the author who said that "nothing is so effectual, as scarifying the gums with a lance," to be repeated as necessary.[30]

Contemporary physicians seldom gave any thought to pharmacology in their use of drugs. Prescriptions were compounded haphazardly and neither chemical purity nor exact dosage were considered important. The same prescription compounded by ten different physicians or pharmacists (physicians usually compounded their own drugs during this period) would probably look, taste, and act differently in each instance.[31]

The effects of the treatments of early nineteenth-century physicians on the patient are difficult for the modern mind to contemplate. John Scudder, an eminent physician of the last half of the century, stated:

One must needs have lived in those days, and have seen the sick, to realize the terrible character of regular medicine. The miserable sinners suffering from disease were tormented continuously by nauseant drugs, by unutterable nausea of the stomach, the torments of physic, the suffering from blisters, and the terrible thirst [from mercury] which . . . cried to heaven from relief. . . . The blister was drawn, clipped, poulticed, and not unfrequently stunk so as to be recognized as soon as the door of the house was opened. Patients were unwashed, clothing and bed-clothing allowed to become dirty—dirt and bad odors, indeed, were characteristic of the treatment.

The mortality was large, ranging from ten to fifty per cent., in the ordinary diseases of the country. . . . Many people refused to call the physician if it were possible to be avoided, preferring to trust nature and domestic remedies. The increased death-rate might have been borne, for the dead are relieved from suffering, but the slow convalescence, and the frequency of chronic disease of the stomach, intestines and liver, following the simple diseases of the country, informed the people that there was a serious wrong in the practice of the day. The wrongs that followed the administration of mercury were of the character that they could not be mistaken—the loss of teeth, carious bones, disease of liver and intestinal canal, mercurial rheumatism, etc.—and the frequency of these unpleasantnesses added to the distrust.[32]

An apt summary of this period of medicine is the description of the death of George Washington in 1799, written by his two attending physicians, one of whom Blanton described as "a successful physician whose services were greatly in demand." Washington's ailment was diagnosed by the physicians as "an inflammatory affection of the upper part of the windpipe," which led to fever and "laborious respi-

[30] Jameson, *American Domestick Medicine*, p. 583; Buchan, *Domestic Medicine*, p. 561; James Ewell, *The Planter's and Mariner's Medical Companion* (Baltimore: 1813), p. 338.

[31] Duffy, *Epidemics in Colonial America*, p. 8.

[32] J. M. Scudder, "A Brief History of Eclectic Medicine," *Eclectic Medical Journal* 39 (1879): 298.

ration" as well as considerable pain and discomfort in the throat. Their report stated:

The necessity of blood-letting suggesting itself to the General, he procured a bleeder in the neighborhood, who took from the arm in the night, twelve or fourteen ounces of blood. . . . [The following day:] Discovering the case to be highly alarming, and foreseeing the fatal tendency of the disease, two consulting physicians were immediately sent for . . . . In the interim were employed two copious bleedings; a blister was applied to the part affected, two moderate doses of calomel were given, an injection was administered which operated on the lower intestines, but all without any perceptible advantage, the respiration becoming still more difficult and distressing. Upon the arrival of the first of the consulting physicians, it was agreed . . . to try the result of another bleeding, when about thirty-two ounces were drawn, without the smallest apparent alleviation of the disease. . . . ten grains of calomel were given, succeeded by repeated doses of emetic tarter, amounting in all to five or six grains, with no other effect than a copious discharge from the bowels. The powers of life seemed now manifestly yielding to the force of the disorder. Blisters were applied to the extremeties, together with a cataplasm of bran and vinegar to the throat. Speaking, which was painful from the beginning, now became almost impracticable, respiration grew more and more contracted and imperfect, till . . . he expired without a struggle [the same evening].[33]

Blanton diagnosed the illness as inflammatory oedema of the larynx, which he stated was frequently fatal in that period. He concluded: "The vigorous therapy resorted to by his physicians may have hastened Washington's death, but it could in no way have caused it."[34]

DISEASE IN EARLY NINETEENTH-CENTURY AMERICA

Had the United States been a basically healthy country, contemporary medical practice might have afflicted only a small part of the population. The country, however, was young and poor, with a considerable amount of illness. Polluted water supplies, unsanitary means of sewage disposal, unhygienic methods of food preparation and transportation, and the lack of any control over mosquitoes, flies, and other insect vectors exposed many people to illness. Among the rural and poor urban inhabitants, malnutrition, poor housing, and exposure to weather grossly intensified the harsh effects of the more general factors. Illness was thus a major part of the lives of Americans, and major epidemics as well as the persistent endemic diseases were characteristic of the period.[35]

[33] Blanton, *Medicine in the Eighteenth Century*, pp. 305–6.
[34] *Ibid.*, pp. 310–11.
[35] Wilson G. Smillie, "The Period of Great Epidemics in the United States (1800–1875)," in C.-E. A. Winslow, *et al.*, *The History of American Epidemiology* (St. Louis: Mosby, 1952), p. 69.

ENDEMIC DISEASES

Malaria was the most common and significant endemic disease in early nineteenth-century America. It was most prevalent in the frontier and southern regions, but was also a major problem in such northern states as Wisconsin and Minnesota in the first half of the century. All these states had numerous marshes and bodies of stagnant water that were ideal breeding grounds for mosquitoes.[36] One English observer commented in 1840 about an inn twelve miles south of Chicago:

The place . . . seemed to be the headquarters of the mosquito tribe; they kept our hands and handkerchiefs in constant motion; and yet they evaded both, so as to cover the faces of most of the parties with large pustules from their bites. They were the largest and most venomous I had ever seen; and the sultriness of the night, the closeness of the place, and the filth of the room in which we were staying, seemed to give them new vigour. I went into the open air, hoping for some relief, but met as large a legion of them without as within, and found there was no escape from their tormenting attacks. One of our Western passengers declared that in a part of the prairie from which he had come, they were so thick that if you held out your naked arm straight for a few minutes, so as to allow them to settle on it, they would be followed by such a cloud of others hovering around them, that if you suddenly drew in your arm, you would perceive a clear hole left in the cloud, by the space which the arm had occupied![37]

The role of mosquitoes as a vector in malaria was unknown, and the dominant theory of the time held that malaria was caused by marsh miasm, the heavy dews and mists arising from "organic decomposition in soils" in marshes, swamps, and jungles. The term malaria itself comes from the Italian, meaning bad air.[38]

Malaria was so prevalent that it was regarded as a natural part of life. It was considered an inevitable part of the "seasoning" of newcomers and people became so accustomed to the "ague" after years of attacks that they no longer considered it a significant illness. Consequently, most cases of malaria were treated by self-medication.[39]

[36] Erwin H. Ackerknecht, *Malaria in the Upper Mississippi Valley 1760–1900* (Baltimore: Johns Hopkins Press, 1945), pp. 75–76; Paul M. Angle, "The Hardy Pioneer: How He Lived in the Early Middle West," *Essays in the History of Medicine* (Chicago: University of Illinois Press, 1965), p. 136.

[37] J. S. Buckingham, *The Eastern and Western States of America* (London, 1842), vol. III, quoted in Angle, "Hardy Pioneer," p. 138. The flies were even more prevalent. Buckingham said that at one meal it was impossible to see the food on the dishes because of the mass of black flies. *Ibid.*, p. 140.

[38] For a good description of the state of knowledge of malaria in the nineteenth century, see W. E. Bloyer, "Malarial Fever," *Eclectic Medical Journal* 46 (1886): 14–18.

[39] Ackerknecht, *Malaria in the Upper Mississippi Valley*, pp. 4–5.

Physicians could do very little for malaria patients because of their ignorance of the proper way to use cinchona or quinine and because of their insistence on administering bloodletting and calomel with it. One physician reminisced:

> The doctors found the ague [malaria], in many instances, more than a match for their skill. It was of the real shaking, quaking variety, the chill lasting not infrequently three or four hours, to be followed by raging fever and intense insatiable thirst. . . . Peruvian bark [cinchona] and calomel would temporarily check the fever, but cold weather seemed to be the only thing that would stop this dreadful scourge, and even this failed in some cases, and the poor invalid either wore himself out or else wore out the disease.[40]

Second only to malaria as endemic diseases were dysentery and diarrhea. Dysentery was an inflammation of the intestines that brought fever, cramps, and a diarrhea with bloody, mucous evacuations which led to its being called the flux or bloody flux. Like malaria, it was more debilitating than fatal and recurred well into the nineteenth century. Chronic diarrhea, the result of lack of sanitation, was a particular problem in the South. J. Marion Sims, an eminent physician who suffered from the disease throughout his life, wrote: "When you see in the South a man in vigorous health and middle life gradually wasting away, and at the end of eighteen months drop as a skeleton into the grave, . . . he has died of chronic diarrhea." These intestinal disorders were most fatal to children, often in the form known as *cholera infantum*, and were the leading cause of infant mortality throughout the nineteenth century.[41]

Respiratory ailments were also major causes of death in this period. Pneumonia and influenza recurred with great frequency. In the urban areas of the northeast, pulmonary tuberculosis soon became the leading cause of death among children and adults. Because the national impact of tuberculosis increased in the second half of the century, it will be discussed in more detail subsequently. Nevertheless, in states like Massachusetts and New York, tuberculosis's greatest contribution to the total mortality occurred before the Civil War.[42]

[40] MacCoy, "Pioneer Physicians of Bartholomew County," pp. 110–11; see also A. B. Shipman, "Professional Matters at the West—Malarious Fever," *Boston Medical and Surgical Journal* 40 (1849): 69–73, 161–64, 238–41.

[41] Duffy, *Epidemics in Colonial America*, pp. 214–22; J. Marion Sims, *The Story of My Life* (New York: Appleton, 1884), p. 252; Smillie, "Period of Great Epidemics," pp. 69–70.

[42] Duffy, *Epidemics in Colonial America*, pp. 200, 238; Wilson G. Smillie, *Public Health: Its Promise for the Future* (New York: Macmillan, 1955), pp. 150–55, 379.

EPIDEMIC DISEASES

Numerous epidemic diseases added to the burden of the endemic diseases in the pre-Civil-War nineteenth century. Although endemic diseases were the principal causes of death in the period, the epidemic diseases struck communities with an abruptness and high mortality which can be compared only to the effects of warfare in the twentieth century.

Cholera was probably the most terrifying of all epidemic diseases. It struck the sufferer so rapidly that it was almost a shock. One victim of an attack stated that as he was walking he felt himself growing stiff from the knees downward. Then, he related, "I felt suddenly a rush of blood from my feet upward, and as it rose my veins grew cold and my blood curdled. My legs and hands were cramped with violent pain." Suddenly, he found himself thrown to the floor "as if shot." William McPheeters, a physician who treated patients during the 1849 St. Louis epidemic, stated that the symptoms were "vomiting freely with frequent and copious discharges from the bowels; at first of slight bilious character, but it soon became pure 'rice water'; cramps in the stomach and lower extremeties and tongue cold; skin of a blue color and very much corrugated; urinary secretions suspended; eyes sunken and surrounded by a livid hue." All this occurred in a few hours, while the patient sunk into a corpselike collapse.[43]

Cholera appeared periodically in the United States in the first half of the nineteenth century, with major nation-wide epidemics in 1832, 1849 (through 1854 in some areas), and 1866. These were frequently so abrupt as to defy easy description. In the 1849 epidemic in St. Louis, the number of deaths from cholera was 68 in March, 131 in April, 517 in May, 1,799 in June, 1,895 in July, and 62 in August. Altogether, in a city which had been reduced to 50,000 persons because of residents who fled the city, 4,557 persons died from cholera in that year. Furthermore, because the disease was most severe "in those parts of the city which were damp and filthy and in which the greatest number of persons were crowded together," the mortality rate among the lower classes must have been appalling. In the 1854 epidemic in New York City, the mortality among hospital patients was so great that on two occasions when an unusually large number of severe cases had been

[43] Lucius H. Zeuch, *History of Medical Practice in Illinois* (Chicago: 1927), I: 166; William M. McPheeters, "Epidemic of Cholera in St. Louis in 1849," in E. J. Goodwin, *A History of Medicine in Missouri* (St. Louis: Smith, 1905), p. 72; Charles E. Rosenberg, *The Cholera Years* (Chicago: University of Chicago Press, 1962), p. 151.

admitted to a ward, physicians found the next morning that all the patients and all the nurses in the ward had died during the night. In the New Orleans epidemic of 1832, the death rate for the population, according to Hoffman, reached the "almost incredible figure of 140.9 per 1,000." This can be compared with New Orleans death rates of 39 in the preceding year, and of 85 in the following year, when cholera was still present.[44]

In these situations, physicians reached the point of pure desperation in their treatments. The rapidity and severity of the epidemics created such a degree of fear, panic, and uncertainty that heroic therapy was pushed to its extreme. McPheeter provided a description of the therapies which he and other physicians used during the 1849 St. Louis epidemic. He tried calomel "faithfully" in hundreds of cases, in doses from two to sixty grains, because it was "regarded by many as the sheet anchor in the treatment of cholera." Even though the patients died anyway, he continued to use calomel throughout the epidemic, but in smaller quantities. He turned to bloodletting, and although his first few cases "seemed rescued from the jaws of death by free blood letting," his later unfavorable experiences led him to abandon it. Other physicians tried external applications like cupping, warm and cold baths, and mustard plasters without success. He cited the case of one patient brought into the hospital, "the soles of whose feet were burnt to a crisp by the application of hot bricks, yet without producing reaction." Another patient lost a limb from gangrene produced by plasters. Eventually, the author settled on a regimen which included repeated doses of calomel, opium, acetate of lead, and a large blister over the abdomen. These were not excessively harsh treatments. Rosenberg has cited examples of even more extreme therapies. Undoubtedly, the danger from the physicians may have exceeded the danger from the disease in many cases.[45]

Yellow fever was comparable to cholera in its dramatic and devastating impact. Between 1702 and 1800, it appeared somewhere in the country thirty-five times, and between 1800 and 1879 it appeared every year with two exceptions. In the famous Philadelphia epidemic of 1793, over 4,000 of the 27,000 residents remaining in the city died in the summer and autumn. The disease was so common in New Orleans

[44] McPheeters, "Epidemic of Cholera," pp. 79, 81; Walsh, *History of Medicine in New York*, I: 110 (the nurses were all male nurses); Frederick L. Hoffman, "American Mortality Progress During the Last Half Century," in *A Half Century of Public Health*, Mazyck P. Ravenel, ed. (New York: American Public Health Association, 1921), pp. 103–4.

[45] McPheeters, "Epidemic of Cholera," pp. 89–91; Rosenberg, *Cholera Years*, pp. 66–67.

that it was almost endemic. Whenever it struck, thousands of residents would flee to neighboring communities and spread the disease throughout the whole region and into neighboring states. Normal business activity ceased, and the major occupations of the residents became caring for the sick and burying the dead, who were often stacked like cordwood in cemeteries. The great New Orleans epidemic of 1853 produced thirty to forty thousand cases, with eight to nine thousand deaths, in a city whose population had been reduced to perhaps two-thirds or one-half of its 150,000 inhabitants.[46]

The treatment for yellow fever appears to have been similar in most places. Early in the century, Buchan advised bleeding eight to twenty ounces two to four times a day after every exacerbation of fever, for as long as seven or eight days. He supplemented this by purging with eight to twelve grains of calomel mixed with a similar amount of jalap or rhubarb, given every four to six hours. While this therapy was a beginning, it was tentative and conservative compared with later treatment. Louisiana physicians prescribed sixty grains of calomel rather than eight or twelve. Cooling water was recognized as desirable, and Duffy has stated: "Here again is reflected the prevailing attitude that one could not get too much of a good thing. If a little cool water reduced fever, then a lot of it would be even more beneficial," and patients were doused with cold sea water for as long as they could bear it. Quinine was also used in the mistaken belief that yellow fever was an intensified form of malaria, which disillusioned many physicians about the value of quinine.[47]

Another epidemic disease starting its fatal course in the first half of the nineteenth century was diphtheria. This children's disease was characterized by a severe sore throat and often the formation of a membrane across the larynx that caused actual suffocation. The mortality rate was very high and several children in the same family often died in the course of an epidemic. The therapy was commensurate with the severity of the disease. Children of three or four years were given calomel in ten-grain doses for several days and were purged with

[46] Ira V. Hiscock, "The Background of Public Health in Connecticut," in Herbert Thoms, ed., *The Heritage of Connecticut Medicine* (New Haven, Conn.: 1942), p. 142; John M. Armstrong, "The First American Medical Journals," *Lectures on the History of Medicine 1926–1932* (Philadelphia: Saunders, 1933), p. 362; Hoffman, "American Mortality Progress," p. 104; John Duffy, *Sword of Pestilence: The New Orleans Yellow Fever Epidemic of 1853* (Baton Rouge: Louisiana State University Press, 1966); Duffy, *History of Medicine in Louisiana*, II: 126, 130–33.

[47] Buchan, *Domestic Medicine*, pp. 221–22; Duffy, *History of Medicine in Louisiana*, I: 279, 274, 276; II: 9, 12–13.

tartar emetic. Venesection from the jugular vein was employed, and blisters were raised and drawn over the throat from ear to ear.[48]

Numerous other epidemic diseases occurred as well, although none were as terrifying as yellow fever or cholera. Typhoid increased in importance when cities grew larger without making efforts to provide clean water to all residents. Even smallpox appeared frequently, introduced by immigrants and fostered by the neglect of vaccination.[49]

Conclusion

Several characteristics of the medical profession in the first half of the nineteenth century can be inferred from these and other data. First, physicians accepted and used the three major medically valid practices of the period described in Chapter 2—smallpox vaccination, cinchona bark, and surgery—to the extent that they were demonstrable and consistent. Most physicians accepted smallpox vaccination early in the century. The usefulness of cinchona bark was limited by diagnostic and pharmacological problems, but by midcentury physicians were agreed on the fundamental validity of the therapy. Although surgery will be examined in detail in a subsequent chapter, it can be observed here that it was also accepted as a medically valid therapy. Even those physicians who opposed heroic therapy and advocated a more passive role for physicians acknowledged the utility of surgery. Jacob Bigelow, the most illustrious of the physicians who opposed heroic therapy, called surgery the "one great exception in favor of artificial and even heroic therapy," although he claimed there were too many "cruel but unavailing operations [which inflicted] pain without corresponding good."[50]

Second, in situations where medically valid therapies were unknown, physicians developed a small number of medically invalid therapies—like bloodletting, calomel, and blisters—that produced consistent and demonstrable changes in the patient's physiological condition. Most regularly trained physicians used these standardized therapies almost exclusively, even though textbooks on therapeutics contained hundreds of alternatives. One physician stated in 1849 that for many physicians "the lancet, mercury, antimony or opium, are the great guns that they always fire on all occasions. . . . whoever sends for

[48] Walsh, *History of Medicine in New York*, pp. 100, 97.

[49] *Ibid.*, p. 96; Smillie, "Period of Great Epidemics," pp. 58, 70.

[50] Jacob Bigelow, *Modern Inquiries* (Boston: Little, Brown, 1867), pp. 229–30; for a history of early nineteenth century surgery, see Courtney R. Hall, "The Rise of Professional Surgery in the United States: 1800–1865," *Bulletin of the History of Medicine* 26 (1952): 231–62.

a physician of this sort expects to be bled, blistered or vomited, or sub-
mitted to some other painful or nauseous medication." In fact, heroic
medication became normative, and those physicians who did not conform were chastized by their colleagues. Jacob Bigelow wrote: "so great
at one time was . . . the ascending of heroic teachers and writers, that
few medical men had the courage to incur the responsibility of omit-
ting the active modes of treatment which were deemed indispensable
to the safety of the patient."[51]

While the medically invalid therapies produced demonstrable
and consistent physiological changes in the short run, in the long run
they were often detrimental to the patient's health, as a few contemporary physicians realized. J. Marion Sims wrote that, shortly after his
graduation from medical school in 1835,

the practice of that time was heroic: it was murderous. I knew nothing
about medicine, but I had sense enough to see that doctors were killing their
patients, that medicine was not an exact science, that it was wholly empirical
and that it would be better to trust entirely to Nature than to the hazardous
skill of the doctors.[52]

About this same time, many patients and some other physicians came
to the same conclusion and rebelled against heroic therapy. Before
describing those events, however, it is necessary to examine the development of the medical institutions which brought about the standardization of medically invalid therapies. The institutionalization of
medical societies, medical licensing programs, and medical schools will
be examined in the next three chapters.

[51] Dan King, "The Evils of Quackery, and its Remedies," *Boston Medical and Surgical Journal* 40 (1849): 373; Bigelow, *Modern Inquiries*, p. 228.
[52] Sims, *Story of My Life*, p. 150.

CHAPTER 4 MEDICAL SOCIETIES AND MEDICAL LICENSING

IT WAS OBSERVED in Chapter 1 that professional societies can be categorized into two different types, exclusive and inclusive. Exclusive societies have restrictive membership policies in which each applicant is evaluated by the medical society itself. Inclusive societies admit any reputable physician who meets certain objective criteria established by the state. At the turn of the nineteenth century, there were few medical colleges, only a small number of medical college graduates, and no effective state licensing laws. Consequently, the profession was heterogeneous in terms of professional education, therapeutics, wealth, and clientele. Under these circumstances, exclusive societies were the only feasible form of professional organization. Local medical societies were formed first, but were soon followed by state societies. Gradually, as the number of medical school graduates and licensed physicians increased, medical societies adopted less restrictive membership policies. The major activity of most medical societies was licensing, used by society members to separate themselves from other medical practitioners. Societies also established fee bills and codes of ethics in order to regulate the conduct of their members, and claimed that they engaged in scientific activities. As a result of the importance of the first of these activities, medical societies grew from an insignificant position at the turn of the century to become the major institution in the profession by midcentury.

THE DEVELOPMENT OF EXCLUSIVE MEDICAL SOCIETIES

RELATIONS AMONG PHYSICIANS

Relations among physicians in the early part of the century can be characterized by one word—factiousness. The *New York Monthly Chronicle of Medicine and Surgery* observed in 1825: "no body of men are less in concert or seem less influenced by the *esprit du corps*, than physicians. . . . the quarrels of physicians are proverbially frequent and bitter, and their hatred, intensity, and duration seem to exceed that of other men. This state of things is in some degree attributable to the nature of the profession."[1] Conflicts over therapies were largely responsible for these quarrels.

The unscientific nature of medical practice made it impossible to prove the validity or invalidity of therapies, and each physician could praise his own therapies and damn those of his competitors without the possibility of any objective resolution to the dispute. Some medical historians have argued that the quarrels were caused by the different theories of disease on which the use of different therapies was based, but, as Daniel Drake observed in 1832, the therapeutic consequences of the theories was the source of the conflict:

Differences of opinion, on the principles of the profession, lead to many of the personal antipathies and controversies which disturb the profession. . . . This results, from the ultimate practical tendency, of every professional speculation. If the theories of medicine, did not influence its practice, and, by that means, the business of its practitioners, conflicting opinions as to the seats, causes and treatment of diseases, would no more excite personal altercation, than disputes on the materiality of light, or the Eleusinian mysteries. As every medical theory, is to stand or fall, by the test of experiment, the opposing partisans, naturally magnify their own, and depreciate each others success; which of course leads to reciprocal charges of misrepresentation; and the conflict of opinion, cannot be long maintained, without engendering personal animosities.[2]

These conflicts led to considerable enmity among physicians. When a patient summoned one physician to replace another, according to an account, "there was sure to be a prompt throwing out of medicine, with an admonition delivered to the patient not to take any more of it unless he courted death." The competition frequently resulted in price cutting, which became another bone of contention.[3]

LOCAL MEDICAL SOCIETIES

Given these kinds of conflicts among physicians, medical societies were successful only when a small number of physicians separated themselves from their competitors and formed exclusive societies. Here the members could agree on therapies, share the prestige of membership, call fellow members in for consultations on difficult cases, and allocate appointments to the faculties of the medical col-

1 George Rosen, *Fees and Fee Bills* (Baltimore: Johns Hopkins Press, 1946), p. 2.
2 Daniel Drake, *Practical Essays on Medical Education and the Medical Profession in the United States* (Baltimore: Johns Hopkins Press, 1952), p. 98.
3 Lucius H. Zeuch, *History of Medical Practice in Illinois*, vol. I (Chicago: 1927), p. 393.

leges and hospitals. The wealthy and best educated physicians were the ones most likely to benefit from membership in these societies: they had the affluent patients needed to make consultations profitable, they provided the capital to establish the medical colleges, they were prestigious and influential enough to be consulted by public authorities about public health problems. They had something to give to benefit the organization, and could also benefit from the organization. The poor physicians, with poor patients and no influence, were of course excluded from these societies. An examination of the early societies formed in the three urban centers of the early nineteenth century—Boston, New York, and Philadelphia—all illustrate this phenomenon.

Physicians in Boston formed a local medical society in 1780, but reorganized it with additional members from elsewhere in the state in 1781 as the Massachusetts Medical Society. An account by one of the early members stated that the Boston founders "were all respectable men in society, and had the best advantages the country could afford. Many of them had spent a part of their time in Europe, and attended practice in the hospitals in London, Edinburgh, etc." The same author said that the original members living outside of Boston were also "eminent men." The founders themselves declared they wished to create an exclusive organization in order "that a just discrimination should be made between such as are duly educated, and properly qualified for the duties of their profession, and those who may ignorantly and wickedly administer medicine whereby the health and lives of many valuable individuals may be endangered, or perhaps lost to the community." In order to assure that the society would not degenerate into a mass organization, its charter limited the membership to seventy. According to a historian of the society, "admission to the fellowship became a proof of distinction which the better educated and higher-minded physicians were proud to attain. This number, furthermore, gave evidence of the comparatively few physicians in the State at that time who were considered worthy of this high distinction." The value of the society to its members and its influence in the community is indicated by the selection of founders of the society as Boston's first three quarantine officers, a position which provided considerable prestige and income.[4]

4 Walter L. Burrage, *A History of the Massachusetts Medical Society* (n.p., 1923), pp. 18–19; Ephraim Eliot, "Account of the Physicians of Boston," *Proceedings of the Massachusetts Historical Society* (Nov., 1863), pp. 180–81; Reginald H. Fitz, "The Rise and Fall of the Licensed Physician in Massachusetts, 1781–1860," *Transactions of the Association of American Physicians* 9 (1894): 3; John B. Blake, *Public Health in the Town of Boston 1630–1822* (Cambridge, Mass.: Harvard University Press, 1959), p. 126.

Although the society was nominally a state-wide organization, Boston physicians dominated it for many years. Meetings were usually held in Boston, even though the city is located at the eastern end of the state. As late as 1848, a committee of the society acknowledged that the society had failed to attract members from areas remote from Boston. Physicians at the extreme western end of the state twice formed their own medical societies.[5]

In Philadelphia, the first stable society of practicing physicians was established in 1787 as the College of Physicians (the terms "college" and "faculty" when applied to physicians often referred to the body of practitioners in a community; no pedagogical associations were intended). It too was formed, according to Shryock, to set some physicians "apart from other practitioners in the community." The organization had 29 members in its first year, but in the next 31 years only 28 other physicians were elected to membership, which reduced the active membership to 18 because of deaths, resignations, etc. Although the rate of election of new members increased thereafter, by 1849 only 180 members had been elected in the organization's 62-year history. Furthermore, in the years from 1792 to 1807, the membership fee was $26.66 and the annual dues $4—sums prohibitive to all but the wealthiest physicians in the city. The prestige of the organization was recognized by the governor and the state legislature, who sought its advice two years after its founding and fairly regularly thereafter.[6]

The history of medical societies in New York City before the Revolutionary War was one of sporadic organization. Shortly after the war, the Medical Society of the State of New York (a misnomer, because all the members were residents of New York City) was formed as a society to which belonged "almost all physicians with any pretension to prominence," according to Calhoun. The society recommended surgeons to the Army and Navy on behalf of the whole profession in the city. In 1794, the society was reorganized as a much smaller organ-

5 Fitz, "Licensed Physician in Massachusetts," p. 13; Peter D. Gibbons, "The Berkshire Medical Institution," *Bulletin of the History of Medicine* 38 (1964): 46.

6 Richard H. Shryock, "The College of Physicians of Philadelphia in Historical Perspective," *Transactions and Studies of the College of Physicians of Philadelphia*, ser. 4, vol. 27 (1960): 152; W. S. W. Ruschenberger, *An Account of the Institution and Progress of the College of Physicians of Philadelphia . . .* (Philadelphia: 1887), pp. 23, 25, 49, 69, 76, 88, 100, 173. In 1789, another medical society was formed in Philadelphia as the Philadelphia Medical Society. Most of its members were medical students and its activities generally catered to their interests. The College of Physicians stood aloof from the other society, "the rather more exclusive nature of its organization and the prestige it acquired seem to have reserved for it from the beginning an uncontested place of its own." Samuel X Radbill, "The Philadelphia Medical Society, 1789–1868," *Transactions and Studies of the College of Physicians of Philadelphia*, ser. 4, vol. 20 (1953): 104.

ization, which prompted some non-members to form a rival society. This rival organization did not last long, but another rival society was founded in 1802. The Medical Society of the State of New York endeavored to cooperate with this society, although it was unwilling to merge with the new organization.[7] Thus, in all three cities, highly exclusive societies were the first stable medical organizations.

The elite societies characteristic of the large cities were not possible in the smaller towns and rural areas, where it was necessary to organize virtually all reputable physicians to support a medical society. Nonetheless, exclusiveness was also the major objective of those societies. Connecticut medical societies provide an example of this type of organization.

The first medical society in Connecticut was organized in 1767 in Litchfield, a town with about 2,500 residents. Most members were from Litchfield and the neighboring town of Sharon, but some were from elsewhere in Litchfield County and other nearby towns, such as Waterbury. The purpose of the society, according to the account of an ex-member, was "to promote a good agreement, and harmony amongst its members, endeavour to be mutually assisting to each other, in the healing art, and to keep out all Quacks, and vain pretenders to Physic. . . . The grand thing . . . is to keep out Quacks, and pretenders." Of course, the society would determine who was or was not a quack. It notified the public through a Hartford newspaper that all physicians coming to the county and all apprentices of county physicians were expected to submit to and abide by the results of an examination by the society "on Pain of the highest Displeasure and Neglect" of its members. The society was short-lived, and suspended activities in 1771.[8]

When a successor society was founded in 1779, its members also felt that the control of quackery was a paramount consideration. A statement issued at the founding meeting read: "One of the greatest evils . . . mankind suffers is disease, and 2dly the miserable, ignorant, and injudicious application of medicine" by quacks, whom they resolved to treat with the "abhorrence and detestation, they justly merit."[9]

In 1784, physicians in New Haven County formed a medical so-

[7] Daniel H. Calhoun, *Professional Lives in America* (Cambridge, Mass.: Harvard University Press, 1965), pp. 28–30.

[8] Byron Stookey, "Found! The Record of the 1767 Medical Society in Litchfield," *Connecticut State Medical Journal* 21 (1957): 353, 346, 192–94.

[9] Walter R. Steiner, "The Date of the Organization of the Litchfield County Medical Association," *Yale Journal of Biology and Medicine* 9 (1936): 128–29.

ciety, the objective of which was "in time [to] answer all the purposes
of reducing the Medical Profession to a regular System, and prevent
the world from the horrid imposition of Quacks, Medicasters and
Vain Pretenders, with which it is now infested." To do this, the society
set up an examination committee to select members in the same way
as the Litchfield County society.[10]

These Connecticut physicians, although constrained by their small
communities to establish relatively broadly based societies, still desired
to establish a more exclusive organization. In 1786 and 1787, a number
of them petitioned the state legislature for a Connecticut Medical
Society with a membership limit of seventy (perhaps influenced by the
same limit in the Massachusetts Medical Society) and with the power
to issue licenses. That this society was not simply a state medical
society is made evident by another provision in the same bill that
organized the county societies in the state into a Medical Convention
without any power to issue licenses. The legislature turned down the
request and the effort was discontinued.[11]

The history of medical societies in most areas of the country,
which were small towns or rural areas, was very similar to the history
of those in Connecticut. The societies included most reputable physicians, but insisted on some self-determined membership policy to
exclude all whom they chose to define as quacks or pretenders. In this
way exclusive medical societies proliferated in the first half of the
century.

STATE MEDICAL SOCIETIES

Because physicians compete in a local market, the most stable and
enduring form of medical organization was the local society. At the
same time, physicians in the same state shared problems which induced
them to form state societies. The most important common problem
was state regulation of medical practice, which will be discussed below.
State societies were established in three different ways: as independent
organizations with a state-wide membership; as nominal state societies
which depended on a single community or local area for the great
bulk of their members; or as federations of local societies. Most of the
earlier state societies were founded on the two former principles.

[10] Creighton Barker, "The Founding of the New Haven County Medical
Association," Connecticut State Medical Journal 5 (1941): 180–81.
[11] Henry Bronson, "Historical Account of the Origin of the Connecticut Medical Society," Proceedings of the Connecticut Medical Society, ser. 2, vol. 4 (1873):
196–97.

State societies established as independent organizations were generally the product of state-wide conventions of physicians called for that purpose. State societies founded in this manner in the smaller states, like New Hampshire (1791), Maryland (1799), Rhode Island (1812), and Vermont (1814), were successful because the physicians in the few populous communities served as the nucleus of the membership. Furthermore, the problems of transportation and communication were not overwhelming in the geographically smaller states. In the larger states, this approach to organizing usually failed until a number of stable local societies had been formed as a foundation for a state society. For example, the Medical Conventions of Ohio was organized as an autonomous state society in 1835, but it led a precarious existence marked by several suspensions. Eventually, it merged with another state-wide body, the Ohio State Medical Society, which was based on a network of local societies and was far more stable than the Conventions.[12]

The second method of forming state societies involved a nominal rather than a real state organization. A local society simply expanded its membership to include a few residents of other areas of the state or adopted the name of a state society. In neither case was there any real effort to establish a society representing physicians from throughout the state. This procedure was very common in the period before the Civil War (Table IV.1). Almost all the societies either disbanded within a few years or reorganized as local societies. Only two of them—in New Jersey and Massachusetts—survived as state societies. They succeeded because they created local societies as subordinate or even co-equal organizations and thus established a foundation of local support for the state society.

The third method of forming state societies was as a federation of local and county societies. This method was first used in Connecticut, where one local and several county societies were established during the 1770's and 1780's. Representatives of these societies obtained a charter for a state society from the state legislature in 1792. This charter created a state society composed of delegates from the county societies, which were also incorporated in the act. The act provided

[12] Histories of the state societies referred to are found in Appendix III; the history of the Ohio state societies is from: Robert G. Paterson, "The Role of the 'District' as a Unit in Organized Medicine in Ohio," *Ohio State Archaeological and Historical Quarterly* 49 (1940): 371; Donald D. Shira, "The Organization of the Ohio State Medical Society and its Relation to the Ohio Medical Convention," *Ohio State Archaeological and Historical Quarterly* 50 (1941): 366–72.

that physicians in each county hold meetings and elect delegates who were to comprise the state society. In this way a state society was created without any independent existence apart from the member county societies.[13] This form of state society was especially stable, and ultimately all state medical societies were organized or reorganized on this basis.

GROWTH OF LOCAL AND STATE SOCIETIES

The best possible measure of the growth of medical societies in the early nineteenth century would be a chronological tabulation of their number and size. However, many medical societies of the period survived only briefly, and most of the others experienced periodic suspensions and reorganizations. Written records are rarely sufficiently detailed to permit accurate tabulations of the number of medical societies in existence at any time. Therefore, selective tabulations have been made (in Appendix I) and summarized (in Table IV.2) of the most important medical societies established before the Civil War in all states which were widely settled by 1840. This includes all states east of the Mississippi River—excluding Florida, Wisconsin, and Minnesota—and also Louisiana and Missouri. These data show that the

TABLE IV.1

PRE-CIVIL WAR LOCAL MEDICAL SOCIETIES DESIGNATED AS STATE MEDICAL SOCIETIES

Date of Founding	Name of Society	Membership Composition
1766	Medical Society of New Jersey	Most of the early members lived in Essex and Middlesex Counties
1781	Massachusetts Medical Society	Society activities and many members in Boston
1789	Medical Society of South Carolina	Limited to Charleston
1791	Medical Society of the State of New York	Limited to New York City
1804	Medical Society of Georgia	Limited to Savannah
1821	Medical Society of Virginia	Most members lived in Richmond
1830	Medical Society of Tennessee	Most members lived in Nashville area
1837	Medical Society of Missouri	Limited to St. Louis, and reorganized as St. Louis Medical Society in 1850
1847	Alabama Medical Society	Limited to Selma, and name changed to Selma Medical Society in 1867

SOURCE: See the appropriate references listed in Appendix III.

13 The act of incorporation of the state society is in *Reprint of the Proceedings of the Connecticut Medical Society from 1792 to 1829, Inclusive* (Hartford: 1884), pp. vi–viii; see also Bronson, "Historical Account."

number of existing state and local societies grew steadily from the 1780's to the Civil War, following the growth of the population of those states. Medical societies were formed before 1800 in most of the states settled during the colonial period, and after 1800 in the midwestern and other southern states.

As the profession grew in the larger cities, the local medical societies either expanded their membership to include more physicians, or were supplemented by new medical societies with more open membership policies. In Boston, the Massachusetts Medical Society was reorganized in 1803 without any maximum membership limit. From 1781 to 1801, the society had admitted a total of 95 physicians, and in 1803 alone it admitted 55. From this period on, the society became a less exclusive body. In New York, the Medical Society of the State of New York was reorganized in 1806 as the society of the County of New York, and immediately began to admit larger numbers of members. In Philadelphia, the Philadelphia County Medical Society was founded in 1849 and became the general medical organization in that city. It should not be thought that elitism in medical organizations had disappeared, for in both Boston and New York, as well as in other cities, elite organizations were soon formed in addition to the exclusive

TABLE IV.2
INCEPTION OF STABLE MEDICAL SOCIETIES IN STATES HEAVILY SETTLED BY 1840

Region	Date of Organization of Stable Medical Society			
	Before 1800	1800–19	1820–39	1840–59
Northeast	Connecticut Massachusetts New Hampshire	Maine Rhode Island Vermont		
Mid-Atlantic	New York Delaware Maryland New Jersey Pennsylvania	District of Columbia		
Southern and Border	South Carolina	Georgia Kentucky	Louisiana Tennessee	Alabama Mississippi Missouri North Carolina Virginia
Midwestern			Indiana Michigan Ohio	Illinois

SOURCE: Appendix III.

ones, and in Philadelphia the College of Physicians remained an elite organization.[14]

MEDICAL LICENSING LEGISLATION

Licensing is generally defined as a mechanism whereby the state grants certain exclusive privileges to individuals meeting the qualifications set down by the state or its legally appointed representatives. The origin of licensing is frequently traced to the guild system of medieval Europe, where guilds were empowered by the state to exercise a monopoly over the practice of their craft, to control admission to it, to determine the prices to be charged, and to regulate many features of guild life. It is often argued that medical licensing in America can be traced to this philosophy of regulation and that the principles of guild regulation were transferred to the American medical profession.

The evidence does not support this position. Medical societies were generally small and rarely influential enough to obtain such important powers for themselves. The rural population, served by few full-time physicians, opposed any stringent licensing measures. The empirics and midwives also resisted all serious efforts to eliminate their livelihoods. Furthermore, there is no evidence that public opinion elsewhere in the least supported such a move. It was shown in Chapter 2 that the public viewed the role of the medical profession with considerable skepticism, if not hostility. Public support for the regulation of medical practice was lacking and, without it, no stringent regulations could have been imposed on the right to practice medicine. Rather, the purpose of virtually all medical licensing during the first half of the nineteenth century was honorific—to provide physicians with some exclusive legal privileges which would enhance their position in the community without depriving other practitioners of the right to practice.

LICENSING IN THE COLONIAL PERIOD

In the colonial period, the most common purpose of licensing was to award some certificate to distinguished or influential physicians to differentiate them from the common herd of practitioners. Colonial legislatures issued licenses of this sort fairly frequently.

In 1721, for example, a number of residents of a small Connecticut community petitioned the colonial legislature for a license for a

[14] Burrage, *Massachusetts Medical Society*, pp. 59, 71–72; Calhoun, *Professional Lives*, pp. 31–35; J. Madison Taylor and Rufus B. Scarlett, "History of the Medical Societies of Philadelphia," in Frederick P. Henry, ed., *Founders' Week Memorial Volume* (Philadelphia: 1909), pp. 881–82.

physician who "had for many years studied the art and method of physic—had made divers experiments, by the blessing of God, with good success, to the satisfaction of those who have been benefited and blessed thereby, besides the judgment and approbation of divers able doctors in the neighboring governments." This petition was refused, but others were not.[15]

Physicians soon recognized that such a licensing system could be used to their own advantage, to separate those whom they considered qualified from those whom they considered quacks, empirics, or other undesirable competitors. Thus, for example, in 1763, a number of physicians in Norwich, Conn., petitioned the colonial legislature "to Distinguish between the Honest and Ingenious Physician and the Quack or Empirical Pretender" by permitting the physicians in the state to establish medical societies with licensing boards. Unlicensed practitioners would be denied the use of the courts to recover debts owed them for services rendered as physicians. Two features of this memorial stand out. First, the petitioners did not try to limit medical practice to licensed physicians, but only to give them legal recognition and exclusive use of the courts to sue for debts—surely an honorific right with little practical importance. Second, the physicians wanted the licenses to be issued by medical societies rather than by a board appointed by the legislature or governor. This would have given physicians complete control over issuing licenses to their own apprentices. The request was denied by the legislature.[16]

The physicians' demands were more ambitious in other localities. In a Pennsylvania county in 1775, they complained to the legislature that the area was "infested with a Set of Men, who taking upon themselves the Offices of Physicians and Surgeons, (though in Reality no better than Empiricks or Quacks) administer Drugs so unskillfully and ignorantly, that some Persons have, in all Probability, thereby lost their Lives, and others been rendered Cripples." These physicians wanted the state to require *all* physicians to obtain licenses before practicing. This request was also refused by the legislature.[17]

Throughout the colonial period, physicians made numerous attempts like the ones just described to obtain licensing legislation. With a few exceptions, discussed in Chapter 2, they were unsuccessful.

15 Joseph F. Kett, *The Formation of the American Medical Profession* (New Haven: Yale University Press, 1968), p. 7; George O. Sumner, "Early Physicians in Connecticut," *Connecticut State Medical Journal* 6 (1942): 464.

16 Charles J. Bartlett, "Medical Licensure in Connecticut," *Connecticut State Medical Journal* 6 (1942): 182.

17 Whitfield J. Bell, Jr., "Medical Practice in Colonial America," *Bulletin of the History of Medicine* 31 (1957): 442.

Most legislatures consistently refused to grant regulatory licensing privileges to physicians.

THE ENACTMENT OF LICENSING LEGISLATION

After the Revolution, legislatures became more receptive to the physicians' requests. By this time, the number of regularly educated physicians had increased, following the establishment of several medical colleges and the growth of the apprenticeship system. Physicians in the larger cities were wealthy and influential men, and the independent practicing physician was becoming increasingly common everywhere. Physicians themselves were becoming more aware of their common professional interests and were establishing local medical societies in the more populous areas. These physicians viewed licensing as a major activity of medical societies. Licensing would give state sanction to the exclusive membership policies of the societies, enable the societies to exert more control over their members, provide income to the societies through licensing fees, and help regulate the supply of physicians in the community.

For these reasons, most licensing legislation in the period immediately after the Revolution was enacted as part of legislation establishing medical societies. Two general forms of such legislation emerged, corresponding to the size and population density of the states involved. In the smaller states, some physicians banded together at a convention or on some other occasion and drafted a petition to the legislature requesting incorporation and licensing authority for themselves as a state society. This occurred in such states as Massachusetts (1781), New Hampshire (1791), Connecticut (1792), Maryland (1799), and Rhode Island (1812). In the larger states, the dispersion of the population made this impractical. In three large states—Pennsylvania, Virginia, and North Carolina—neither stable state medical societies nor licensing laws were established until the middle of the century. In most of the others, a small number of unrepresentative physicians (whose names are in many cases unknown), acting without ascertaining the amount of professional interest in the matter throughout the state, convinced the legislature to incorporate a state medical society and grant it licensing authority, even though few or no medical societies existed in the state. The physicians who obtained passage of these laws obviously sought to induce their colleagues to form state societies and enforce the licensing laws.

This kind of hot-house germination of medical societies had an obvious drawback: while some of the leaders of the profession were interested in medical societies and licensing legislation, the majority of physicians in most states were not, and even the lure of already established licensing powers did not induce them to participate.

The only successful application of this strategy occurred in New York State. While physicians in New York City had been successful in organizing societies, physicians elsewhere in the state were unable to do so. N. S. Davis, an important member of the medical profession during the middle of the century, stated that around 1800 the "great mass" of the profession in New York State "were alike unsocial and ungoverned by ethical laws." When 21 physicians in Saratoga County established a medical society in 1796, "so discordant were their feelings and modes of thought" that it did not survive the year.[18] This state of affairs continued for another decade, with only the New York City physicians having any medical societies. Then in 1806, a group of un-organized physicians in three upstate counties, including Saratoga, obtained passage of legislation which empowered physicians in the state to establish state and local medical societies and to issue licenses. The New York City physicians did not participate in this venture, and looked upon such broad-based legislation with some disfavor. The new law was remarkably effective, however, because within two years county societies were established in most inhabited parts of the state on a stable basis, and the state society was functioning satisfactorily. In this way, according to Davis, "two great and all important objects were accomplished, viz.: a thorough organization of the profession in a manner most favorable to its advancement and elevation, and the provision for having all candidates examined before admission, by practitioners, themselves, without the intervention of any other class."[19]

Five years later, physicians in Ohio attempted a similar plan, but it failed. A law was passed in 1811 creating five licensing districts, with three physicians actually named in the act to serve in each. Apparently, the physicians failed to carry out their duties; in 1812 the law was repealed, and another passed that created seven licensing districts, the same number of district societies, and a state medical society consisting of 120 physicians named in the act. This also failed, and in 1813 the law was repealed and a law enacted similar to the 1811 law. This law was amended several times during the next decade and apparently was ineffective. In 1824, another law was passed creating medical societies, but this also failed. Finally, according to a historian, "in 1833, the disgusted legislators, with the consent of the thoroughly

18 N. S. Davis, *History of Medical Education and Institutions in the United States* (Chicago: S. C. Griggs, 1851), pp. 84–85.

19 Calhoun, *Professional Lives*, p. 31; Davis, *History of Medical Education*, p. 88.

disillusioned medical profession, repealed all laws pertaining to the practice of medicine." In this case the laws had gone so far as to name the physicians who were to be members of the societies and the dates and places of the organizational meetings in some instances; yet the societies were never organized and the licensing laws never enforced.[20]

The early experiences of physicians in Illinois and Indiana were very much like those of Ohio physicians, and the same may have been true in other frontier states. The failure of these laws was undoubtedly due to the sparse population, the widely scattered settlements, the difficulty of traveling long distances, and, above all, the small number of physicians in any community who could profit by the existence of a medical society.[21]

CONTENT OF THE LICENSING LAWS

While legislatures were generally willing to grant licensing powers to medical societies, they were unwilling to enact laws which would have seriously deterred unlicensed practitioners. This is clearly indicated by the laws themselves. Appendix II provides a tabulation of all important licensing legislation in practically all of the states whose medical societies were tabulated in Appendix I. Several generalizations can be made from these and other data. First, most of the licensing laws placed licensing powers directly in the hands of the medical societies. Second, few licensing laws gave the societies the right to revoke licenses after they had been awarded. Third, the penalties for unlicensed practice were generally nonexistent or insignificant. The most common differentiation between licensed and unlicensed practitioners was that only licensed practitioners had the right to sue for uncollected fees in court. This was no deterrent to unlicensed practitioners; licensed physicians themselves complained of being unable to collect their fees even with the aid of the courts. The famous Shattuck report of the Massachusetts Sanitary Commission estimated in 1850 that the average Massachusetts physician charged fees amounting to $800 annually, but collected only $600 as his annual earnings. A less common penalty was a fine, which was usually so small that it had little deterrent effect. Furthermore, the imposition of a fine required a jury trial, and juries were often reluctant to convict unlicensed practitioners. Last, apothecaries, midwives, and botanical practitioners were often

[20] Shira, "Ohio State Medical Society," p. 366; Paterson, "Role of the 'District'," pp. 369–70.
[21] Louis G. Caldwell, "Early Legislation Regulating the Practice of Medicine," *Illinois Law Review* 18 (1923): 244.

exempted from the licensing requirements. A broad definition of these vocations would have completely nullified the regulatory aspects of the licensing laws.[22]

In the rare instances when medical societies actively sought to strengthen the licensing regulations, either the legislatures or public opinion refused to permit it. In New York, for example, the original 1806 law prohibited unlicensed practitioners to sue for debts. When this penalty was increased to a $25 fine in 1807, a clause was inserted in the law exempting botanic practitioners and a number of others. The net result was probably a weaker law than the original one. In 1825, the New York state medical society undertook a campaign to strengthen the law. The president of the society complained in that year:

While the regular physician is made subject to several years of study, a set of imposters, whose impudence is only equalled by their ignorance, are allowed to rob and murder the good citizens under the pretence of using only herbs and roots, the product of the country, although it is well known that they deal in the most powerful drugs in the shops, however ignorant, as they must be, of their composition and qualities.[23]

As a result of the subsequent efforts of the society, in 1827 the New York state legislature made the unlicensed practice of medicine a misdemeanor, subject to fine and imprisonment. The significance of this change was not in the penalty, but in the fact that enforcement of misdemeanors rested with the law-enforcement agencies, and police officials would be responsible for ridding communities of unlicensed practitioners. It is not known whether the law was enforced to any degree, but a New York physician of the period wrote that "it was represented as oppressive," and in 1830 the law was repealed and the previous law reenacted in its place.[24]

These and similar experiences of physicians in other states convinced the profession that licensing laws and penalties were ineffective in regulating the number of practitioners. In Maryland, the society's board of censors (licensing examination committee) stated in 1811 that they were unable to bring violators to justice or induce judges to convict them. A committee of the Albany, New York, medical society concluded several decades later that it was "entirely impossible" to enforce the laws in that state: "For many years they have been in existence,

22 *Ibid.*, p. 235; Massachusetts Sanitary Commission, *Report of a General Plan for the Promotion of Public and Personal Health* (Boston: 1850), p. 59.

23 Florence A. Cooksley, "A History of Medicine in the State of New York and the County of Monroe," *New York State Journal of Medicine* 36 (1936): 1682.

24 Charles B. Coventry, "History of Medical Legislation in the State of New York," *New York Journal of Medicine* 4 (1845): 156–57.

and yet men have practiced under our eyes openly and avowedly in violation of them, and in no one instance has the penalty been enforced." In Ohio, the president of the Ohio State Medical Society reported in 1849 that "all enactments upon the subject of medicine or prescriptions under fines, penalties, or the like, are extremely difficult of execution and have impracticability and soon become a dead letter." A committee of the Louisiana State Medical Society came to the same conclusion in 1850. As late as 1877, a committee of the Mississippi state society concluded that "it would be difficult to have any law enforced which would deprive the people of the inestimable privilege of being poisoned in their own chosen way. . . . until the necessity for such legislation shall be appreciated by the masses of the people, the passage of any such laws will be premature, and they will remain dead letters on the statute books."[25]

Once physicians realized that the licensing laws were totally unenforceable, they began to have second thoughts about retaining or enacting the laws. The Louisiana committee referred to above considered recommending imprisonment for violators as a means of enforcement, but abandoned the idea because the public would never "consent to the enactment of a penal statute for the protection of this or any other science." Physicians in Chicago in 1844 and 1858 were opposed to the enactment of any new licensing laws because they believed that their enactment would only increase public sympathy for unlicensed physicians. Many leaders of the profession counseled patience and held that physicians should rely upon their superior knowledge and skill to gain public support. One of the earliest advocates of this view was Nicholas Romayne, one of the most influential physicians of his time and a president of the New York state medical society. He stated in 1810 that, inasmuch as the public was opposed to restrictive licensing legislation, physicians could successfully eliminate quackery only by providing therapies which were demonstrably superior to those of other practitioners. He asserted that "when Practitioners of Medicine are diligent and judicious in the exercise of their professions, they manifest to men of any discernment, their superior skill and success in the cure of diseases; and will show in a striking point of view, the difference between the well educated Physician and Surgeon, and the

25 Kett, *American Medical Profession*, pp. 21–22; Jonathan Forman, "Organized Medicine in Ohio, 1811 to 1926," *Ohio State Medical Journal* 43 (1947): 58; John Duffy, ed., *The Rudolph Matas History of Medicine in Louisiana* (n.p.: Louisiana State University Press, 1962), II: 113; Felix J. Underwood and R. N. Whitfield, *Public Health and Medical Licensure in the State of Mississippi 1798–1937* (Jackson, Miss.: 1938), p. 141; see also Madge E. Pickard and R. Carlyle Buley, *The Midwest Pioneer* (New York: Henry Schuman, 1946), p. 262.

mere pretender to professional knowledge."[26] As it turned out, physicians had little choice but to console themselves with the opinions of men like Romayne. None of the licensing laws in this period was ever effective, and ultimately, for reasons to be discussed in a subsequent chapter, most of them were repealed.

LICENSING BOARDS AND REGULAR PHYSICIANS

Even if licensing laws had been enforceable, the regular physicians and their societies were confronted with so many problems operating the licensing boards that they would have been unable to enforce the penalties under any circumstances. Most licensing laws authorized county societies to establish licensing boards and issue licenses valid for the entire state. An applicant who was turned down by one board could therefore try his luck in a neighboring county. This would not have been a major problem, except that the societies relied on the fees obtained from issuing licenses for partial support of their activities. Refusing an applicant meant losing the license fee that would probably go to the board in a neighboring county. According to Davis, this competition among licensing boards produced "an universal laxity in the examination of students, instead of a uniform rigidity and exactitude." Consequently, the possession of a license offered little assurance that the licentiate was a competent physician.[27]

Given all these dilemmas, it may be asked why physicians did not give up licensing boards altogether. They aroused public hostility, they were ineffective in maintaining any standards of competence in the profession, they demonstrated the weakness and ineffectiveness of the medical societies. With all these disadvantages, it might be expected that the boards would have fallen into disuse and neglect. They did not, because in spite of all their shortcomings, they were still of considerable benefit to physicians. In this period most physicians were educated as apprentices. When the graduated apprentice sought to open his own practice, his only evidence of professional training was a letter of commendation from his tutor, which was meaningful only if the client knew the tutor. A license, on the other hand, represented the collective judgment of a board of censors recognized by law, and was therefore a more useful formal recognition of the apprentice's

[26] Duffy, *Medicine in Louisiana*, p. 113; Thomas N. Bonner, "The Social and Political Attitudes of Midwestern Physicians 1840–1940: Chicago as a Case History," *Journal of the History of Medicine and Allied Sciences* 8 (1953): 134–35; James J. Walsh, *History of the Medical Society of the State of New York* (n.p.: 1907), pp. 100–101.

[27] N. S. D[avis], "National Convention," *New York Journal of Medicine* 6 (1846): 288.

attainments. Tutors also found licensing useful, especially when their apprentices received sympathetic treatment before the licensing boards. The revenue produced by licensing boards was an important source of income to the local societies. The total income of the state medical society of Maryland in 1831 was $1240, 27 percent of which came from licenses.[28] In addition, membership on a licensing board became coveted because the members obtained the prestige of the position and could easily attract apprentices, who could then expect little difficulty in obtaining licenses. According to Daniel Drake, these positions were often a source of discord in the profession:

The office of censor is essentially one of rotation, and generally, becomes an object of ambition. Its acquisition is often attended with circumstances of management, that are discreditable to the profession; and its administration, still oftener, perhaps, so conducted, as to offend the feelings of those, who have an immediate interest, in the admission or rejection of such candidates, as are their own pupils. Thus feuds are generated, and a whole district is degraded, by reciprocal changes of malfeasance in office; which, whether true or false, disturb the harmony of a profession. . . .[29]

Licensing therefore, whatever its intrinsic inadequacies, was useful to the profession in providing income to the societies, adding greater formality to the apprenticeship system, and giving prestige to physicians who served on the boards. For these reasons, licensing remained important to the profession for several decades.

REGULATION OF THE CONDUCT OF MEDICAL SOCIETY MEMBERS

In addition to their licensing activities, medical societies undertook to regulate the behavior of members by means of fee bills (lists of minimum fees to be charged for specified services) and codes of ethics. The significance of fee bills and codes of ethics as activities of medical societies can be illustrated by a unique example. The Medical Society of the District of Columbia was organized in 1817 under a Congressional charter which permitted the society to license members and undertake scientific endeavors, but prohibited fee bills and codes of ethics. By the 1820's, conflicts within the profession in the city had become so rife that the society became moribund and lost its charter. In 1833, a number of physicians founded an unchartered medical organization which could and did establish a fee bill and a code of ethics—the Medical Association of the District of Columbia. Although the Society was reorganized in 1838, the Association became and re-

28 Davis, *History of Medical Education,* p. 105; Eugene F. Cordell, *Medical Annals of Maryland* (Baltimore, Md.: 1903), p. 92.
29 Drake, *Practical Essays,* p. 92.

mained, until their merger in 1911, the more powerful and important medical society in the District.[30] This example illustrates the great significance of regulation of economic activities in all local medical societies.

The efforts made by medical societies to regulate economic competition among their members were rarely successful. Three major factors—lack of sanctions to impose on deviant members, lack of control over non-members, and impractical or unenforceable regulations —hampered their efforts. The only sanctions that members could impose on deviants were expulsion from the society and denial of informal favors, like consultations and appointments to hospitals or medical schools. Expulsion from the society was almost self-defeating, because the society then lost all influence over expelled members. Denial of favors was ineffective to the extent that the deviant did not depend on them for his livelihood, which generally enabled a physician to become a deviant in the first place. Lack of control over non-members was a problem primarily because society members were forced to violate the fee bills and codes to compete with them. The tendency of medical societies to adopt unenforceable or impractical regulations can best be ascertained from an examination of the nature of fee bills and codes of ethics themselves.

FEE BILLS

Given the lack of any restraints on entrance into the profession, competition over fees was a major problem. A New York medical journal commented in 1825: "amongst the most prominent of the sources of discord, is the subject of fees. . . . We are far from desiring that the physician should demand the same compensation from the rich and the poor . . . but . . . let him charge a proper fee, and then make such deduction as the pecuniary circumstances of his patient require and not openly profess to practice medicine at half price."[31] Undercutting was common in this period because, according to Drake, it was profitable:

Undercharging, is a source of personal difficulty among physicians. . . . when a physician charges less than the customary fees of the place in which he lives, he . . . generally, augments the demand for his services, till he more than compensates the reduction of price. In this proceeding, he cannot be met by his more reputable brethren; because the public sentiment of the profession, does not tolerate such debasing competition; nor, if they once

[30] John B. Nichols, et al., History of the Medical Society of the District of Columbia, Part II, 1833–1944 (Washington, D.C.: 1947), pp. 10–11, 45, 54–55.
[31] Rosen, Fees and Fee Bills, p. 2.

reduced their fees, could they afterward, without difficulty raise them to the proper standard.[32]

For these reasons, virtually every medical society adopted fee bills which listed minimum fees for treatments, office visits, house calls, night house calls, and mileage charges for out of town visits. In many cases, fee bills covered only the more common treatments; in others, they were extraordinarily detailed.

Practitioners who were excluded from the societies felt no compunction to adhere to the fee bills, and their undercharging created major problems for society members. A postscript to one fee bill complained, "There are always quacks putting themselves forward, and doing what they do for half price, and some men think more of the almighty dollar than their family's lives, and it seems as though we are blest with a goodly number of that class here." Medical society members were sometimes forced to retaliate in kind, often making fee bills totally ineffective in urban or other areas with many practitioners outside the societies. A Philadelphia medical journal, for example, stated that fee bills were disregarded in litigation compared with the attested evidence of physicians, and that most physicians in Philadelphia did not even know of the accepted fee bill.[33]

CODES OF ETHICS

The other major regulatory mechanism adopted by medical societies was a code of ethics. This term was actually a misnomer, because the codes included matters of professional etiquette as well as ethics. Austin Flint differentiated the two by stating that ethics "have a moral weight. Medical etiquette, on the other hand, consists of the forms to be observed in professional intercourse. These are conventional. They have not the binding force of ethical rules; nevertheless, they claim observance." Virtually all codes adopted by American medical societies were based, in whole or in part, on the code published in 1803 by Thomas Percival, an English physician.[34]

The codes of the various societies varied significantly in detail and content, but two major activities appeared in virtually all of them. One was professional consultations, which at that time were a very important part of the medical practice of the wealthier physicians.

---

[32] Drake, *Practical Essays*, p. 100.

[33] Rosen, *Fees and Fee Bills*, pp. 55–56, 49; and Wilhelm Moll, "Medical Fee Bills," *Virginia Medical Monthly* 93 (1966): 657–64.

[34] Austin Flint, "Medical Ethics and Etiquette," *New York Medical Journal* 37 (1883): 286; Donald E. Konold, *A History of American Medical Ethics 1847–1912* (Madison, Wis.: State Historical Society of Wisconsin, 1962), pp. 9–10.

The AMA code, adopted in 1847, stated: "consultations should be promoted in difficult or protracted cases, as they give rise to confidence, energy, and more enlarged views in practice."[35] At the same time, they were a major source of conflict among physicians, according to Drake:

Consultations are copious sources of personal difficulty in the profession. . . . Great reliance is, generally, placed by the patient, or his friends, on the consulting physician, because the other is presumed to have exhausted his skill. Should the patient die, it is often supposed, that he might have lived, if the consultation had been held earlier. Thus the consulting physician, has nothing to lose, and much to gain. . . . The consulting physician, moreover, is often questioned, apart from the other [physician], on the past treatment and the probable issue of the case; when, if deficient in honor, he is apt to say, or look or insinuate, such things, as he knows will operate to the injury of his colleague; who of course resents the insidious attack on his character should he discover it. . . . The principles of treatment must be discussed; but this may end in controversy instead of concert.[36]

In order to resolve these conflicts, many codes attempted to regulate each minute detail of professional etiquette in consultations, specifying which consulting physician should speak first, what should be done if the consulting or family physician was delayed or failed to make an appearance, who should speak to the patient, etc. Probably the most important part of the code provisions dealing with consultations limited permissible consultations to members of the same society, or otherwise defined who was and who was not an acceptable consultant. Physicians viewed the code clauses involving consultations as being of particular importance. For example, when the Medical Society of the State of New York developed its first code in 1823, the drafting committee was instructed to give special attention to consultations. Nichols stated in his history of the Medical Association of the District of Columbia that the consultation provisions "came to acquire almost the force of a moral principle and a point of honorable conduct in the ideology of the members. . . . Lists of members were frequently issued, to show who were entitled to the privilege of consultations."[37]

The other widespread code provision prohibited the use or sale of secret nostrums by physicians. Because of the absence of laws requiring patent medicines to list their ingredients, patent medicine manufacturers rarely divulged the contents of their medicines, making every patent medicine a secret one. The effect of the code prohibition was

35 Flint, "Medical Ethics," p. 341.
36 Drake, *Practical Essays*, p. 101.
37 Calhoun, *Professional Lives*, p. 36; Nichols, *Medical Society of the District of Columbia*, p. 29.

thus to deny physicians the use of many drugs which were readily accessible, often inexpensive, and probably as good as those made up by pharmacists. It is not surprising, therefore, to find that this clause was disregarded by most physicians. It was probably the most frequently violated provision of the codes, and the most common cause of expulsion from medical societies during this period.[38]

Like the fee bills, the codes of ethics were a source of much contention within medical societies, and were probably an even more divisive force than fee bills. The effort spent on these controversies, like that spent on enforcing fee bills, was often fruitless.[39]

SCIENTIFIC ACTIVITIES OF MEDICAL SOCIETIES

Many medical societies of the period claimed to be a boon to scientific investigation and the diffusion of new medical knowledge. However, an examination of their activities does not reveal much concern with scientific investigation. It has already been observed that the Medical Society of the District of Columbia devoted itself to scientific investigation and was unsuccessful. In Massachusetts, the Massachusetts Medical Society concerned itself primarily with licensing, according to a historian, and delegated professional scientific work to the district societies. The district societies, however, appear to have been equally lax. When a number of physicians in Boston formed a small society for scientific investigation, the *Boston Medical and Surgical Journal* urged in 1835 that additional similar societies be formed, because scientific societies had to be small to be effective. In many other large cities, scientific societies similar to the Boston one were formed and will be described below, but here it need only be noted that they, rather than the regional societies, undertook the study of medical science.[40]

As the profession became larger, wealthier, and more influential, medical societies grew and prospered. By the second quarter of the century, they were the dominant institution in American medicine. During the same period, however, another institution, the medical school, developed and disrupted the patterns of professional life organized around the societies and their licensing agencies.

38 Henry Burnell Shafer, *The American Medical Profession 1783 to 1850* (New York: Columbia University Press, 1936), p. 222.

39 *Ibid.*, p. 221.

40 Davis, *History of Medical Education*, pp. 83–84; J. Collins Warren, "Medical Societies: Their Organization and the Nature of their Work," *Medical Communications of the Massachusetts Medical Society* 12 (1881): 481–82; "Boston Society for Medical Improvement," *Boston Medical and Surgical Journal* 12 (1835): 225.

CHAPTER 5 MEDICAL EDUCATION

MEDICAL SCHOOLS replaced the apprenticeship system as the dominant mode of medical education during the second quarter of the nineteenth century. Because medical schools were operated as commercial enterprises, physicians tended to open new ones whenever they found it profitable to do so, which increased the number of schools considerably. The ensuing competition for students forced the schools to lower their entrance and graduation requirements, which in turn lowered the quality of medical education. As schools became larger and more prosperous, their power and influence in the profession increased.

APPRENTICESHIP

Most early nineteenth-century medical students obtained their education by apprenticing themselves to a physician, called a preceptor, for a period of time. As apprenticeship became institutionalized, medical societies adopted a number of rules to govern the relationship between preceptors and apprentices. The standard apprenticeship program was three years, at a fee to the preceptor of $100 per year modified according to the preceptor's reputation. The preceptor furnished all the books and equipment required and provided the apprentice with a certificate when the term of instruction was completed.[1]

The course of apprenticeship had two major parts. The first part, called "reading medicine with a doctor," generally included anatomy, chemistry, botany, physiology, materia medica (drugs and their action), pharmacy, and clinical medicine. Dissection was often performed with human or animal cadavers. The student began by reading basic texts and performing simple chores. Daniel Drake said his "first assigned duties were to read [John] Quincy's *Dispensatory* and grind quicksilver into unguentum mercuriale; the latter of which, from previous

[1] Frederick Clayton Waite, *Western Reserve University Centennial History of the School of Medicine* (Cleveland: Western Reserve University Press, 1946), pp. 5–6.

practice on a Kentucky hand-mill, I found much the easier of the two." Gradually, as the apprentice became more skilled, he helped with office calls, performed bloodletting, opened abscesses, dressed wounds, and in general acted as a pharmacist and nurse. In the second phase of the education, called "riding with the doctor," the apprentice accompanied the doctor on house calls and sometimes assisted in surgeries. This constituted the clinical part of his education.[2]

Because any physician could serve as a preceptor if he could find apprentices willing to study with him, the education of apprentices was often deficient. For one thing, many preceptors were themselves poorly trained, especially in the basic medical sciences. For another, many preceptors did not take their pedagogical responsibilities seriously. Daniel Drake stated in 1832 that "the physicians of the United States, are culpably inattentive to the studies of their pupils; and ... this is one of the causes which retard the improvement, and arrest the elevation of the profession. Exceptions ... are frequently met with, especially in the great cities; but still they are *only* exceptions." Preceptors often used the apprentices who boarded with them as cheap labor. Because there were few pharmacists during this period, most physicians had to gather the roots and herbs and grind and mix their own drugs. Apprentices often spent many hours at these menial tasks and in routine household chores.[3]

Apprentices, on their part, usually took advantage of the situation to evade many of their responsibilities, especially when they did not board with their preceptors. Drake complained in 1844 about "the almost total absence of discipline in the period of private pupilage; the preceptor seldom laying down any rules, and the student, for the most part, coming and going at his pleasure, not even making his intended absence known to his preceptor; reading on one topic to-day, and, leaving it unfinished, taking up another tomorrow."[4]

At the end of the allotted time, the apprentice was given a certificate from his preceptor. Daniel Drake's read as follows:

> I do hereby certify, that Mr. Daniel Drake has pursued under my direction, for four years, the study of Physic, Surgery and Midwifery. From his good Abilities and marked Attention to the Prosecution of his studies, I am

[2] Daniel Drake, *Practical Essays on Medical Education and the Medical Profession in the United States* (Baltimore: Johns Hopkins Press, 1952), p. viii; Waite, *Western Reserve School of Medicine*, pp. 6–7.

[3] William Frederick Norwood, *Medical Education in the United States before the Civil War* (Philadelphia: University of Pennsylvania Press, 1944), p. 380; Drake, *Practical Essays*, p. 41; Harry B. Ferris, "Some Early Medical Teachers in Connecticut," in Herbert Thoms, ed., *The Heritage of Connecticut Medicine* (New Haven, Conn.: 1942), p. 34.

[4] Daniel Drake, *Physician to the West*, ed. Henry D. Shapiro and Zane L. Miller (Lexington: University Press of Kentucky, 1970), p. 297.

fully convinced that he is qualified to practice in the above branches of his Profession.

Wm. Goforth, Surgeon General,
1st Division Ohio Militia.[5]

Given what has been stated above, such a certificate obviously meant little to anyone who did not know the preceptor. One can easily understand why licensing became so popular, and how useful it was to the apprentice-trained physician as a means of making known his competence.

The standards of the apprenticeship system were nominally maintained by the medical licensing laws. Licensing itself applied only to apprentice-trained physicians in the many states whose licensing laws exempted graduates of medical schools. The licensing laws usually required all applicants for licenses to be 21 years of age and to have completed a minimum term of apprenticeship (three years in most states). The laws also required that the board of censors examine all applicants to insure that their education was satisfactory. These provisions were probably as ineffective as the other aspects of the licensing laws.

Not all preceptors were incompetent, and not all medical students were lackadaisical about their education: some good physicians were educated under the apprenticeship system. Nonetheless, as the body of medical knowledge advanced in the second quarter of the nineteenth century, even the best preceptor was incapable of providing a superior education to his apprentices. Thus the educational value of apprenticeship was limited not only by the indifference of the parties to the relationship, but also by the growing complexity of medical knowledge. Apprenticeship survived because it was popular with physicians, who used it to augment their income and obtain a supply of cheap labor, and acceptable to students, who did not have to pay very much or travel very far to obtain their education. Apprentices also had the advantage of close personal contact with their preceptors, which could have been of considerable value in clinical training. Nevertheless, as a means of training physicians, apprenticeship was generally unsuccessful.

MEDICAL SCHOOLS

THE INCEPTION OF MEDICAL SCHOOLS

As the number of medical students in a community increased, the local preceptors realized that it would be more economical and time-saving for them and better for the students if the academic subjects were taught in classrooms, rather than from each preceptor to each

[5] Drake, *Practical Essays*, p. ix.

apprentice. When this occurred, physicians in the larger cities undertook to add a medical school to the local liberal arts college, or at least to add some courses to the college curriculum for the benefit of their own students. For instance, an informal local medical society was formed in Boston in 1780. At one of its first meetings, according to the reminiscence of a physician who was an apprentice at the time, a member "made a proposition to the club, that, as there are nearly a dozen pupils studying in town, there should be an incipient medical school instituted here for their benefit." The local liberal arts college agreed to award the degrees, members of the society were offered courses to teach, and in this way the medical school of Harvard University was formed. Some years earlier, similar medical colleges had been appended to the University of Pennsylvania (which had a full medical school faculty in 1769 but first offered courses in 1765) and Columbia University (1767).[6]

In communities where no liberal arts college existed or where affiliation was otherwise impossible, the physicians petitioned the state legislature for a charter to establish a corporation to operate a medical school and grant degrees. The first school of this type was founded in Baltimore in 1807 as the University of Maryland. Whenever the legislature refused to give the physicians a charter, as sometimes occurred when a medical school already existed in the community, the physicians usually managed to convince a liberal arts college elsewhere in the state or in a nearby state to permit them to use the college's charter to grant degrees. Liberal arts colleges were often receptive to these overtures because the medical schools made no financial demands on them and gave them added prestige. Regardless of whether the medical school was independent or legally affiliated with a liberal arts college, all medical schools of the period were proprietary in that they were financially autonomous. This greatly restricted the influence of the liberal arts colleges over the actions of the medical schools.[7]

THE CURRICULUM OF THE MEDICAL SCHOOLS

The educational program of early nineteenth-century medical schools was characterized by three major features. First, the lecture was the sole pedagogical method used in all courses, except practical anatomy. Clinical, tutorial, or laboratory instruction was rare, even in subjects like chemistry. Second, the quality of instruction, even at the

---

[6] Ephraim Eliot, "Account of the Physicians of Boston," *Proceedings of the Massachusetts Historical Society* (Nov. 1863), pp. 181–82; Waite, *Western Reserve School of Medicine*, p. 12.

[7] *Ibid.*, p. 26; Norwood, *Medical Education*, pp. 384–85.

best schools, could be no better than the state of medical knowledge, and was consequently deficient in all aspects. Third, formal medical education complemented rather than replaced the apprenticeship system. Clinical subjects were supposed to be taught by the preceptor, and scientific subjects by the medical school faculty.

The curriculum of medical schools was divided into courses along somewhat different lines at different schools, but it was widely agreed that a complete faculty of a medical school should have seven members. Most colleges did not reach this number, and usually two courses, like anatomy and physiology, were combined into one for purposes of instruction. Four faculty members were considered a minimum for a medical school.[8]

A full course of instruction in all medical schools of the period required attendance at two four-month terms, preferably in successive years. The terms were not graded by subject matter or level of difficulty, however: a student attended lectures on every subject offered in a term, returned the next year, repeated all of them, and received an M.D. degree if he passed a final examination. This procedure maximized the earnings of the faculty members, but it obviously placed a considerable strain on the student, who was advised to concentrate his attention on the basic sciences in his first term, and on the more advanced subjects in his second term.[9]

The medical school curriculum covered three broad fields: the basic sciences, the theory and diagnosis of disease, and the treatment of disease.[10] In each of these areas, the utility of medical education was greatly hindered by both the pedagogical methods of the schools and the state of medical science.

The most basic of the sciences was chemistry. Chemistry was divided into two parts: the study of heat, light, and other subjects today considered part of physics; and inorganic chemistry. Organic chemistry was not taught until late in the period. Because pharmacy was taught in another course, the actual utility of this course to the physician was extremely limited. A few schools also taught such other sciences as physics, botany, mineralogy, and zoology.

The most basic medical sciences were anatomy and physiology, for as Daniel Drake said, "diseases consist either in alterations of struc-

8 Frederick Clayton Waite, *The Story of a Country Medical College* (Montpelier, Vt.: Vermont Historical Society, 1945), pp. 23–24.

9 John Brooks Wheeler, *Memoirs of a Small-Town Surgeon* (New York: Garden City, 1935), p. 2.

10 The discussion below is based on Henry Burnell Shafer, *The American Medical Profession 1783 to 1850* (New York: Columbia University Press, 1936), pp. 63–72; and Drake, *Physician to the West*, pp. 153–55.

ture, or in disordered and irregular movements in the function of that structure; and in both cases, without an acquaintance with the *healthy* condition, no degree of genius can enable us to understand the *morbid.*" At first, these two courses were often combined into a single course which covered human and comparative anatomy (describing human and animal bones and organs), and pathological anatomy (describing the same in their diseased state). The study of the organs and systems of organs was later placed in a separate physiology course. The large lecture classes in both these subjects were often ineffective because the students were unable to examine the bones and organs at close range. The faculty members who taught the anatomy and physiology courses were almost always practitioners, because of the lack of trained anatomists and physiologists at the time. Their interest in and knowledge of a subject so removed from their other professional concerns must have been small.[11]

Clinical dissection was taught in another course called practical anatomy. Practical anatomy was rarely required for graduation because of anti-dissection laws and public opposition to dissection. Nevertheless, virtually all schools offered the course either openly or surreptitiously, depending on the local laws and the state of public opinion. The schools obtained cadavers in a variety of legal and illegal ways, although the public was usually told that cadavers were obtained from distant places or great seaports. Each student paid a "demonstrator" a fee for his assistance in the dissecting room, which was concealed in a remote part of the building. Although many cadavers were simply disinterred from nearby cemeteries, others were shipped in brine from elsewhere to appease public opinion. By the time of actual dissection, the latter were often so deteriorated that they were useful only for the grossest analysis. Thus the actual educational value of the practical anatomy course was limited by both the difficulty of obtaining clinical material and the absence of direct personal instruction by the faculty.[12]

The second broad grouping of courses concerned the etiology and diagnosis of disease, and included pathology and the theory of medicine. Until about 1845, most of the texts in the theory of physic, as the

11 *Ibid.*, p. 153. In his survey of American medical schools in 1891, a British physician commented on the inadequacy of using practitioners to teach the basic medical sciences; undoubtedly the same problem existed in the first half of the century. Norman Walker, "The Medical Profession in the United States," *Edinburgh Medical Journal* 37 (1891): 241.

12 Waite, *Country Medical College*, pp. 70–71; Charles B. Johnson, "Getting My Anatomy in the Sixties," *Bulletin of the Society of Medical History of Chicago* 3 (1923): 110.

etiology course was sometimes called, followed the systems of such eighteenth-century medical theorists as Sydenham, Cullen, Boerhaave, and Rush. These speculative and unempirical systems were a serious detriment to medical education in turning the student's attention away from empirical observation toward rationalistic nosologies. Because both histology and bacteriology were in their infancy, and because the microscope was rarely used in the educational program, the study of pathology also suffered from the lack of scientific observation.

The third group of courses concerned the treatment of disease. The basic course in this sequence was called the practice of physic, and was often combined with the course in theory of physic. The direct relationship between theory and treatment thus obtained is sufficient to make evident the unscientific approach to treatment in these courses. Nonetheless, this course contained much of the practical knowledge which the physician would use during his professional life. Other courses in this broad area included materia medica, which Daniel Drake defined as the study of the "facts and principles which relate to the operation of the various medicinal agents on the human body, both in health and disease; together with their natural history and pharmacological preparation." This course classified and described treatments applied both internally and externally. (Bloodletting, however, was considered part of surgery.) The compilation of rationalistic schemes of classification was a constant challenge to early nineteenth-century medical scholars, who usually grouped drugs according to their effect on the organism (e.g., reduced fever, caused emesis, raised blister, etc.). A comprehensive course in materia medica would also cover medicinal botany, mineralogy, and even zoology, the latter to study leeches and other parasites. This was obviously a course of considerable practical value, but the absence of laboratory and field work must have made it less effective than the same material taught by a capable preceptor.[13]

Surgery was another part of this group of courses. This was also taught as a lecture course, despite the obvious necessity of clinical instruction. Minor operations were sometimes performed before large lecture classes, where few if any students could obtain a close examination of the procedures involved. Surgery textbooks of the period rarely discussed such elementary matters as preparing the patient and dressing and bandaging the wound. Undoubtedly, it was assumed that such matters as well as most of surgery would be taught by the student's preceptor.

[13] Drake, *Physician to the West*, p. 153; Frederick Clayton Waite, *The First Medical College in Vermont* (Montpelier: Vermont Historical Society, 1949), p. 120.

The last major part of this group of courses was midwifery, which was often combined with diseases of women and children into a single course. Because social values of the period precluded student attendance at obstetrical deliveries, most medical students became physicians without ever witnessing the birth of a child.[14]

Gradually, other courses were added to the curriculum. The most common of these was medical jurisprudence, which examined such questions as insanity, toxicology, and medical ethics. Other new courses were invariably specialty courses, such as ophthalmology. These were usually instituted in the second half of the century, and will be discussed later.

Although clinical instruction was considered the domain of the apprenticeship program, urban medical schools began to incorporate it into their curriculum in the second quarter of the century. They established clinics or dispensaries where students could observe ambulatory patients, or built hospitals for invalids. While dispensaries rapidly assumed an important role in clinical medical education, hospitals were less important in the first half of the century because of their expense and because of the unwillingness of patients to place themselves in hospitals. Consequently, hospitals were rarely incorporated into the educational program in the first half of the century.[15]

It may be concluded from the above that the weaknesses of medical education were due only in part to the inadequacies of the faculty and the proprietary nature of the institutions. Their deficiencies were largely those of medicine itself. Medical education could improve only as medical knowledge increased and received greater professional and public support and sympathy.

Preceptors remained important to medical schools for many years in the nineteenth century. The schools obtained many students through referrals of apprentices by preceptors and consequently maintained an educational program which gave a major role to apprenticeship. The requirements for a degree in most schools specified attendance at two four-month terms and evidence of having studied with a preceptor for three years (including the eight months of formal education). Thus the student spent 28 months with his preceptor, vacations included, where he was supposed to receive the clinical experience which was

[14] Waite, *Western Reserve School of Medicine*, p. 7.

[15] Michael M. Davis, Jr. and Andrew R. Warner, "The Beginning of Dispensaries," *Boston Medical and Surgical Journal* 178 (1918): 714–15; Samuel Annan, "Remarks on the Proceedings of the National Medical Convention," *Western Lancet* 6 (1847): 127–28.

not provided in the medical school. In theory, this arrangement was useful both for the student and the preceptor: the student had the benefit of close personal contact in his clinical instruction, and the preceptor had the use of the student's services.[16] In practice, the relationship between student and preceptor frequently became a nominal one in which the student paid his preceptor the necessary fees but spent little or no time with him.

THE PROLIFERATION OF MEDICAL SCHOOLS

During the first half of the nineteenth century, the number of medical schools in the country increased dramatically (Table V.1). Between 1800 and 1820, the number of schools more than trebled, and between 1820 and 1850, they trebled again. One reason for this proliferation was the vast territory of the country and the inadequate means of transportation to the northeast, where the first five medical schools were established.[17] After 1820, the majority of the new medical schools were located in the southern and western states to accommodate students in those areas who were unable to travel to the northeast.

TABLE V.1

REGULAR MEDICAL SCHOOLS PROVIDING INSTRUCTION ON A DEGREE-GRANTING BASIS, BY YEAR, 1770–1860

Year	All Schools	Schools in New England, New York State, and Philadelphia*
1770	2	2
1780	2	2
1790	3	3
1800	4	4
1810	6	5
1820	13	10
1830	22	14
1840	30	16
1850	42	17
1860	47	16

SOURCE: Table calculated from data in William Frederick Norwood, *Medical Education in the United States Before the Civil War* (Philadelphia: University of Pennsylvania Press, 1944).

* No medical schools were founded in New Jersey or elsewhere in Pennsylvania in this period.

[16] Waite, *Country Medical College*, pp. 20–21.
[17] Shafer, *American Medical Profession*, p. 42.

Another reason, and undoubtedly a more important one, was that medical schools were inexpensive to operate and often quite profitable to their faculty. The only equipment required to open a medical school was a faculty of four or more physicians; a classroom and a back room to conduct dissections; students; and legal authority to confer degrees. The few necessary teaching aids, like skeletons and apparatus for performing chemistry experiments, were provided by the faculty. The capital expenses of the building were not large, and public and private support in the form of lotteries, state appropriations, gifts, and loans frequently covered a considerable part of it.[18]

Operating expenses were met totally out of student fees. Two general methods were used to divide up the fees. In one system, the student paid a matriculation fee of three to five dollars, which was used to cover some of the janitorial and administrative expenses. He then paid each faculty member a fee of about fifteen dollars for a ticket which enabled him to attend and receive credit for that faculty member's lectures.[19] One student recalled his experience in this way:

Very well do I remember the first Monday in November, 1830. I then entered the Medical College of Ohio [in Cincinnati] as a student. All of the professors, that morning, at 9 o'clock, were sitting around a long, wide table. Commencing at one, paying fee and taking ticket, every student continued until he had made the entire round. To the best of my recollection, each professor, that morning, got about six hundred dollars.[20]

These fees constituted the earnings of the faculty members. Each student was required to take a final oral examination in order to receive a degree. If he passed the examination, usually by majority vote of the examination committee, he paid a graduation fee of fifteen to twenty dollars which went to the school; if he failed the examination, he paid nothing. As in the county licensing boards, the fee undoubtedly affected the decisions of the examining committees.[21]

Toward the end of the period, another method became more common and eventually replaced the older system. In this method, all fees, ranging from $150 at rural schools to from $200 to $285 at urban ones, were paid in a lump sum. The operating expenses and interest on the debt for the building were paid from these fees first. The remainder went into a fund from which the faculty drew their income. Each faculty member's fraction depended on the amount of his teach-

[18] Waite, *Country Medical College*, p. 48; Norwood, *Medical Education*, pp. 388–89.

[19] *Ibid.*, p. 392.

[20] Otto Juettner, *Daniel Drake and His Followers* (Cincinnati: Harvey, 1909), p. 63.

[21] Norwood, *Medical Education*, pp. 391, 394, 406.

ing and his reputation, which was considered to be a factor in attracting students to the school. Evaluations of reputations often led to controveries, and on occasion the meetings to divide up the fund broke up in disorder or were broken up by the police.[22]

Most operating costs of a medical school were independent of the number of students. Consequently, the more students who attended the school, the more profitable it was to the faculty. Some medical school faculty members became wealthy men in this way. Members of the faculty at the University of Maryland in Baltimore each earned $4,000 per year from student fees in good years. At the College of Physicians and Surgeons in New York City around 1826, the professors earned about $2,000 each per year. At rural medical schools, incomes were smaller, and at one school the faculty earned $1,000 each in 1823. Many faculty members held optional tutorials for students in their classes for an additional $5 or $10 per student, which increased their earnings considerably. Some of these faculty members related class grades to attendance at tutorials to encourage students to pay the additional fees. Faculty members often accepted students as apprentices, and the students were quick to realize the obvious advantages of such an arrangement. One well-known New York City physician earned over $27,000 from 1795 to 1826 in this way. Furthermore, all these physicians retained their private practices, which were often enhanced by their reputations as medical school faculty members and by the consultations offered them by their former students. It would not be unreasonable to assume that a popular and enterprising faculty member of a successful urban school could expect to earn at least $10,000 in a good year, and his less popular colleagues well over $5,000 annually. Around this same time, $1,000 was considered an adequate annual income for a practicing physician, and $2,000 was considered large for practitioners in small towns.[23]

Relations between medical school faculty members and other physicians in the community were often strained because of the private practices maintained by faculty members. Daniel Drake observed:

If the professors, withdrew from practice, on being appointed, they would be viewed with very different feelings, by their brethren. But a professorship, is a passport to business; and the increase that follows an appointment, is of

22 Waite, *Western Reserve School of Medicine*, pp. 131–32.
23 George H. Callcott, *A History of the University of Maryland* (Baltimore: Maryland Historical Society, 1966), pp. 51, 52, 129; David Cowen, *Medical Education: the Queen's-Rutgers Experience 1792–1830* (New Brunswick, N.J.: State University Bicentennial Commission and the Rutgers Medical School, 1966), pp. 19–20, 24; Waite, *First Medical College*, p. 97; Allen Kerr Bond, *When the Hopkins Came to Baltimore* (Baltimore, Md.: Pegasus Press, 1927), pp. 45, 50; Shafer, *American Medical Profession*, pp. 167–69.

course at the expense of those who surround the school; an effect, under which, although pride or prudence may keep them quiet, they cannot be expected to cherish the most friendly or pacific sentiments.[24]

COMPETITION AMONG MEDICAL SCHOOLS

The faculties' strong vested interest in the prosperity of their schools and in their own positions in the schools usually led to great rivalry and conflict both within and among medical schools. Daniel Drake, who was himself personally involved in more than one such dispute, stated:

The establishment of medical schools is a prolific source of discord in the profession. In this there is nothing remarkable. When a faculty is to be made up, there are in general many candidates, and of course many disappointed men, who harbour a secret feeling of dislike, towards the successful aspirants. Moreover, there are at the present time, nearly a hundred medical professors in the United States, and at least a thousand physicians, who in their own and the opinion of their friends, are as well, or better qualified, to fill professorial chairs, as the existing incumbents. These two great classes, of course, stand in a relation to each other, which predispose them to hostility.[25]

The ensuing proliferation of medical schools soon produced an extensive competition to attract students, especially among the rural schools which had no large local population from which to draw students. Students and faculty members often spent part of the period before each semester touring the countryside for new students, and students who were successful in attracting new students had their fees reduced. Faculty members often gave free lectures in the area to spread and enhance the reputation of their schools. Preceptors were made "fellows" of the schools or even granted honorary degrees to induce them to send their apprentices to the schools.[26] These efforts, however, were only the beginning of the struggle. N. S. Davis stated:

The rapid multiplication of medical schools . . . also exerted a very material bearing upon the organization of the colleges themselves, by placing a direct barrier in the way of allowing their competition and rivalry to be based entirely upon the question of which should present the most perfect and extended facilities for acquiring an education, in the form of another question, which experience has shown to be far more powerful in its influence, both upon the students and the colleges, namely, at which college can the student obtain his diploma that is to be his license to enter the profession, with the least expenditure of time and money?[27]

[24] Drake, *Practical Essays*, p. 99.
[25] *Ibid.*, pp. 98–99.
[26] George H. Weaver, "Beginnings of Medical Education in and near Chicago," *Bulletin of the Society of Medical History of Chicago* 3 (1925): 374; Waite, *First Medical College*, pp. 67, 110.
[27] N. S. Davis, "Address on the Present Status and Future Tendencies of the Medical Profession in the United States . . . ," *Journal of the American Medical Association* 1 (1883): 35.

The competition among the medical schools thus led to reduced graduation requirements and shorter terms. The original inclusion of Latin and natural philosophy (physics) in the curriculum and the thesis requirement were often minimized or disregarded altogether. The final oral examination, according to a teacher, was "not unduly severe as to the questions which were asked, nor as to the manner in which the answers were marked." The apprenticeship requirement was also reduced or disregarded. An AMA survey of 30 medical schools in 1849 showed that only 4 required certification of apprenticeship for the full three-year period, 19 others required certification of some apprenticeship without any specification of time, and 7 did not require any certification of apprenticeship.[28] The requirement of attendance at two terms of lectures was not violated outright as frequently as the others because of its direct effect on the income of the schools. Instead, it was often evaded in such a way that the student paid for two terms, but was allowed to minimize his attendance. This was often done by permitting the student to register after the term began and to leave before it ended. Davis stated:

It would be useless to extend the college term, for it was now a notorious fact, that scarcely half the students could be kept together through a term of four months, and much less would they attend six. It was even said, and truly, too, that very many do not now arrive at the college until the term is nearly half gone, and others leave a month or six weeks before its close. Now, there is a very plain reason why these things are so. It is simply because the colleges keep their matriculating books open until the middle of their terms and credit students for full courses who leave before three-fourths of the lectures have been given.[29]

Another way of reducing the time required was to permit the student to take both terms in the same year, inasmuch as many schools held two different terms in the same year anyway. This was common as late as the 1870's. Some schools even took the ultimate step of discounting the price of their lecture fees. Drake said of these schools, "the real motive is, the acquisition of students, by the only means they are competent to wield."[30]

THE ROLE OF THE MEDICAL SCHOOL IN THE PROFESSION

Medical schools were now becoming a powerful part of the profession of their time. One reason was that most state licensing laws made a diploma from a medical college equivalent to a license from a

[28] Norwood, *Medical Education*, pp. 404–5; Wheeler, *Memoirs*, p. 2.
[29] N. S. Davis, *History of Medical Education and Institutions in the United States* (Chicago: S. C. Griggs, 1851), p. 181.
[30] Waite, *Country Medical College*, pp. 98–99; Wheeler, *Memoirs*, pp. 3–4; Drake, *Practical Essays*, p. 46.

society and enabled the graduate to practice with full legal privileges. This enabled the schools to disregard the medical societies in their activities. Another reason was the great increase in the number of medical school students and graduates. The data in Table V.2, drawn from catalogues of the schools,[31] show that the number of graduates of medical schools increased many times over during the period. This augmented the resources and enhanced the political and social influence of the medical schools in their communities and states.

A third reason for the increased power of the medical schools was the decline in the number of rural medical schools. One of the unique characteristics of American medical education was the development of rural medical schools, which were popular in the first decades of the nineteenth century. Before the Civil War, 28 of the 85 medical schools established in the United States were in rural areas. Furthermore, Waite has estimated that almost one third of the physicians who attended a medical school before the Civil War did so at a rural school. Rural medical colleges were easy to establish because of their low capital and operating expenses, and were attractive to students because of their low tuition and living expenses. Rural schools had several weaknesses, however. Because no small town had enough resident physicians to constitute a faculty, the rural medical schools relied on visiting professors, some of whom taught at several medical schools in

TABLE V.2
GRADUATES OF MEDICAL SCHOOLS IN THE UNITED STATES, 1769–1868

Years	Number of Graduates
1769–1799	221
1800–1809	343
1810–1819	1375
1820–1829	4338
1830–1839	6849
1840–1849	11828
1850–1859	17213
1860–1868	16717

SOURCE: John S. Billings, "Literature and Institutions," in Edward H. Clarke et al., *A Century of American Medicine* (Philadelphia: Lea, 1876), p. 359.

31 Billings's method of calculation left some margin for error. It was quite common for schools to exaggerate the number of their students. Speaking complimentarily of Yale's medical school in 1839, the *Boston Medical and Surgical Journal* commented: "This school has not been guilty of the dishonesty practised by some in this country, of magnifying its patronage by the addition of fictitious names to the annual catalogue and circular." ("Medical School of Connecticut," in vol. 20 (1839): 16.)

different periods in the same year. The rural schools had to stagger their terms to avoid overlap with the urban schools, where many of these visiting faculty members also taught.[32] Thus, unlike the urban schools with their permanent faculty, the rural schools did not have a base of resident faculty to support and strengthen the institution, to attract students, and to be concerned with its growth and prosperity. Rural schools also were unable to have clinical instruction, because the small local populations did not provide enough cases of illness to support dispensaries and hospitals at the medical schools.

The students attracted to rural schools were primarily those who could not afford the greater expenses of the urban schools, those who would otherwise, as one physician said, "either make but humble attainments, or seek other channels for the business of life." After the depression of the late 1830's and early 1840's, the importance of the lower costs of the rural schools diminished, and improved means of transportation made the urban schools more accessible to the rural students. In addition, clinical instruction was being inaugurated at the urban schools, which gave them a further advantage in the competition for students. By the middle of the century, therefore, the rural medical schools declined in number and importance.[33]

As the urban schools prospered at the expense of their rural counterparts, they increased their power in the profession and their position in the community. For example, when urban medical schools began to provide a significant amount of clinical training, they opened free dispensaries and clinics and advertised to attract large numbers of patients. The local practitioners whose business was affected received this very critically. The New York Academy of Medicine passed two resolutions in 1852 condemning the clinics of the New York City medical schools. One read:

Whereas, the cliniques now held at the medical colleges as at present conducted, are or may be made tributary to the private interests of the professors at the expense of other and younger members of the profession, depriving them by an odious monopoly of practice and operation and often to fees to which they are justly entitled, therefore resolved, as the sense of this Academy, that to prescribe for or to operate upon the legitimate patients of any other physician, knowing them to be such, although done gratuitously at a clinique, is equally unwarrantable and unprofessional . . . and . . . is a violation of the code of medical ethics adopted by this body.[34]

---

[32] Waite, Country Medical College, pp. 9–10, 24–26.

[33] M. Paine, "Medical Education in the United States," Boston Medical and Surgical Journal 29 (1843): 333; Waite, Country Medical College, p. 139.

[34] Philip Van Ingen, The New York Academy of Medicine (New York: Columbia University Press, 1949), p. 60.

Another resolution condemned advertising in any way by clinics and schools. Neither had any impact on the schools: clinics soon became very popular, and advertising by medical schools was very common during the entire nineteenth century.

CONCLUSION

Medical schools served an important role in early nineteenth-century medicine. They revolutionized medical education and made it readily accessible to masses of students, thereby making possible the growth of the profession; they motivated prominent physicians to write new textbooks and thus contributed to the advancement and spread of medical knowledge of the period;[35] they helped standardize the medical practice of the period by promulgating a set of doctrines through these texts which became the basis of the medical practice of the students; and they established many clinics and dispensaries which provided medical care for the poor and indigent. As a result, the medical societies, once foremost in the profession, now had to share their influence and power with this new and dynamic institution. A conflict between the two institutions was inevitable.

[35] For example, one writer has stated that the major development in pediatrics around the middle of the nineteenth century in America was the increased number of textbooks which promulgated the latest knowledge in the field to medical students. Ernest Caulfield, "The General State of American Pediatrics in 1855 with Particular Reference to Philadelphia," *Pediatrics* 19 (1957): 461.

CHAPTER 6 RELATIONS BETWEEN MEDICAL SCHOOLS AND MEDICAL SOCIETIES

THE GROWTH of formal medical education meant that there now existed two major institutions in the medical profession—medical schools and medical societies—whose economic interests differed in two important ways. The medical societies, representing the interests of the rank-and-file of the profession, approved of the apprenticeship and licensing systems; the medical schools viewed them as hindrances to their growth. The societies wanted to limit the supply of new physicians to raise their members' earnings; the schools wanted to enroll and graduate as many students as possible to increase their incomes. One consequence of this conflict was the formation of the American Medical Association.

THE REACTIONS OF PHYSICIANS TO THE MEDICAL SCHOOLS

Physicians reacted critically to the proliferation of medical schools throughout the country. Occasionally, one could find favorable comments, but generally the medical journals were filled with forebodings about the decline of the profession due to the self-serving machinations of medical schools. The bulk of the criticism was directed at the quality of the graduates of the schools. Daniel Drake wrote in 1832:

. . . the ranks of the profession are in a great degree filled up with recruits, deficient either in abilities or acquirements—too often indeed in both—who thus doom it to a mediocrity, incompatible with both its nature and objects. . . .

The profession abounds in students and practitioners, who are radically defective in spelling, grammer, etymology, descriptive geography, arithmetic, and, I might add, book-keeping. . . . what is still more humbling to the pride of the profession, not a few of us never learn to spell the names, either of the medicines which we administer, or the diseases which we cure. Were this confined to unauthorized members of the profession, it would be an affair of little magnitude; but extending to many of the graduates of *all* our Universities, it calls for unreserved exposure and unqualified reprehension.[1]

While these and other criticisms of medical schools were valid, they failed to address the immediate problems. The pressing issue facing the profession was the relationship between formal medical education and apprenticeship: were formally educated physicians superior to apprentice-trained ones, and if so, should the apprentice-trained physicians be granted licenses and admitted to the medical societies? The answer to the first question was clearly that formally educated physicians were much better educated than their apprentice-trained counterparts. One reason was that medical-school faculty members were far better qualified to teach students than were most preceptors. Any physician could serve as a preceptor if he could find students willing to be his apprentices. Even incompetent physicians were motivated to take apprentices, who brought them income and were useful in pharmaceutical and nursing tasks. By comparison, most medical-school faculty members were experienced and generally well educated teachers. Furthermore, the teaching at medical schools was considerably more current and thorough, especially in the basic subjects such as anatomy, physiology, pharmacology, etc. Clinical instruction would have benefited from close contact with a well-qualified preceptor, but most preceptors were neither well qualified nor sufficiently motivated to devote the necessary time to clinical instruction.[2]

Autobiographies of physicians of this period often mentioned the superiority of formal medical education to apprenticeship. For example, a distinguished physician of his time, Charles Caldwell, who studied with a preceptor about 1790, complained that his preceptor, although an intelligent and attentive teacher, had "no library, no apparatus, no provision for improvement in practical anatomy, nor any other efficient means of instruction in medicine." J. Marion Sims, who became a world-famous gynecological surgeon, stated that his preceptor, like Caldwell's, had no facilities for medical education, that his period of apprenticeship in 1830 was of no value, and that he "was very glad" when he could "attend medical lectures." Another physician of somewhat less talent said that his study with a preceptor about 1855 was "time wasted."[3]

[1] Daniel Drake, *Practical Essays on Medical Education and the Medical Profession in the United States* (Baltimore: Johns Hopkins Press, 1952), pp. 5, 11–12.

[2] Frederick Clayton Waite, *The First Medical College in Vermont* (Montpelier: Vermont Historical Society, 1949), p. 52.

[3] Charles Caldwell, *Autobiography* (Philadelphia: Lippincott, Grambo, 1855), p. 77; J. Marion Sims, *The Story of My Life* (New York: Appleton, 1884), pp. 116–17; George J. Monroe, "When I Studied Medicine," *Cincinnati Lancet-Clinic* n.s. vol. 48 (1902): 374.

The leaders of the medical schools made the same observations repeatedly. The dean of the Starling Medical College in Ohio spoke about medical education in this manner in 1848:

The condition of a portion of the profession in Ohio has been, and still is to some extent a disgrace to us. A very considerable proportion of the practitioners of medicine in our state, have never received a regular medical education, or obtained a degree. Some of them (and the practice is still to some extent carried on) entered a physician's office, and after studying from a few months to two or three years . . . more or less started out with a certificate from their preceptor in their pockets, hoisted their "shingle" in some backwoods settlement, and were thenceforth, past all redemption or recall, dubbed *doctors*. . . .

The time has been when *necessity* could be pleaded in extenuation, but that has passed. If a young man commencing study at the present day, with our largely increased facilities for imparting instruction [medical schools], and the readiness and cheapness with which they are attainable, can not obtain a tolerable medical education before commencing practice, he can not possess sufficient energy and perseverance to succeed in any profession. . . . we know many excellent physicians, who are an honor to the profession, who are entirely self-educated. . . . None are more deeply sensible than themselves of the disadvantages under which they labor. At the close of the first session of the Starling Medical College in this city, the degree of M.D. was conferred upon 32 gentlemen, more than half of whom have been practitioners of medicine from four to twenty years, and we presume the proportion of the same was very considerable, if not as great, in the other Ohio schools. This is strong evidence of a desire for better things.[4]

Even the leaders of the societies and the movement to regulate medical schools had to concede the schools' numerous advantages. N. S. Davis, who was undoubtedly the most vocal and well known critic of the policies of medical schools, admitted in 1851 that their graduates left "the colleges tolerably well versed in the ordinary details of medical and surgical practice." He argued that medical education was grossly deficient only in the "less directly practical branches" of medicine, like the basic sciences and medical jurisprudence,[5] areas where preceptors were even more deficient.

Given the demonstrable fact that medical education in the first half of the nineteenth century was a marked improvement over the apprenticeship system, it must be asked why physicians reacted to this great institutional innovation—surely more important for the quality of medical care than any other innovation in the first half of the century—in such a negative manner. Medical schools were a great contribution to medical education, a contribution evident immediately

[4] John Butterfield, quoted in Jonathan Forman, "Organized Medicine in Ohio, 1811 to 1926," *Ohio State Medical Journal* 43 (1947): 279.

[5] N. S. Davis, *History of Medical Education and Institutions in the United States* (Chicago: S. C. Griggs, 1851), p. 178.

to all, and yet physicians reacted by finding fault with most aspects of the educational program of the colleges. If their only motive in making these criticisms was a concern for better education for medical students, the most useful and logical first step would have been to do away with the apprenticeship system, and to encourage all medical students to attend medical schools. One practical step would have been to require all applicants to medical societies to have medical-school degrees. Motions to limit AMA membership to medical-school graduates were defeated by the association in 1855 and again in 1858.[6] No important medical society of the period is known to have restricted its membership formally to medical-school graduates. Thus, the reaction of physicians to the growth of the medical school system must have been due to factors in addition to or besides their concern with the quality of medical education. Two other factors were especially important in shaping their attitudes toward the schools: the effect of the schools on the licensing system, and on the supply of physicians.

THE CONFLICT OVER LICENSING

The first major conflict between medical societies and medical schools developed over the question of licensing. Societies had received the power to license from the states, but most states also made diplomas equivalent to licenses, which exempted medical school graduates from the licensing requirement. Medical societies wanted all physicians beginning practice to obtain licenses; the schools of course felt that their diplomas were adequate. The issue arose in Massachusetts at the inception of the medical school at Harvard in the 1780's. The school had begun operation with a single faculty member, who in 1788 sent his only two students to be examined by the board of censors (licensing committee) of the Massachusetts Medical Society. The board feared that licensing the students would encourage the school's proponents to expand its curriculum and grant degrees. It therefore rejected the students, even though a local physician who observed the affair, Ephraim Eliot, claimed that "the candidates . . . had dissected much, and were probably far better qualified than any who had presented themselves" to the censors before. The medical-school faculty member had been waiting for this opportunity, and began a course of lectures, intending to award degrees to the students at the next commencement. The society members urged the president of Harvard and

---

6 Donald E. Konold, *A History of American Medical Ethics 1847–1912* (Madison, Wis.: State Historical Society of Wisconsin, 1962), p. 16.

some members of the board of overseers of the school to halt the courses, but to no avail. At the end of the term, a public examination was held at which, according to Eliot, the candidates "were thoroughly sifted; and they afforded much gratification to all who were present." The society members realized they would soon be confronted with a *fait accompli* in the matter, and held a re-examination of the two men in the week before the commencement, at which "a few questions were asked, and they were passed." At the commencement, the two men received the degree of Doctor in Physic, which established the school's rights once and for all.[7]

Thus the issue was resolved in Massachusetts clearly in favor of the medical school, whose degrees were thereafter considered equivalent to the society's licenses. However, the second medical school founded in Massachusetts, the Berkshire Medical Institution, was forced to obtain legislation (enacted in 1837) to grant its graduates the same privileges as those of Harvard.[8]

In Connecticut, at the Medical Institution of Yale College, the matter was resolved in another way. When the medical school was incorporated in 1810, the state legislature created an examining board consisting of an equal number of faculty members and members of the Connecticut Medical Society, with the President of the society empowered to cast the deciding vote in case of a tie. Thus both parties were involved in issuing all medical degrees given by the school until 1884, when the board was dissolved by mutual consent. Similar arrangements may have been adopted in other states.[9]

Elsewhere, the societies had no effective control over the graduation policies of the medical schools. To be sure, some medical schools appointed delegates from the medical societies to sit on their examining committees, and often the delegates were also members of the boards of censors of the societies, but this was an informal arrangement, established and maintained at the option of the schools. Generally, however, physicians could only condemn a situation which, they believed, produced an excessive number of physicians. In 1826, for example, the president of the Medical Society of the State of New York observed that "so long as the emoluments of teaching depend on the

[7] Josiah Bartlett, *A Dissertation on the Progress of Medical Science in the Commonwealth of Massachusetts* (Boston: 1810), p. 25; Ephraim Eliot, "Account of the Physicians of Boston," *Proceedings of the Massachusetts Historical Society* (Nov. 1863), pp. 183–84.

[8] Peter D. Gibbons, "The Berkshire Medical Institution," *Bulletin of the History of Medicine* 38 (1964): 54.

[9] Charles J. Bartlett, "Medical Licensure in Connecticut," *Connecticut State Medical Journal* 6 (1942): 184–85.

number of pupils, they must continue to be of injurious tendency." He suggested that either the mode of compensation of faculty members be changed, or the license be separated from the degree, and the latter made "simply a professional distinction" without any legal privileges.[10]

The significance of the problem increased in the second quarter of the century, as fewer medical students obtained licenses from the societies and more received diplomas from the schools. For example, in New York State in 1820, only 38 students received the M.D. degree from colleges in the state, while over one hundred received licenses from the state and county societies. By 1846, the number of graduates had climbed to 246, while the number receiving licenses had declined to fewer than ten. In Maryland, the state medical society granted an average of 28 licenses a year from 1820 to 1834, and only six a year from 1834 to 1850. In Connecticut, the decline in the number of licenses began in the 1820's. In New Jersey, the decline occurred after 1830, and in an effort to stem the tide, the society obtained a new charter from the state in 1863 enabling it to issue M.D. degrees instead of licenses; in all likelihood, it had little effect.[11]

The major reason for this trend was that the prestige of a diploma was considerably greater than that of a license. Daniel Drake stated in 1832:

What is a license but a certificate of inferiority? A licentiate may be a good physician, and become a great man, but still there is an original technical difference between him and a graduate, which everybody recognizes; and, as far as testimonials are concerned, he is one, who has not made the attainments, which entitle him to a doctorate.[12]

The relegation of licenses to a secondary status in the profession and among the public had major ramifications within the profession. First, medical societies no longer controlled access to the more prestigious elements of the profession: the M.D. degree was available to anyone approved by the medical schools. Second, the decline of the

[10] Lyman Bartlett How and Henry O. Smith, *The Story of the New Hampshire Medical Society* (Nashua, N.H.: Phaneuf Press, 1941), pp. 29–30; Waite, *First Medical College in Vermont*, pp. 144–46; Byron Stookey, *A History of Colonial Medical Education* (Springfield, Ill.: Thomas, 1962), pp. 201–2.

[11] Davis, *History of Medical Education*, pp. 116–17; Eugene F. Cordell, *Medical Annals of Maryland* (Baltimore, Md.: 1903), p. 737; Francis Bacon, "The Connecticut Medical Society," *Proceedings of the Connecticut Medical Society* (1892), p. 199; William Pierson, "Historical Narrative," *Transactions of the Medical Society of New Jersey; Centennial Meeting* (1866), pp. 95–96, 102–3. It should not be thought that all licentiates were apprentice-trained physicians. Many medical school graduates also obtained licenses where they practiced.

[12] Drake, *Practical Essays*, pp. 92–93.

traditional apprenticeship system eliminated a valuable source of cheap labor for many physicians. Third, diplomas created discord within the profession, according to a committee report presented to the 1826 convention of the Medical Society of the State of New York:

The course of medical education has varied greatly during the last quarter of a century. At the commencement of that period, it was generally the custom (with, however, exceptions) to complete the required term of study in the office of some respectable practitioner, and then in a very small proportion of cases, if pecuniary and other circumstances favored, to attend lectures at some of the widely scattered medical institutions. The preliminary attendance for the degree of doctor of medicine, was expensive; the time to be consumed in its attainment was deemed too valuable; and as it was not sought for, except among the residents of our larger and more populous cities, so its absence was not considered as a mark of the want of medical knowledge. The number of gentleman who held the degree of M.D. in this State, thirty years ago, probably did not exceed twenty.

Now, however, from the number of medical schools, and the requisitions of the laws throughout nearly the whole of the United States, demanding attendance as a preliminary requisite for the practice of medicine and surgery; and above all, from the force of public opinion, which justly views a proper education as indispensable in this as in every other profession, nearly two-thirds of the medical students in the United States attend lectures, and of these a number every year obtain the degree of doctor of medicine. They go into practice, and settle by the side of those who have only a license, although the latter in their day complied with all the legal requisities— availed themselves of all the advantages which their situation at that time permitted to them. . . .

That some unpleasant feeling should result from this state of things is natural. . . . The young man, with the degree of doctor of medicine, may presume on his newly obtained honors, while the aged physician, practicing under a license only, may be disposed to depress or underrate his youthful competitor.[13]

The decline in the popularity of licenses also weakened the medical societies. It deprived them of a considerable proportion of their income and forced them to curtail many of their activities. In addition, those physicians who joined medical societies to seek sympathetic treatment for their apprentices or to restrict the number of physicians in their communities lost interest in the societies. Consequently, many local societies suspended their activities during this period.[14]

Once medical societies lost interest in the licensing system, organizations of empirics were able to obtain repeal or virtual nullification of the licensing laws in most states. Medical societies rarely contested

[13] T. Romeyn Beck, "To the Hon. the Regents of the University," *Transactions of the New York Medical Society* (1826; reprint ed., Albany: 1868), pp. 329–30.

[14] Davis, *History of Medical Education*, p. 117.

these repeal campaigns. By the Civil War, the medical licensing system had been destroyed or abandoned in virtually all states.[15]

MEDICAL SCHOOLS AND THE SUPPLY OF PHYSICIANS

The proliferation of medical schools produced a convenient and accessible form of medical education which attracted many students to the profession and greatly increased the supply of physicians. It was shown in Table V.2 that the number of graduates of medical schools increased over fifty times from the first decade of the century to the 1850's. Even though the number of apprentice-trained physicians declined, the total number of physicians grew from a few thousand at the beginning of the century to over 40,000 by mid-century. Considering that the population of the country increased less than five times during the same time span, the effect in many communities was to intensify competition within the profession markedly. This was true even on the frontier. A Mississippi correspondent of the *Boston Medical and Surgical Journal* advised his readers in 1843:

Many young graduates . . . have come to this part of the country with the idea they could make a fortune in a few years, that they could at once step into a lucrative practice, that physicians were greatly needed, and that practice was waiting to receive them. But, alas! they have been badly disappointed—mistaken, perhaps, when it was too late for their good. They little knew or thought that there were twice the number of doctors here that the community needed. . . . I consider a good N. England practice quite as good as the same in Mississippi.[16]

One of the first AMA committees, the committee on standards of medical education, reported in 1847 that the country's twenty million inhabitants were cared for by forty thousand regular physicians and a "long list of irregular practitioners who swarm like locusts in every part of the country." "No wonder," the committee concluded, "that the profession of medicine has measurably ceased to occupy the elevated position which once it did; no wonder that the merest pittance in the way of remuneration is scantily doled out even to the most industrious in our ranks."[17] Here too, however, any analysis must be

[15] For the attitudes of New York and Massachusetts physicians, see: Charles B. Coventry, "History of Medical Legislation in the State of New York," *New York Journal of Medicine* 4 (1845): 158; Reginald H. Fitz, "The Rise and Fall of the Licensed Physician in Massachusetts, 1781–1860," *Transactions of the Association of American Physicians* 9 (1894): 11–12. The activities of the empirics will be described in Chapter 7.

[16] George Rosen, *Fees and Fee Bills* (Baltimore: Johns Hopkins Press, 1946), p. 18.

[17] "Proceedings of the National Medical Convention," *New York Journal of Medicine* 9 (1847): 115.

comparative. The AMA committee chose to compare American conditions with those in Europe, where they claimed the ratio of physicians to population was substantially lower than it was in the United States. However, the committee did not observe that midwives were widely used in European countries while physicians performed most obstetrical cases in America, that there were many more pharmacists in Europe than in America, that hospitals were much more common in Europe than in America, and that the population density was much greater in Europe than in America. Given the great differences between European and American conditions, more physicians per capita would be expected in America because of the relative lack of auxiliary personnel and institutions.

As the graduates of the medical schools swelled the ranks of the profession, physicians became convinced that something had to be done to control this flow. Most physicians believed that the answer to the problem was either to require medical school graduates to obtain licenses or to force medical schools to raise their preliminary (admission) and graduation requirements. Inasmuch as the licensing system was defunct, physicians were compelled to adopt the latter alternative.

Although many physicians spoke repeatedly of the need to increase medical school standards substantially, few of them spoke openly of the consequences of this for the profession. One of the few to do so was Martyn Paine, a professor at a New York City medical college. In at least two addresses, in 1843 and 1846 (N. S. Davis said that the latter was "widely circulated throughout the Union"), he defended the existing system of medical education.[18]

Paine argued that each nation should endeavor to provide "for the diffusion of medical knowledge as far commensurate with the vastness and difficulties of the science ... as the circumstances of each society will admit." The ability of any nation to do this was limited by its wealth: "Where wealth abounds, as in the various states of

[18] M. Paine, "Medical Education in the United States," *Boston Medical and Surgical Journal* 29 (1843): 329–33; Martyn Paine, *A Defence of the Medical Profession of the United States*, 7th ed. (New York: Wood, 1846); [Nathan S. Davis], "History of the American Medical Association," *New Jersey Medical Reporter* 7 (1854): 42. Davis's series of articles, which spanned the 1854 and 1855 volumes of the *New Jersey Medical Reporter*, were published anonymously, but they were reprinted as the *History of the American Medical Association* (Philadelphia: Lippincott, Grambo: 1855), with Nathan S. Davis listed as the author. He admitted in the preface to the book that he had published the articles anonymously because "I had so frequently furnished communications in relation to the Association and its objects, that I might be charged with making it too much a 'hobby,'" but he added that he did not want the book to be published anonymously (*ibid.*, p. vii).

Europe, medical education should be carried" to the maximum extent possible, such that it "should insure to every country in Europe an overflowing profession conversant with every useful department of science, and accomplished in the philosophy of medicine.[19]

Schools of this kind, Paine continued, with their extremely high preliminary requirements, long terms, and exhaustive graduation requirements, were possible only in a wealthy country, with a wealthy population to support them and wealthy students to attend them. The United States, however, was not a wealthy country and could support only a very small number of these elite institutions, while Europe could support a large number. If the standards of American schools were raised to the level of the European schools, many American schools would be forced to cease operation.

Furthermore, the United States is a democratic country: "our institutions go for the equality of man, and legislation proceeds upon this conciliatory, however unfounded, principle." These democratic principles would not permit legislation limiting the right to practice to a small elite of the profession. In the United States, men would practice medicine with or without an education.[20] If the poorer students were not provided with a decent, inexpensive medical education, they would practice without an education, as empirics:

Exact from our physicians the intellectual culture, and rear in this land the high standard of medical acquirements which are so noble and fascinating in some of the schools of Europe, and quackery will reign almost universal from one end of the continent to the other. . . . do not all our Medical Colleges hold out the temptation of moderate fees, and give, in their annual announcements, a conspicuous place to the humble charges for the necessaries of life? But what are these compared with the expenses attendant on the prolonged and higher grades of academic and medical learning in some of the European States? And who does not see the inconsistency that would hold in one hand professions of cheapness to allure the student through our present system of medical discipline, and threaten with the other augmented fees and an impossible exaction upon time? The same principle runs through all our primary schools, our academic, collegiate, legal, clerical and political institutions. Cheapness of education, and a corresponding adaption of time, are found indispensable to the general condition of society. . . .

He, who, in America, aims at the profession of medicine . . . comes from a class where the blandishments of [wealth] have no existence. He has worked his way from elementary schools through the higher departments of academic learning, under the frigid discipline of poverty, and he enters our halls of medical education with little else than the hope that his career may not be arrested by insane exactions. . . .

Raise, therefore, beyond a certain limited poise, our standard of absolute

[19] Paine, "Medical Education," pp. 330–31.
[20] Ibid., p. 331.

requirements, and . . . we shall turn from our medical schools most of their aspirants into more humble channels, or into the walks of empiricism. The exigencies of American physicians demand an early application to the business of life.[21]

Given that these were the predictable consequences of a significant increase in the standards of medical education, why should some physicians advocate these changes? Paine argued:

And now, perhaps, we shall have no difficulty in understanding why it is so earnestly desired to extend the term of instruction in our Medical Colleges and also as a preliminary requisite to admission into these institutions. There is an *aristocratic* feature in this movement of the worst omen. . . . It is oppression towards the poor, for the sake of crippling the principal Medical Colleges. You, and all of us know, as I have already said, that the "great mass" of professional men in this country, Lawyers, Divines and Physicians, belong to the poorer class of society; and should the wirepullers effect an extended term of education it must exclude a large proportion of the "great mass" from the advantages of collegiate instruction; whilst the aristocratic features will be rendered still more offensive by limiting the attendants at Medical Colleges to the few who may spring from families of wealth.[22]

Thus, Paine presented two alternative systems of medical education in the United States. One would have a number of schools, varying in quality from a few equal to the best in Europe down to the humble country schools. The best schools would provide a superior education for "the aristocrats of our profession; made so through the difference of a few dollars, by those noble attainments which that little disparity in fortune qualifies them to bestow upon themselves." The bulk of the schools would provide a decent medical education at low cost for the many poor students.[23]

The other system, according to Paine, would have forced all schools to raise both their entrance and graduation requirements, which would have significantly reduced the number of M.D.'s. Because a large number of physicians were "needed in our immense extent of territory, to allievate the physical woes of humanity," according to the editor of the *Boston Medical and Surgical Journal*, the number of empirics and apprentice-trained physicians would have increased. Thus the profession would have consisted of two classes with a wide gulf between them—a small elite, drawn from the wealthy, and a large number of physicians with little or no formal education. The validity of this argument was recognized and supported by at least two impor-

21 Paine, *Defence of the Medical Profession*, pp. 8–9.
22 *Ibid.*, p. 15.
23 Paine, "Medical Education," p. 333.

tant medical journals of the period, the *Boston Medical and Surgical Journal*, and the *New York Journal of Medicine*.[24]

Oddly enough, although Paine's articles were widely circulated and well known, no direct attempt to rebut them has been found. N. S. Davis, the most outspoken of the founders of the AMA, made several statements contradicting Paine's argument, but these were not expressed in any systematic form. Davis argued that Paine's comments about the differences between European and American medical education were of no consequence: "The only true questions . . . are, whether our system contains important defects; and if so, whether they admit of being remedied." Furthermore, Davis felt that raising the entrance requirements would not have had a major impact on the medical schools: "in our country of school-houses and almost unlimited facilities for acquiring a knowledge of, at least, the ordinary branches of learning," any student who could not acquire a satisfactory preliminary education did not have sufficient "mental energy and perseverance . . . to do justice to a profession as extensive, intricate, and arduous as" medicine. Last, Davis was particularly concerned about the state of the medical societies, and felt that "their universal dissolution is near at hand, unless some *reform* is adopted by which they are re-animated with new vigor and efficiency," and placed their improvement above the prosperity of the medical schools.[25]

Although it is hardly likely that most American physicians sought to turn the profession into an aristocracy, it is equally undeniable that physicians were far more concerned with competition from medical-school graduates than from lesser-trained men or empirics. Most physicians must have recognized that reducing the number of physicians would have led to an increase in the number of empirics, but they were willing to countenance this form of competition as less threatening than competition from medical-school graduates. It must be concluded therefore that Paine's argument, while exaggerated, set forth the two major philosophies of the organization of the medical profession of the time.

Any attempt to ascertain the actual validity of these contrary arguments must examine two questions: (1) was medical education a source of social mobility for many students who would have been un-

[24] "Medical Education," *Boston Medical and Surgical Journal* 29 (1843): 343; "National Convention," *New York Journal of Medicine* 6 (1846): 432. The latter journal did recommend some standards of medical education for "some of the older and wealthier States."

[25] N. S. D[avis], "Medical Reform," *New York Journal of Medicine* 9 (1847): 402; Davis, "History of the American Medical Association," p. 178; N. S. Davis, "Mr. Editor," *New York Journal of Medicine* 8 (1847): 120.

able to obtain a formal medical education if the schools had raised their standards, and (2) were the proposals of those advocating reform in medical education so extreme that their adoption would have drastically reduced the number of students?

In an attempt to answer the first question, the limited amount of information available on the previous education of medical school students can be used as an estimate of their social class backgrounds. Frederick Waite carefully analyzed the previous education of a large number of students who attended a rural medical college in Vermont from 1830 to 1856. By examining the alumni catalogues of all colleges of arts in New England and New York State, where 1296 of the 1407 students had lived, he found that 7 percent of the students had obtained the degree of Bachelor of Arts and another 10 percent had matriculated at a liberal-arts college prior to attending medical college. Allowing for unreported alumni and other types of error, Waite estimated that about 20 percent of the medical students had had some prior liberal-arts college education.[26]

Another study was carried out by Charles W. Eliot, the president of Harvard College. He examined the catalogues of several medical schools for 1870–71 and tabulated the number of students who had received the degree of Bachelor of Arts (Table VI.1). It is difficult to say how much his data were affected by the Civil War, which reduced the number of students at liberal-arts colleges during the war, and therefore would have reduced the number of graduates in medical colleges after the war.

TABLE VI.1
MEDICAL STUDENTS WITH BACHELOR OF ARTS DEGREES AT SELECTED MEDICAL SCHOOLS, 1870

Medical School	Number of Students	Percentage of Students with B.A. Degrees
Harvard (Cambridge, Mass.)	301	19%
Dartmouth (Hanover, N.H.)	44	9
Bowdoin (Brunswick, Maine)	88	15
Columbia (New York, N.Y.)	327	19
Bellevue Hospital (New York, N.Y.)	436	3
Pennsylvania (Philadelphia, Pa.)	310	0
Northwestern (Evanston, Ill.)	100	0
Michigan (Ann Arbor, Mich.)	315	1

SOURCE: Charles W. Eliot, *Forty-Sixth Annual Report of the President of Harvard College, 1870–1871* (Cambridge, Mass.: 1872), p. 20n.

[26] Frederick Clayton Waite, *The Story of a Country Medical College* (Montpelier, Vt.: Vermont Historical Society, 1945), pp. 122–24.

Eliot's data supported Waite's in showing that the New England schools, as well as one New York school, had remarkably large numbers of students with bachelor's degrees, especially considering the extremely small proportion of Americans with such degrees at the time. In the other New York school, in the Philadelphia school, and in all the midwestern schools, the number of medical students with bachelor's degrees was insignificant. In interpreting these data, it should be observed that the schools examined by Eliot were, in his words, "much above the average of American Medical Schools." The data suggest that, in the Northeast, a core of medical students had considerable preliminary education and were probably from well-to-do families. The remainder of the students there and virtually all the students elsewhere were unable to obtain a high level of preliminary education because of their low social class backgrounds and, in many cases, the inaccessibility of higher education on the frontier. Thus it may be concluded that many medical students were socially mobile and would have been deterred from a career in medicine if the standards of medical education had been raised significantly. The specific proposals of the reformers will be described below, and additional comments will be presented there.

THE FOUNDING OF THE AMERICAN MEDICAL ASSOCIATION

The most important movement to deal with the problems of medical education was initiated by physicians in the Medical Society of the State of New York in 1844, when they tried to raise the standards of medical education in their state. The New York State medical schools pointed out that if they raised their standards while the schools in the surrounding states did not, students would abandon New York State schools for those of the other states. Thus it became evident to the leaders of the society that national action was required. The society put out a call in 1845 for a national convention of medical societies and medical schools, to be held in New York in 1846.[27]

Because the actions of the New York state society in 1844 had aroused considerable resentment in the medical schools, many schools refused to attend the 1846 meeting. Davis stated that only eleven colleges were represented at the convention, about one-third of the total number. He attributed this to a "feeling of distrust in regard to the *motives* of those who issued the call for the Convention. There was

[27] Davis, "History of the American Medical Association," pp. 29–31. In the late 1820's, an effort was made to form a similar organization in New England, but it was short lived. Byron Stookey, "Origins of the First National Medical Convention," *JAMA* 177 (1961): 133–40.

a feeling of apprehension . . . that the whole movement originated in a spirit of radicalism and enmity to the Schools. And though such a feeling was without the shadow of a foundation in fact, yet it was evidently the chief cause of preventing the attendance of delegates from a majority of the Medical Colleges in the Union."[28]

The major action of the 1846 convention was the decision to establish a permanent national medical society, which was created at a second convention held in Philadelphia in 1847. This convention was attended by almost 250 delegates, representing more than forty medical societies and 28 medical colleges. The new organization was called the American Medical Association and consisted of delegates from medical societies, medical colleges, and other medical institutions.[29]

The 1847 convention also passed a number of resolutions establishing standards of medical education for both preceptors and medical colleges. Preceptors were urged (1) to require each apprentice to meet certain specified standards of preliminary education, (2) to issue a written certificate to each apprentice stating his possession of the required preliminary education and the length of his apprenticeship, and (3) to advise their apprentices to attend only medical schools meeting the AMA's standards. The standards proposed for medical schools can be conveniently divided into two categories: those which merely codified existing medical school practices and those which would have required changes in the medical schools. The AMA standards in the former category consisted of a list of subjects to be included in the medical-school curriculum, and a recommendation that degree requirements consist of attendance at two courses of lectures and three years of total medical education including apprenticeship certified by a preceptor. The AMA standards in the latter category required medical schools to provide clinical instruction at a hospital "whenever it can be accomplished," to make dissection compulsory, to lengthen the school term from four to six months, and in effect to adopt certain preliminary education requirements which were to be certified by the preceptors. An AMA committee's survey of 19 of the 33 existing medical schools (the others did not reply to the questionnaire) showed that only 12 schools required clinical instruction (and then probably at a clinic and not a hospital), and only 5 required

28 Davis, "History of the American Medical Association," pp. 47–48. For the reaction of a New York medical school faculty member to the actions of the New York state society, see Charles B. Coventry, "Remarks on some of the Proceedings of the New York State Medical Society," New York Journal of Medicine 7 (1846): 192–99.

29 Davis, "History of the American Medical Association," pp. 48–49, 176, 181.

dissection. The length of the terms in the schools varied from 13 to 18 weeks, with most colleges offering 16-week terms. No information was obtained about the preliminary education of the medical students.[30]

The proposals which sought to change medical-school policies were wholly ineffective in achieving their objectives. The reaction of the medical schools is exemplified by their response to the AMA proposal that the terms be extended from four to six months. Davis stated that the schools were not generally opposed to the increased term per se, but declared "that they were ready to comply with the request so soon as it shall appear that *all* the other colleges will do so. Thus it is . . . in plain English, because each college fears to lay a single item of burthen on the student, even in the way of affording him greater facilities for obtaining knowledge lest some neighboring college, by failing to add such burthen, should prove a more successful rival."[31] Thus the AMA was no more successful than the New York state medical society, because neither organization could impose effective penalties on substandard medical schools. The AMA, furthermore, was unwilling to impose penalties on preceptors who did not adhere to the AMA standards when they selected apprentices. The New York state society proposed to the AMA in 1848 that boards of censors be established in every county in the nation to approval all students before they were accepted by preceptors. Each board would issue its own certificates, and no preceptor could accept a student who did not have a certificate from the board in his area. The AMA rejected this proposal, and Davis complained in 1854:

[There is] a disposition to look to the Medical Colleges for too large a share of the action necessary for the accomplishment of the objects desired.

Instead of regarding these institutions as mere schools for Medical Instruction, and demand of them such action only, as was calculated to render their courses of instruction more systematic and complete, they have been looked to for the practical execution of almost every specific recommendation which has been made by the Association on the subject of education. Thus, of the seven resolutions adopted at Boston [in 1849] . . . four directly related to the action of the Medical Colleges, two to the further organization and action of the State Medical Societies, and one, couched in very general terms, was addressed to the individual members of the profession generally. . . . [The New York state resolution] was a specific plan, fully within the control of the local profession everywhere, eminently practical in its nature, and well calculated to secure the end proposed; and yet, the Association . . . rejected this plan, and in its place adopted the very general and vague recommendation, "that physicians generally . . . be advised and requested to

---

[30] *Ibid.*, pp. 177–79; "Proceedings of the National Medical Convention," pp. 114–15.

[31] Davis, *History of Medical Education*, pp. 180–81.

require of those wishing to become their pupils, *evidence of a proper general education*, before admission into their offices." By such action, the Association directly refused to provide or recommend any regular mode, by which the student was to procure the very certificate, which the Medical Colleges were advised to require of him [by another resolution]. . . . it is well known that nine-tenths of all the students, first enter the office of some practitioner, and there pursue their studies from six months to two years, before they attend any Medical College. When they come to the College, they bring to the Faculty letters of introduction from their preceptors. . . . Suppose it is soon ascertained that one half of them are sadly deficient in their general education. . . . Now, is it reasonable to suppose that the Colleges will ever go back of the private preceptors, and take the responsibility of shutting such students out of their Halls? Certainly not. But they will continue, as they have done, to claim that the responsibility of exacting proper preliminary education is with the profession at large. . . . In this the Colleges are right, and the sooner the members of the profession can be made to feel their individual responsibility in the matter, the better for all parties. . . .

It is a very easy matter for men to assemble in Conventions and Societies, and declare abstract truths in formal resolutions. . . .

But so long as they not only feel no *individual* responsibility in the matter, but return to their homes and send directly from their own offices, young men to the Colleges, who are grossly deficient in almost all the elementary branches of knowledge, they must . . . expect to see their resolves unheeded.[32]

The AMA's rejection of the proposal was undoubtedly due to the members' direct economic interest in maintaining an open apprenticeship system. First of all, many physicians profited by the fees they charged apprentices. Second, according to Samuel Annan, a Lexington, Kentucky medical-college professor who wrote a first-hand account of the 1847 convention: "physicians engaged in an extensive practice, hold out inducements to the youths in their respective neighborhoods to enter their offices as students, because it relieves them from a great deal of labor, to have some one to put up medicine from their prescriptions." In order to obtain such assistance, physicians even waived the apprenticeship fee. Annan concluded that these physicians would not be willing to make extensive demands as to the preliminary education of their apprentices: "We opine that Latin, and Greek, and Algebra will be as feathers in the scale, when weighed against convenience and interest."[33]

Even if the medical schools had been willing to comply with the AMA's proposals, some of the standards were attainable only by a few of the elite schools. The most demanding of the AMA standards estab-

[32] Davis, "History of the American Medical Association," pp. 347–50.
[33] Samuel Annan, "Remarks on the Proceedings of the National Medical Convention," *Western Lancet* 6 (1847): 125.

lished preliminary educational requirements for apprentices. Preceptors were instructed to verify their apprentices' attainments in certificates which medical schools were supposed to demand of all entering students. These standards included "a good English education, a knowledge of Natural Philosophy, and the elementary Mathematical Sciences, including Geometry and Algebra, and such an acquaintance, at least, with the Latin and Greek languages as will enable them to appreciate the technical language of medicine, and read and write prescriptions."[34]

To assess the potential impact of these requirements on medical schools, it is necessary to understand the educational system of the country at the time.[35] Most students obtained their primary education in the common or elementary schools which existed in most communities. These schools taught none of the subjects recommended by the AMA, except English. Students seeking a higher level of education attended private academies, which existed in most towns and cities and often received some public assistance. Public high schools existed only in Massachusetts and a few cities elsewhere in 1847. All the subjects required by the AMA were taught in most academies and high schools. Colleges and universities at that time did not form a distinct third level of education. College entrance requirements did not include graduation from a secondary school, and many of the subjects taught in colleges were also available in secondary schools. (Indeed, some private academies provided education from the elementary grades through several years of college.) The major difference between colleges and secondary schools was the greater amount of classical studies available in colleges, which was irrelevant for medical education. Therefore, a college education was not a useful preliminary education for medical students, and no medical organization or school ever established this as a preliminary requirement.

The subjects recommended by the AMA were all readily available in most secondary schools of the period. Because they were radically different from the entrance requirements of liberal-arts colleges (which required much more Latin and Greek, and did not require either

[34] Davis, "History of the American Medical Association," p. 177.

[35] The following sources were used in gathering this data: Alexander James Inglis, *The Rise of the High School in Massachusetts* (New York: Teachers College, Columbia University, 1911); Emit Duncan Grizzell, *Origin and Development of the High School in New England Before 1865* (New York: Macmillan, 1923); George F. Miller, *The Academy System of the State of New York* (1922; reprint ed. New York: Arno Press, 1969); Walter John Gifford, *Historical Development of the New York State High School System* (Albany: Lyon, 1922); Edwin Grant Dexter, *A History of Education in the United States* (New York: Macmillan, 1904).

geometry or natural philosophy), it was extremely unlikely that many secondary school students would have studied all the courses recommended by the AMA. There is some direct evidence on this point. An analysis of the courses studied by students in a number of Massachusetts public high schools in and shortly after 1847 showed that only a very small proportion of the students in these institutions studied all the subjects proposed by the AMA. Very few students in any of the high schools studied Greek. In some schools, only a few students studied geometry, although a large number studied natural philosophy; in other schools the reverse was true.[36] In the better private academies, which were basically college preparatory schools, a larger proportion of students would have studied Greek, but because neither geometry nor natural philosophy were college entrance requirements, it is unlikely that many students would have studied both of them. Thus it may be concluded that the number of students who would have met all the AMA requirements was so small as to make the proposals grossly unrealistic.

Nevertheless, it is possible to interpret the AMA's standards more loosely and ask how many white male students (virtually no females or non-whites attended medical school in this period) would have had a reasonable amount of secondary school education of any kind at mid-century. There are no readily available data on this matter, but some estimates can be made. As late as 1870, only two percent of the 17-year old white population had received secondary school degrees. In 1850, the proportion must have been much smaller, because the period after 1850 was one of great growth in secondary education. Allowing for greater attendance of males than females at secondary schools and for the students who attended secondary school for several years but did not receive a degree, it may be estimated that less than four percent of the 23-year old population (the median age of those entering one medical school) would have had two years or more of secondary school education. Numerically, making the most liberal estimates, this amounts to less than eight thousand white males in the United States at the time. In 1850 about 1,500 students entered all medical schools. Thus it is inconceivable that medical schools could have maintained their enrollments even had they significantly reduced the AMA standards.[37]

Furthermore, there is evidence that the practice of medicine was not a popular vocation among the better-educated young men of the

36 Inglis, *Rise of the High School*, pp. 88–93.
37 U.S. Bureau of the Census, *Historical Statistics of the United States* (Washington, D.C.: 1960), p. 207; Waite, *Story of a Country Medical College*, p. 124.

period. A survey in 1864 of the 1854–64 graduates of one secondary school, the New York (City) Free Academy, revealed the following distribution of occupations: teachers, 20 percent; lawyers, 20 percent; clergymen, 10 percent; physicians, 6 percent; military vocations, 6 percent; bankers, 6 percent; architects and engineers, 6 percent; and the remainder scattered. In 1850 the AMA's Committee on Medical Education analyzed the careers of the graduates of Harvard, Yale, Dartmouth, Brown, Princeton, Union, Amherst, and Hamilton Colleges, from about 1800 to about 1850, with slight differences in periods for different institutions. Of the 12,400 graduates of all schools, 26 percent became clergymen, about the same number became lawyers, and less than 8 percent became physicians. With respect to the academic honorary fraternity, Phi Beta Kappa, at Harvard, Yale, and Hamilton, a smaller proportion of members than non-members became physicians. The committee concluded that medicine attracted a small number of graduates and generally the academically inferior ones.[38] This situation was undoubtedly as well known to the physicians who established the AMA standards as it was to many other physicians of the time. Samuel Annan, for example, observed that the AMA proposals were hopelessly impractical:

Young men thus prepared, are not to be found. If all who obtain the degree of Bachelor of Arts, from Literary Institutions, should study medicine, they would scarcely supply the demand for physicians; and it is known that a large majority engage in the study of divinity and law, or become merchants and farmers. . . .

It is requiring an impossibility to insist that all the physicians of our new, thinly populated, and as yet, in many parts, rude and unenlightened country, shall be men of high scholarship.[39]

Only one conclusion is possible from these data: rigid enforcement of the AMA's preliminary education standards would have closed down practically every medical school in the country, and would have depleted the ranks of formally educated physicians in a few years. The medical schools never considered the proposal seriously. It must be concluded, therefore, that the AMA's recommended preliminary education requirements were, at best, ill considered, and, at worst, a crude attempt to destroy most of the medical colleges.

As a result of these activities of the AMA, many medical colleges regarded the Association simply as an attempt to reduce the number

[38] Gifford, *New York State High School System*, p. 77; W. Hooker *et al.*, "Report of the Committee on Medical Education," *Transactions of the American Medical Association* 4 (1851): 421–22.
[39] Annan, "National Medical Convention," pp. 125–26.

of physicians by destroying medical schools, and as an organization with little or no interest in actually improving medical education. Annan wrote the following about the 1847 AMA convention:

> In the reports of the committees, and more especially in the speeches of the members of the convention, there were numerous and strong professions of regard for the interests of suffering humanity. . . . Loud and melancholy were the lamentations over the injury done to society by the crowd of imperfectly educated young men, who are pressing into the ranks of the profession. The rapid increase of the number of students who attend the medical colleges, attracted by the facility with which degrees are obtained, it was said, was well calculated to produce mournful forebodings in the mind of every philanthropist. While this was the general tenor of the remarks, . . . one old gentleman . . . took a very singular view of the subject. He insisted that it was the injury done to the doctors themselves by the host of young and active competitors who are continually sent out by the medical colleges, with the highest honors of the profession, to contend with them, and too often successfully, for that patronage, on which they depend for the support of themselves and families, which is the chief grievance. . . . In the opinion of this venerable father, it is necessary to apply some check to the rapid multiplication of physicians, not that the community may be saved from destruction, but that those engaged in practice may remain undisturbed in the possession of the public confidence. It is, however, but simple justice to state that this gentleman was regarded as eccentric and indiscreet.[40]

The medical colleges became less interested in the activities of the Association after its creation. The number of delegates from medical colleges (two were permitted from each college) averaged 52 at the AMA conventions of 1847–49, and 34 at those of 1850–52. During the same years, the delegates from the societies varied randomly around 200.[41]

Other motives behind the formation of the AMA broadened its appeal to the profession, but these will be discussed in a later chapter. For the present, it may be concluded that the AMA served as a force behind which the societies and their advocates could coalesce, but at the same time made the schools and their advocates realize that they could not look to the rest of the profession for wholehearted support. For the remainder of the nineteenth century, relations between the schools and the societies were estranged, and each institution developed independently of the other. The schools, rather than the local, state, and national societies, had the greater impact on the profession and on medicine.

40 *Ibid.*, pp. 120–21.
41 Davis, "History of the American Medical Association," *New Jersey Medical Reporter* 8 (1855): 391.

PART III THE REBELLION AGAINST THE REGULAR MEDICAL PROFESSION

"THE PEOPLE of this state have been bled long enough in their bodies and pockets, and it was time they should do as the men of the Revolution did: resolve to set down and enjoy the freedom for which they bled."

A NEW YORK STATE LEGISLATOR
advocating repeal of the licensing laws

CHAPTER 7 THE THOMSONIAN MOVEMENT

THE PROLIFERATION of medical schools brought about the standardization of regular medical therapeutics as a few dozen medical schools, using a smaller number of textbooks, replaced thousands of preceptors, each of whom taught his own idiosyncratic practices. The schools inculcated in their students the regimen of bloodletting, cathartics, blistering, and all the other therapies characteristic of heroic medicine. Eventually an aroused public rebelled against this form of medical practice.[1] The major beneficiary of their ire was an itinerant root and herb doctor, Samuel Thomson, who developed his own system of botanical practice and promulgated it through his book on domestic medicine. Public support for his system led to the development of a significant social movement which included local and national voluntary associations, lay medical journals, and the rudiments of a medical sect. The Thomsonian movement caused the regular profession considerable difficulty and was the major force behind the repeal of the medical licensing laws.

THE SECTARIAN NATURE OF REGULAR MEDICAL PRACTICE

The major limitation of formal medical education in the first half of the nineteenth century was the absence of any practical clinical and laboratory training. Newly graduated physicians simply had no practical experience with most drugs and no sustained direct observation of patients. N. S. Davis complained that medical education could never be of much value until the student "actually engages with scalpel in hand, in a patient practical study of anatomy and physiology...; chemistry in the laboratory; materia medica and medical botany in the fields and forests; and clinical practice by the bed-side

[1] See the epigraph above; as quoted by Henry Burnell Shafer, *The American Medical Profession 1783 to 1850* (New York: Columbia University Press, 1936), p. 210.

of his preceptor's patients."[2] This, however, was rarely done by either the medical schools or the preceptors.

Consequently, the average graduate was often completely ignorant of medical practice. J. Marion Sims, an eminent gynecologist and surgeon of his day, wrote: "When I graduated [in 1835] I presume I could have gone into the dissecting room and cut down upon any artery, and put a ligature around it, but I knew nothing at all about the practice of medicine." In his first case as a physician—an infant suffering from gastroenteritis (called cholera infantum, but unrelated to cholera), a very common cause of infant mortality in that period when nothing was known about pasteurization of milk or sanitation— Sims related:

. . . I examined the child minutely from head to foot. I looked at its gums, and, as I always carried a lancet with me and had surgical propensities, as soon as I saw some swelling of the gums I at once took out my lancet and cut the gums down to the teeth. This was good so far as it went. But, when it came to making up a prescription, I had no more idea of what ailed the child, or what to do for it, than if I never studied medicine. I was at a perfect loss what to do. . . .

I hurried back to my office, and took out one of my seven volumes of Eberle, which comprised my library, and found his treatise on the "Diseases of Children." I hastily took it down, turned quickly to the subject of "Cholera Infantum," and read it through, over and over again, to the end most carefully. I knew no more what to prescribe for the sick babe than if I hadn't read it at all. But it was my only resource. I had nobody else to consult but Eberle. . . . At the beginning of his article . . . there was a prescription. . . . So I compounded it as quickly as I knew how [and it was administered]. . . . [When I next saw the child] I saw that as the medicine had done no good it was necessary to change it. . . . I turned to Eberle again, and to a new leaf. I gave the baby a prescription from the next chapter. Suffice it to say, that I changed leaves and prescriptions as often as once or twice a day.[3]

To his regret, the infant died. Sims continued, "my feelings can well be imagined at the idea that I had lost my first patient. I attended the funeral; I was the chief mourner of all. Certainly its father and mother did not feel so badly over the loss of their child as I did at the loss of my first patient." While every new practitioner may not have had Sims's bad luck—his second patient had the same illness with the same result—"Again I had to be the chief mourner at the funeral of another little lost citizen of Lancaster"—the absence of detailed practical in-

2 N. S. D[avis], "National Medical Convention," *New York Journal of Medicine* 6 (1846): 132.

3 J. Marion Sims, *The Story of My Life* (New York: Appleton, 1884), pp. 140–42.

struction was a critical limitation of the system of formal medical education of the day.[4]

Because of their ignorance, physicians were forced to use a few remedies as panaceas, which led to a dreary and often fatal routine unenlightened by adequate practical knowledge. Davis stated that a few physicians rose above this routine:

> But far otherwise is it with the great mass; the ninety-nine out of every hundred. With no *practical* knowledge of chemistry and botany; with but a smattering of anatomy and physiology, hastily caught during a sixteen weeks' attendance on the anatomical theatre of a medical college; with still less of real pathology; they enter the profession having mastered just enough of the details of practice to give them the requisite *self-assurance* for commanding the confidence of the public; but without either an adequate fund of knowledge or that degree of mental discipline, and habits of patient study which will enable them ever to supply their defects. Hence they plod on through life, with a fixed routine of practice, consisting of calomel, antimony, opium, and the lancet, almost as empirically applied as is cayenne pepper, lobelia, and steam, by another class of men.[5]

In this way regular medicine turned into a sect, whose members were generally ignorant, dogmatic, and committed to heroic therapy.

As this routine became more prevalent with the increased number of graduates of the medical schools, hostility to heroic practice increased. Eventually public opposition to its excesses reached what some physicians considered truly alarming proportions. One physician advised his colleagues in 1835:

> It is but the other day that I saw a case of gastroenteritis, in which calomel was pushed till the countenance exhibited a most frightful appearance, owing to the excessive swelling of the cheeks, lips, tongue, fauces, and throat, while the saliva flowed in streams.
>
> It is the observation of this injudicious use of mercury, by the common people, at the instigation of interested quacks, and unprincipled men in our own profession, that has caused such a hue and cry, such an inveterate and overweening prejudice in the minds of a vast multitude, against it; which has produced a war for its utter and entire destruction and annihilation, that rages in many parts of our country with as much venom, fury, and heat, as ever did feudal war or party politics. . . . It is this, more than any one, and perhaps all causes combined, that has produced, does continue, and will perpetuate (unless obviated), the fear, jealousy, and suspicion, that exist between what may be called the anti-calomel part of the community, and the profession at large. . . .
>
> Under these circumstances, is it not better to conciliate the prejudices of the people, and inspire their confidence and support, by dispensing with

---

[4] *Ibid.*, pp. 143–45.

[5] N. S. D[avis], "National Medical Convention," *New York Journal of Medicine* 5 (1845): 418.

its use, and substituting in its stead vegetable articles, in all cases in which it would not be attended with too much risk to the welfare and safety of the patients? . . .

Instead of this course of conciliation and forbearance, many members of our profession pursue a directly opposite course; and instead of humoring the prevailing whims and prejudices, are intolerant and overbearing. And if any [patient] have the boldness or temerity to doubt their infallibility, and the necessity of administering a medicine, the bad effects of which they so often see (or think they see), [these physicians], in the plentitude of their wisdom and power, are determined to inflict summary vengeance on them for their temerity and doubt, by a ten times more frequent and greater use of the article in question, than they otherwise would have done.[6]

Thus the battle lines were drawn. In one camp were the swelling ranks of the regular profession, emerging from the medical schools imbued with an abiding faith in calomel, bloodletting, and all the other therapeutics of their heroic art. In the other camp, the ranks were not so well defined. Many people opposed the regular profession, but they had no more knowledge of how to remedy its deficiencies than did the regular physicians. They found many aspects of regular medicine repugnant, but they did not know why or how they were undesirable. The public could only choose among the alternatives available at the time.[7]

Of the various alternatives to regular therapy, only botanical medicine was widely used and understood by the public. The "root and herb" and "Indian" doctors had long offered themselves to the public as critics of and alternatives to regular medicine. Both botanical practitioners and nostrum venders often used the slogan "no calomel" in their advertising and name plates. These men, however limited their training and formal education, based their practice on the long tradition of botanical medicine in America and on hostility to regular medicine.[8] Consequently, many people turned to botanical practitioners when they became dissatisfied with regular medicine.

SAMUEL THOMSON AND THE BOTANICAL MOVEMENT

The greatest single beneficiary of these forces was Samuel Thomson (1769–1843), a self-made man who rose to great prominence in this period due largely to a system of medicine he described in his book,

[6] G. C. Howard, "On Calomel in Gangrenopsis," *Boston Medical and Surgical Journal* 12 (1835): 411–12.

[7] Cf. Lester S. King, *The Medical World of the Eighteenth Century* (Chicago: University of Chicago Press, 1958), p. 54.

[8] A detailed account of the widespread use of botanical medicines and the prevalence of botanical practitioners during this period is provided in: Madge E. Pickard and R. Carlyle Buley, *The Midwest Pioneer* (New York: Henry Schuman, 1946), pp. 35–97.

New Guide to Health: or, Botanic Family Physician, containing a Complete System of Practice, on a Plan Entirely New; with a Description of the Vegetables made use of, and Directions for Preparing and Administering Them, to Cure Disease, to which is Prefixed, a Narrative of the Life and Medical Discoveries of the Author.[9]

Thomson's own life and early career epitomized the influence of rural botanical medicine. He was born to poor parents in 1769 in an isolated part of New Hampshire. He soon developed an interest in botanical medicines, which he cultivated with the aid of a local root and herb doctor:

I was very curious to know the names of all the herbs which I saw growing, and what they were good for; and, to satisfy my curiosity was constantly making inquiries of the persons I happened to be with, for that purpose. . . . There was an old lady . . . lived near us, who used to attend our family when there was any sickness. At that time there was no such thing as a Doctor known among us, there not being any within ten miles. The whole of her practice was with roots and herbs, applied to the patient, or given in hot drinks, to produce sweating; which always answered the purpose. . . . By her attention to the family, and the benefits they received from her skill, we became very much attached to her; and when she used to go out to collect roots and herbs, she would take me with her, and learn me their names, with what they were good for. . . .[10]

On one occasion, Thomson badly lacerated his ankle with an axe while clearing some virgin land with his father. After a number of treatments, including soaking it in turpentine, he ended up at the home of one Dr. Kitteridge:

The doctor soon came home, and on entering the room where I was, cried out in a very rough manner, who have you here? His wife answered, a sick man. The devil, replied he, I want no sick man here. I was much terrified by his coarse manner of speaking, and thought if he was so rough in his conversation, what will he be when he comes to dress my wound; but I was happily disappointed, for he took off the dressing with great care, and handled me very tenderly. On seeing the strings that were in the wound [setons], he exclaimed, what the devil are these halters here for? My father told him they were put in to keep the sore open. He said he thought the sore open enough now, for it is all rotten. Being anxious to know his opinion of me, my father asked him what he thought of my situation. What do I think? said he, why I think he will die; and then looking very pleasantly at me, said, though I think young man, you will get well first. . . . I have been more particular in describing this interview with Dr. Kitteridge, on account of his extraordinary skill in surgery, and the great name he acquired, and justly deserved, among the people throughout the country. His system of practice

---

[9] Third edition, (Boston: 1832). The *New Guide to Health* and the *Narrative* were published and paginated separately, but bound together.
[10] Thomson, *Narrative*, pp. 15–16.

was peculiarly his own, and all the medicines he used were prepared by himself, from the roots and herbs of our own country. . . .[11]

Some years later, Thomson made what he considered to be his greatest discovery: the therapeutic value of *Lobelia inflata*, an emetic herb. He stated in his *Narrative*:

. . . when mowing in the field with a number of men one day, I cut a sprig of [lobelia], and gave to the man next to me, who eat it; when we had got to the end of the piece, which was about six rods, he said that he believed what I had given him would kill him, for he never felt so in his life. I looked at him and saw that he was in a most profuse perspiration, being as wet all over as he could be; he trembled very much, and there was no more colour in him than a corpse. I told him to go to the spring and drink some water; he attempted to go, and got as far as the wall, but was unable to get over it, and laid down on the ground and vomited several times. He said he thought he threw off his stomach two quarts. I then helped him into the house, and in about two hours he ate a very hearty dinner, and in the afternoon was able to do a good half day's labour. He afterwards told me that he never had any thing do him so much good in his life; his appetite was remarkably good, and he felt better than he had for a long time. This circumstance gave me the first idea of the medical virtues of this valuable plant, which I have since found by twenty years experience, in which time I have made use of it in every disease I have met with, to great advantage, that it is a discovery of the greatest importance.[12]

Thomson was forced to resign himself to the existence of a rural farmer, an occupation he disliked intensely. He soon began having difficulty with the local physicians who treated his family. His mother became ill and died: "the doctors gave her over, and gave her disease the name of galloping consumption, which I thought was a very appropriate name; for they are the riders, and their whip is mercury, opium and vitriol, and they galloped her out of the world in about nine weeks."[13] His wife also became ill after the birth of her first child, and Thomson related:

Her fits continued and grew worse; there were six doctors attended her that day, and a seventh was sent for; but she grew worse under their care; for one would give her medicine, and another said that he did wrong; another would bleed her, and the other would say he had done wrong, and so on through the whole. I heard one of them say that his experience in this case was worth fifty dollars. I found that they were trying their practice by experiments; and was so dissatisfied with their conduct, that at night I told

---

[11] *Ibid*, pp. 22–23. Thomson's description of Kitteridge as famous appears to be correct. In a history of New Hampshire medicine written about this time (1780–85), Lyman How referred to the "celebrated Thomas Kitteridge," who was probably the same man. Lyman Bartlett How and Henry O. Smith, *The Story of the New Hampshire Medical Society* (Nashua, N. H.: Phaneuf Press, 1941), p. 26.

[12] Thomson, *Narrative*, p. 27.

[13] *Ibid.*, pp. 40, 24.

them what I thought; and that I had heard them accusing each other of doing wrong; but I was convinced that they had all told the truth, for they had all done wrong. They all gave her over to die, and I dismissed them. . . .[14]

He then brought in two root and herb doctors, under whose care his wife recovered.

Shortly thereafter, Thomson resolved to treat himself and his family, using the botanical remedies with which he was familiar, as well as another common treatment of the period, steam baths. He gave up his farm about 1805 to become an itinerant herb doctor and practiced with considerable success in the area around southern New Hampshire, southern and eastern Maine, and northeastern Massachusetts. In the course of his practice, he developed his "system" of medical therapeutics, utilizing a number of botanical remedies in a predetermined order. The turning point in his career came when he went to Eastport, Maine, in 1811. There he taught his mode of practice to some residents, whom he organized into a society pledged to use his methods of treatment and to aid each other. He provided the residents with a stock of medicine, and in effect set them up as a lay medical society for their mutual care and treatment, establishing a pattern he later used with many other groups. In the following year, 1812, he published a "medical circular" describing his system, and then patented the system itself in 1813. Thomson expanded the pamphlet several times and, with the aid of an educated clergyman, published it in 1822 as a book. The book soon became extremely popular and went through thirteen editions, including one translated into German for the Pennsylvania Germans. Thomson stated in 1839 that 100,000 copies of his book had been sold.[15]

An analysis of the Thomsonian movement must therefore be divided into several parts. First, there was the book itself, the *New Guide to Health*, which was surely sold to many people who never participated in the societies. Second, there were the societies set up by Thomson and his followers and agents. Third, there were the professional botanical practitioners who adopted Thomson's system or incorporated its major features into their own practice.

THOMSON'S *New Guide to Health*

Like any other book, the *New Guide to Health* (including the *Narrative*) had an existence independent of that of its author. Thomson and his many authorized agents sold copies to thousands of fami-

14 *Ibid.*, p. 25.

15 *Ibid.*, pp. 112–16; Frederick C. Waite, "American Sectarian Medical Colleges Before the Civil War," *Bulletin of the History of Medicine* 19 (1946): 148–49.

lies, who undoubtedly used it like any other volume on domestic medicine: to prevent and cure illness in their families without reliance on outsiders. For this reason, the book can be analyzed independently of the rest of the Thomsonian movement.

The system described by Thomson in his book was basically a variant of the evacuants and tonics system so popular in the regular profession. Thomson prescribed an ordered course of medicines, which cleaned out the system with emetics and restored it with tonics. His basic theory was quite simple:

Heat, I found was life; and Cold, death. . . . Our life depends on heat; food is the fuel that kindles and continues that heat. . . . By constantly receiving food into the stomach, which is sometimes not suitable for the best nourishment, the stomach becomes foul, so that the food is not well digested. This causes the body to lose its heat; then the appetite fails; the bones ache, and the man is sick in every part of the whole frame.

This situation of the body shows the need of medicine, and the kind needed; which is such as will clear the stomach and bowels, and restore the digestive powers. When this is done, the food will raise the heat again, and nourish the whole man. All the art required to do this is, to know what medicine will do it, and how to administer it, as a person knows how to clear a stove and the pipe when clogged with soot, that the first may burn free, and the whole room be warmed as before.[16]

His "course" of medicines began with an emetic, which he called *Number 1*. Thomson used lobelia, which was designed "to cleanse the Stomach, overpower the cold, and promote a free perspiration." If lobelia were insufficient to do this, steam baths must be used: "In all cases where the heat of the body is so far exhausted as not to be rekindled by using the medicine and being shielded from the surrounding air by a blanket, or being in bed, and chills or stupor attend the patient, then applied heat by steaming, becomes indispensably necessary. . . ." Lobelia, he found, "would not hold [the heat] long enough to effect the desired object, so but that the cold would return again and assume its power." Thus the patient moved on to *Number 2*, which was cayenne pepper in the form of one-half to one teaspoon in sweetened hot water, to be repeated as needed. This, he felt, would restore the desired internal heat. *Numbers 3* and *4*, used to "correct the Bile and restore Digestion," were simply teas and tonics made from local roots, leaves, barks, and berries. *Numbers 5* and *6*, "to strengthen the Stomach and Bowels, and restore weak patients," were basically brandy or wine mixed with some herbs, barks, etc. In addition to these six, Thomson recommended the use of a number of teas, all made from the leaves of local plants, such as spearmint, pep-

16 Thomson, *New Guide to Health*, pp. 7–8.

permint, mayweed, wormwood, etc. This, in essence, was the sum total of Thomson's system. The user could easily make his own remedies, and Thomson gave detailed advice and instructions on how to obtain good quality ingredients and how to prepare them. Thomson and his agents sold both crude ingredients and prepared remedies in a number of stores throughout the country.[17]

The book also contained useful advice on medical problems not involving drugs. For example, in an era when most physicians believed that most diseases were transmitted by odors in the air, Thomson stated:

While I was in New York [in 1806], I took particular notice of their manner of living; and observed that they subsisted principally upon fresh provisions, more particularly the poorer class of people; who are in the habit in warm weather of going to market at a late hour of the day, and purchasing fresh meat that is almost in a putrid state, having frequently been killed the night previous, and being badly cooked, by taking it into the stomach, will produce certain disease. . . . If people would get into the practice of eating salt provisions in hot weather and fresh in cold, it would be a very great preventive of disease. One ounce of putrid flesh in the stomach is worse than the effect produced by a whole carcass on the air by its effluvia.[18]

Thomson was particularly concerned with midwifery, and devoted much attention to it. He argued that a great change had occurred in the practice of midwifery. "Thirty years ago the practice of midwifery was principally in the hands of experienced women, who had no difficulty, [but the doctors] have now got most of the practice into their own hands . . . [These] young, inexperienced doctors . . . have little knowledge, except what they get from books, and their practice is to try experiments," so that the death of mother or child is the not infrequent result. In addition, they use forceps with such force that "they often not only crush the head of the child, but also the neck of the bladder." Thomson was probably correct in this, inasmuch as most physicians began practice without ever having seen an obstetrical delivery.[19] Thomson's own recommendations were full of common sense and sound advice:

It is very important to keep up the strength of women in a state of pregnancy, so that at the time of delivery, they may be in possession of all their natural powers; they should be carried through a course of the medicine

[17] Ibid., pp. 38, 20; Thompson, Narrative, p. 44, and New Guide to Health, pp. 52, 59, 62, 66–68; Alex Berman, "The Thomsonian Movement and its Relation to American Pharmacy and Medicine," Bulletin of the History of Medicine 25 (1951): 520–28.

[18] Thomson, Narrative, p. 58.

[19] Thomson, New Guide to Health, pp. 130–34; Frederick Clayton Waite, The First Medical College in Vermont (Montpelier: Vermont Historical Society, 1949), p. 122.

several times, particularly a little before delivery, and keep them in a perspiration during and after delivery, which will prevent after pains, and other complaints common in such cases. Beware of bleeding, opium, and cold baths; invigorate all the faculties of the body and mind, to exert the most laborious efforts that nature is called upon to perform, instead of stupifying, and substituting art for nature.[20]

Thomson spent a large part of the book attacking the regular profession and "their instruments of death, Mercury, Opium, Rats-bane [arsenic], Nitre, and the Lancet."[21] He attacked bleeding in the following manner:

The practice of bleeding for the purpose of curing disease, I consider most unnatural and injurious. Nature never furnishes the body with more blood than is necessary for the maintenance of health.... If the system is diseased, the blood becomes as much diseased as any other part; remove the cause of the disorder, and the blood will recover and become healthy as soon as any other part; but how taking part of it away can help to cure what remains, can never be reconciled with common sense. . . . .

When in Philadelphia, Thomson visited a faculty member of the University of Pennsylvania medical school:

I stated to him pretty fully my opinion of the absurdity of bleeding to cure disease; and pointed out its inconsistency, inasmuch as the same method was made use of to cure a sick man as to kill a well beast. He laughed and said it was strange logic enough.

While in the city of Philadelphia, I examined into their mode of treating the yellow fever; and found to my astonishment that the treatment prescribed by Dr. [Benjamin] Rush was to bleed twice a day for ten days. It appeared to me very extraordinary to bleed twenty times to cure the most fatal disease ever known; and am confident that the same manner of treatment would kill one half of those in health. This absurd practice being followed by the more ignorant class of the faculty, merely because it has been recommended in some particular cases by a great man, has, I have not the least doubt, destroyed more lives than has ever been killed by powder and ball in this country in the same time.[22]

He also strongly attacked blistering:

There is no practice used by the physicians that I consider more inconsistent with common sense, and at the same time more inhumane than blistering, to remove disease; particularly insane persons, or what the doctors call dropsy of the brain; in which cases they shave the head and draw a blister on it. Very few patients, if any, ever survive this application. . . . I have witnessed many instances where great distress and very bad effects have been caused by the use of blisters; and believe I can truly say that I never knew any benefit derived from their use. . . .

20 Thomson, *New Guide to Health*, p. 131.
21 *Ibid.*, p. 9.
22 *Ibid.*, pp. 18–19; Thomson, *Narrative*, pp. 125–26.

I never could see any reason why a scald on the head or body, done on purpose, should have a tendency to effect a cure, when the person is sick, and the same thing happening to them by accident, when well, should destroy their health or cause their death. If a person should have their head or stomach so badly scalded as to take off the skin, we should consider them in the most dangerous condition; but nothing is said about it when drawn on purpose. I shall leave it to the reader to reconcile, if he can, this inconsistency.[23]

Thomson condemned the use of all poisons, whether mineral or vegetable. He quoted extensively from "standard medical works," showing that their authors, on the one hand, cited the lethal effects of large doses of calomel, arsenic, antimony, nitre, and opium and, on the other hand, recommended their use in small doses.[24] He concluded:

During thirty years practice, I have had opportunity to gain much experience on this subject, and am ready to declare that . . . there can be no possible good derived from using in any manner or form whatever, those poisons. . . . the greatest difficulty I have had to encounter in removing the complaints which my patients [with chronic diseases] laboured under, has been to clear the system of mercury, nitre or opium, and bring them back to the same state they were in before taking them. It is a very easy thing to get them into the system, but very hard to get them out again.

Those who make use of these things as medicine, seem to cloak the administering them under the specious pretence of great skill and art in preparing and using them; but this kind of covering will not blind the people, if they would examine it and think for themselves, instead of believing that every thing said or done by a learned man must be right; for poison given to the sick by a person of the greatest skill, will have exactly the same effect as it would if given by a fool.[25]

Thomson was not an unqualified critic of all regular physicians. He attacked heroic medical practice, but spoke sympathetically of those physicians who shared his opposition to heroic treatment, even if they also rejected his system:

Among the practising physicians, I have found, and I believe it to be a well known fact, that those who are really great in the profession and have had the most experience, condemn as much as I do, the fashionable mode of practice of the present day, and use very little medical poisons, confining themselves in their treatment of patients to simples [medicines composed of a single drug] principally, and the use of such things as will promote digestion and aid nature; and many of them disapprove of bleeding altogether. Those of this description, with whom I have had an opportunity to converse, have treated me with all due attention and civility.[26]

[23] Thomson, *New Guide to Health*, pp. 19, 99.
[24] *Ibid.*, pp. 27–31.
[25] *Ibid.*, pp. 26–27.
[26] Thomson, *Narrative*, p. 41.

From this account of the *New Guide to Health*, it must be concluded that Thomson was neither a crude empiric nor a demagogue intent on destroying the regular profession. Rather, his criticisms of the medical profession were generally well taken and his suggestions frequently sound and full of common sense. The fact that his system was of little value is not an overwhelming weakness; when used as suggested in the book, it did little harm, and it was far superior to the heroic therapy which it replaced.

Regardless of the manner in which the book would be judged today, the question must be asked: why was it so popular at the time? Contemporary readers did not have the knowledge of medicine available in the twentieth century; the readers who approved of Thomson's system must have done so because it appealed to them, given their knowledge of medicine.

The first point to be made is that there was nothing strange or foreign in any part of Thomson's approach. Books on domestic medicine were popular in early nineteenth-century America. William Buchan's *Domestic Medicine*, for example, was published in several editions in America in the late eighteenth and early nineteenth centuries and was both popular and esteemed. There were also a number of botanical books on domestic medicine, such as Peter Smith's *The Indian Doctor's Dispensatory*, originally published in 1813. This volume was very similar to Thomson's, even to the extent of numbered remedies. Smith also opposed the use of calomel, although he did recommend bloodletting. Therefore, Thomson's book was directed at a public well acquainted with volumes on domestic medicine.[27]

Thomson limited his practice to botanical medicines, which were widely known and accepted in many parts of the country as being particularly beneficial. Even the specific remedies that Thomson used were well known. A regular physician, in denouncing the system in 1835, stated:

> The principal [treatments] are, lobelia or Indian tobacco, which is an emetic, and . . . I have no doubt, a very valuable remedy properly used, and which is or may be in the hands of every physician; steaming, which, it is well known, is not new, it having been used in domestic practice from the earliest periods, is common to barbarian nations, was found in use among the aborigines of our own country, and, of course, does not exclusively belong to the Thomsonian system; the bark of the root of bay or myrtle bush, the hemlock bark, white pond lily, peach kernels, raspberry leaf tea, and a

27 Frederick Clayton Waite, *Western Reserve University Centennial History of the School of Medicine* (Cleveland, Ohio: Western Reserve University Press, 1946), pp. 38–39; Peter Smith, "The Indian Doctor's Dispensatory," *Bulletin of the Lloyd Library of Botany, Pharmacy and Materia Medica*, No. 2, Reproduction Ser. No. 2.

few other common, domestic, old woman remedies, the most of which are and have been in use where Thomson's book was never seen; with cayenne pepper, which . . . is the most important remedy of the whole, and enters largely into most of those famous numbers. . . .[28]

Thomson himself claimed credit only for lobelia, but it also had been used before the nineteenth century by settlers.[29] Furthermore, ipecac, a vegetable emetic that was quite similar to lobelia in its effects, was widely used by regular physicians of the period. Thomson's only real contribution to therapeutics was to arrange the drugs into a "course" and to recommend doses. The previous popularity of the elements of his system was undoubtedly a major basis of its appeal to lower-class rural constituents, who would have distrusted anything novel.

A second reason for the popularity of Thomson's book was that the *Narrative* as literature was an excellent example of the virtue-triumphant-over-adversity school of writing so popular in the nineteenth century, and exemplified in the Horatio Alger stories written years later.[30] The *Narrative* was basically a highly moral, although not religious, work. Thomson stated his basic theme in these words:

I found I had enemies on every hand, and was in danger of falling by some one of them. Every thing seemed to conspire against me; but I had some friends who have never forsaken me; my courage remained good, and my spirits were never depressed; and it appeared to me that the more troubles I had to encounter, the more firmly I was fixed in my determination to persevere unto the last.[31]

One quotation will serve to illustrate the literary quality of the book:

While I remained in this place, . . . I was called on to attend several cases, in all of which I was very successful; most of them were such as had been given over by the doctors. One of them was the case of a young man, who had cut three of his fingers very badly, so as to lay open the joints. Dr. French had attended him three weeks, and they had got so bad that he advised him to have them cut off as the only alternative. The young man applied to me for advice. I told him if I was in his situation, I should not be willing to have them cut off till I had made some further trial to cure them without. He requested me to undertake to cure him, to which I consented

[28] Dr. Williams, "The Thomsonian National Infirmary," *Boston Medical and Surgical Journal* 12 (1835): 203.

[29] J. U. Lloyd and C. G. Lloyd, "Life and Medical Discoveries of Samuel Thomson, and a History of the Thomsonian Materia Medica," *Bulletin of the Lloyd Library of Botany, Pharmacy and Materia Medica*, No. 11, Reproduction Ser. No. 7, 1909, p. 88 (second set of page numbers).

[30] The Horatio Alger stories contained many of the same themes prevalent in Thomson's autobiography, and one writer has attributed Alger's success to his depiction of these themes. R. Richard Wohl, "The 'Rags to Riches Story' " in Reinhard Bendix and Seymour Martin Lipset, eds., *Class, Status, and Power* (New York: Free Press, 1966), 2nd ed., pp. 501–6.

[31] Thomson, *Narrative*, p. 122.

and began by clearing the wound of mercury, by washing it with weak lye; I then put on some drops, and did it up with a bandage which was kept wet with cold water. While I was dressing the wound, a young man, who was studying with Dr. French, came in and made a great fuss, telling the young man that I was going to spoil his hand. I told him that I was accountable for what I was doing, and that if he had any advice to offer I was ready to hear him; but he seemed to have nothing to offer except to find fault, and went off, after saying that Dr. French's bill must be paid very soon. I continued to dress his hand, and in ten days he was well enough to attend to his work, being employed in a nail factory. Soon after, I saw him there at work, and asked him how his fingers did; he said they were perfectly cured; he wished to know what my bill was for attending him. I asked him what Dr. French had charged, and he said he had sent his bill to his mother, amounting to seventeen dollars; I told him I though that enough for us both, and I should charge him nothing. His mother was a poor widow depending on her labour and that of her son for a living.[32]

This is surely magnificent writing. It is succinct, unaffected, exploits the popular prejudice against physicians so prevalent at the time, draws each character in a few concise strokes, has a moral, and promotes virtue. One need only imagine these passages read aloud at a country hearth in the evening to realize their effect. Furthermore, the story is basically about a country boy who finds himself beleaguered by regular physicians, befriending knaves who betray him, being gullible and suffering for his errors, yet, all in all, achieving success through initiative and effort. Surely the *Narrative* itself had some part to play in the appeal of Thomson's book.

The last and probably the major reason for the system's success was its exploitation of public concern over rising medical expenses. No theme was more prevalent in Thomson's book than the burdensome fees of regular physicians. He continually and repetitiously spoke of physicians "who fare sumptuously every day; living in splendour and magnificence, supported by the impositions they practice on a deluded and credulous people."[33] Thomson said of midwifery:

[The midwife's] price was one dollar; when the doctors began to practise midwifery in the country [rural areas], their price was three dollars, but they soon after raised it to five; and now they charge from twelve to twenty. If they go on at this ratio, it will soon take all the people can earn, to pay for their children. . . . should the child be born, fortunately for the mother and child both, before the arrival of the doctor, he even then, instead of the price of a common visit, considers himself entitled to a half fee; that is, ten dollars. . . . Then dismiss the doctor; restore the business into the hands of women, where it belongs; and save your wife from much unnecessary pain,

32 *Ibid.*, pp. 60–61.
33 *Ibid.*, p. 34.

your children, perhaps, from death, and at all events, your *money*, for better purposes.[34]

The popular concern with high medical fees to which Thomson appealed with such success was illustrated by the public reaction to the fee bill and code of ethics established by the Medical Association of the District of Columbia immediately after its formation in 1833. Laymen denounced the new organization as a conspiracy to increase medical costs and oppress the poor, and condemned the fee schedule as "exhorbitant, unjust and oppressive." Public meetings were held, people were urged to blacklist the members, and physicians elsewhere were invited to settle in Washington. The issue was resolved shortly, but the intensity of the public reaction revealed the depth of their sentiment about medical costs.[35]

Public discontent with high medical costs seemed rather incongruous at the same time when physicians were bitterly complaining about their inability to collect fees, about fees being too low, and about the poor economic condition of the profession in general.[36] The answer must lie in what Thomson described as occurring. Although physicians' competition with each other had forced them to lower their fees, they had apparently driven out of practice many midwives and other part-time practitioners who were not able to compete with the more prestigious M.D.'s. This enabled physicians to raise their prices well beyond what the part-time practitioners charged.

Thomson's solution to the problem was for patients to "depend more upon themselves, and less upon the doctors," especially in cases of "trifling sickness," by purchasing his book and using it for self-instruction.[37] The nominal fee for the book and the right to belong to the Societies was twenty dollars, an enormous sum among the rural population of that day. However, many, if not most, persons never paid that much. Thomson stated in his *Narrative*:

In selling family rights, I have always been as liberal to purchasers as they could wish, particularly where I was convinced their circumstances made it inconvenient for them to pay the money down; and have been in the habit of taking notes payable at a convenient time. This has occasioned me

---

[34] Thomson, *New Guide to Health*, pp. 131–34.

[35] John B. Nichols, *et al.*, *History of the Medical Society of the District of Columbia, Part II, 1833–1944* (Washington, D.C.: 1947), p. 15; a Thomsonian journal of the time featured an article about the citizen's committee organized to protest the fee bill, which was also listed. "Washington City," *Thomsonian Recorder* 1 (1833): 347–50.

[36] See, for example, George Rosen, *Fees and Fee Bills* (Baltimore: Johns Hopkins Press, 1946), pp. 7–10.

[37] Thomson, *Narrative*, p. 32.

considerable loss; but in most cases the purchasers have shown a disposition to pay if in their power, have treated me with a proper respect, and have been grateful for the favour; with these I have been satisfied, and no one has had reason to complain of my want of generosity towards them. There have been some, however, who have taken a different course, and have not only refused to comply with their contract, but have, notwithstanding they have continued to use the medicine, turned against me and have tried to do me all the harm in their power. Such conduct has caused me some considerable vexation and trouble.[38]

Thomson undoubtedly had as much difficulty collecting his fees as the regular physicians had collecting theirs.

THOMSON'S ORGANIZATION

Samuel Thomson was not only a botanical physician; he was also an entrepreneur of considerable talents. After his book was published, he developed a marketing program whereby his system was widely distributed throughout the nation and became extremely popular. One part of his system was his Friendly Botanical Societies. Purchasers of his book automatically became members of the Friendly Botanical Society (the book and the membership together constituting a "right"), and were permitted to converse with other owners "for instruction and assistance in sickness, as each one is bound to give his assistance, by advice or otherwise, when called on by a member." Local chapters of the society were formed in each community by Thomson's agents, who constituted the second part of his program. Thomson appointed numbers of agents whose job it was to sell books and rights, instruct the people, and set up the societies. In 1833, he employed 167 agents throughout the United States.[39]

This plan was carried out quite diligently, and the movement soon became institutionalized in a number of other ways. The *Boston Medical and Surgical Journal* editorialized in 1837:

If half the effort were made by scientific practitioners of medicine throughout the United States, to elevate the profession, that is exerted by those speculating adventurers in the healing art . . . there would hardly be a single quack from Maine to Georgia. The Thomsonians are busily organizing, holding annual conventions, publishing circulars, issuing pamphlets and circulating their successes, and evince a determination to make the world know they are in being. . . . One of their periodicals, which has an extensive circulation, contains double the number of original reported cases which are found in our pages. But the course they are pursuing is admirable, for it tends to improve them individually; yet unless a counteracting influence is

[38] *Ibid.*, p. 170.
[39] *Ibid.*, p. 147; Berman, "Thomsonian Movement," pp. 416–17.

put in motion, there is reason to fear that in the interior of the country they will eventually become the dominant party.[40]

The Thomsonian movement spread rapidly in the East and into the midwestern and southern states. In the late 1820's, a Boston physician estimated that one sixth of the city's sixty thousand inhabitants used Thomson's system. Although most of the eastern supporters of Thomsonism were lower class, according to a physician in eastern Pennsylvania, the system was popular with all social classes in the midwest and south. In 1829, the *Boston Medical and Surgical Journal* stated: "The support of a number of intelligent and disinterested persons, has given currency to the claims of these Thomsonian practitioners, and, under this sanction, their business has become very extensive, particularly in the [mid]western states." Thomsonians claimed that one-half of the population of Ohio supported Thomsonism, while regular physicians conceded one-third of the state's population to the movement. In the south, the governor of Mississippi claimed in 1835 that one-half of the population of his state were supporters of the system.[41]

Thomson's great success in the Midwest and South led him to emphasize those areas in his activities. In 1833, he employed 41 agents in Ohio, 29 in Tennessee, 21 in Alabama, 11 in Indiana, and only 8 in New York State and 14 in all of New England. In addition, the first four national conventions of the Friendly Botanical Society were held in Columbus, Pittsburgh, Baltimore, and Richmond respectively, four cities located within 250 miles of each other and all in close proximity to the western and southern frontiers.[42]

THE PROFESSIONAL BOTANICAL PRACTITIONERS

Professional botanical practitioners soon realized that the widespread appeal of Thomson's system could be turned to their own benefit. They had been using botanical drugs for years, and easily associated themselves with Thomson's movement by adopting his system or some of his remedies. Even Thomson's agents often became his competitors. Once they learned his system, according to Thomson,

---

[40] "Thomsonian Conventions," *Boston Medical and Surgical Journal* 17 (1837): pp. 322–23.

[41] Reginald H. Fitz, "The Rise and Fall of the Licensed Physician in Massachusetts, 1781–1860," *Transactions of the Association of American Physicians* 9 (1894): 8–9; Sumner Stebbins, *Address in Refutation of the Thomsonian System of Medical Practice* (West Chester, Penn.: 1837), p. 36; "The Patent Thomsonian Practice of Physic," *Boston Medical and Surgical Journal* 2 (1829): 366; Berman, "Thomsonian Movement," p. 407.

[42] *Ibid.*, pp. 417–20.

they "attempted to get the lead of the practice into their own hands, and deprive me of the credit and profits of my own discovery."[43] Thomson removed and replaced any agent caught in these activities, which only served to increase the number of his competitors.

These botanical practitioners, who constantly denigrated regular therapies, nevertheless practiced what could only be termed heroic botanical medicine. They used large and frequent doses of lobelia, and steamed their patients until almost parboiled. Thomson referred contemptuously to a "competitor" who gave one woman nineteen courses of his treatment in six weeks "and then left her in a very weak and low condition (No wonder)." He accused these "speculators" of "crowding their patients with unnecessary courses of medicine, one after another, . . . for the sake of sponging out of them . . . three or four dollars for each course." Thomson himself, however, appears to have been more vigorous in his therapeutics than the *New Guide to Health* would indicate. This is suggested by his self-medication during his terminal illness, when he took enemas and emetics far beyond anything called for in his book.[44]

THE INSTITUTIONALIZATION OF THOMSONISM

As the number of Thomsonian societies and full-time agents increased, and as greater pressures were placed on the movement by botanical practitioners outside the fold, both the professional and lay segments of the movement became increasingly institutionalized. Professional Thomsonian practitioners opened local "infirmaries" which provided facilities for steam baths and other treatments. In at least one state, New York, a Thomsonian society established a formal distinction between professional and lay members. Under the leadership of John Thomson, one of Samuel's sons, the New York (State) Thomsonian Medical Society, founded in 1835, created two grades of membership, one for all owners of rights and the other consisting of those who exhibited "such testimonials of ability, understanding, and other necessary qualifications, as shall secure to him a diploma from the officers of this society. . . ."[45] As will be shown below, this differentiation was designed to legitimate the professional Thomsonian practitioners affiliated with the society.

43 Thomson, *Narrative*, p. 134.

44 Frank G. Halstead, "A First-Hand Account of a Treatment by Thomsonian Medicine in the 1830's," *Bulletin of the History of Medicine* 10 (1941): 680–87; Lloyd and Lloyd, "Life of Samuel Thomson," pp. 86–88; Samuel Thomson, "To the Public," *Thomsonian Recorder* 4 (1836): 388.

45 Berman, "Thomsonian Movement," pp. 530–31.

Beginning in 1832, national conventions of the Friendly Botanical Society were held, partly to urge repeal of existing licensing laws, partly as general social gatherings, partly to boast of the movement's success. At the second convention, the first steps were taken to turn the Thomsonian movement into a medical sect. A resolution was enacted providing for the establishment of a national Thomsonian Infirmary in Baltimore, and efforts were made to legitimate the other infirmaries. These measures were only way-stations to the ultimate goal of the full-time practitioners—Thomsonian medical schools. At the 1835 convention, the body resolved to establish a medical school together with the national infirmary.[46]

Thomson himself saw a great danger in all this. He believed that formal medical education was unnecessary, and that while the study of anatomy, for example, might be "pleasing and useful," it was "no more necessary to mankind at large, to qualify them to administer relief from pain and sickness, than to a cook in preparing food to satisfy hunger and nourishing the body." Not only was it unnecessary, according to Thomson, it was in many ways dangerous: "the moment you blend the simplicity of my discoveries with the abstruse sciences, such as chemistry and other discoveries that have nothing to do with medicine, that moment the benefit of my discoveries will be taken from the people generally, and, like all other crafts, monopolized by a few learned individuals. . . ."[47] The belief that specialized knowledge could be used to obtain a monopoly over the practice of medicine was at the root of his fear of infirmaries and medical schools:

. . . as long as people can go to Infirmaries, or else have a doctor come into their families, they do not see the importance of trying to obtain the knowledge [of the principles expounded in the *New Guide*] for themselves; not thinking, perhaps that in time, Thomsonian doctors may become as bad as any other doctors, and take the advantage of them as such. It gives the superintendents of these Infirmaries, if they are so disposed—and if there be nothing to check it, in time they will be, [the power] to make monopoly of it, and to go into all manner of speculations concerning it.[48]

Thus, once again, the issue was joined between those who sought to limit medical practice to a small number of practitioners and those who wanted to open it to a large number. The full-time botanical practitioners, like the regular medical societies, wanted to limit medical practice to a small number of practitioners approved by them; Thom-

46 *Ibid.*, pp. 418–19, 533–34, 425.
47 Thomson, *New Guide to Health*, pp. 11–12; Berman, "Thomsonian Movement," p. 246.
48 *Ibid.*, p. 424.

son, like the regular medical schools, believed in making medical knowledge available to all who wished to study it. Thomson and the medical schools would not have agreed completely, because the regular medical schools wanted some limitation on the right to practice and Thomson wanted none. Yet the conflict between an open and a closed profession existed both in the Thomsonian movement and in the regular profession.

MEDICAL LICENSING AND THE THOMSONIAN MOVEMENT

The regular profession reacted to the growing popularity of Thomsonism by trying to use the licensing laws to discredit Thomsonian practitioners or, if possible, to deprive them of the right to practice. In 1835, for example, a suit was brought in New York State against John Thomson as a botanical practitioner, and the state Supreme Court eventually ruled that he could not sue for debts in court. Most of these efforts were fruitless. Samuel Thomson, who often complained of harassment against himself and his movement, wrote: "This has caused me a great deal of trouble and expense, and has been of no great benefit to them. It has been like whipping fire among the leaves, which only tends to spread it the faster."[49]

The growing popularity of Thomsonism soon provided its leaders with an opportunity to respond to the harassment of the regular physicians. The first national convention was called in part to deal with this problem. Many of the professional botanical practitioners, but not Thomson, wanted to solve the problem by amending the licensing legislation to permit them to obtain licenses equivalent to those of the regular physicians. They did not want repeal of all licensing laws. John Thomson and the New York Thomsonian Medical Society advocated this view. It has already been mentioned that his society had two grades of membership, which served to separate the professional and lay members of the movement. When a committee was appointed by the New York State legislature to consider repeal of the licensing laws, John Thomson testified before it in 1840. He stated that his society wanted licensing expanded only enough to include persons who "studied and practiced in company with a member of this Society one year, and [have] undergone an examination before the board of censors [of the society], and received a diploma as evidence thereof."[50] These procedures were already incorporated in the So-

[49] "Botanical Physicians Supreme Court," *Boston Medical and Surgical Journal* 14 (1836): 306–7; Thomson, *Narrative*, p. 181.

[50] "Report of the Minority of the Select Committee to which were referred numerous petitions asking a change of the laws towards Thomsonian physisians . . . , May 12, 1840," *Transactions of the Medical Society of the State of New York* (1841; reprint ed. Albany: 1868), p. 246.

ciety's constitution. In speaking of those who owned rights obtained by purchasing the *New Guide to Health*, John Thomson stated:

We do not consider them fit, as general practitioners; they have merely the right to compound their own medicines, and practice in their own families, and have no right or business to practice on community, they are not presumed to be acquainted with disease or medicine, and should not be tolerated to practice, or to collect their pay for their services; community is in danger from these unskillful practitioners.[51]

This scheme was actually put into effect in at least one state. In Connecticut, the licensing law was never repealed, but a Botanico-Medical Society was chartered by the state in 1848 and allowed to grant licenses equivalent to those of the regular licensing board.[52]

Most lay members of the societies, as well as Thomson himself, wanted outright repeal of all licensing legislation. This was the case even in New York State, where in 1840 the leaders of the movement presented the legislature with petitions advocating repeal signed by more than 36,000 persons. The petitions themselves were rather jumbled: some of them were as much as ten years old, some included the names of deceased persons (critics implied that the deaths of some of the signers antedated the dates of their signatures), and different petitions advocated different proposals. In any event, they sufficed to influence the legislative committee considering the repeal measures. The committee recommended in 1841: "Men cannot be legislated out of one religion and into another; nor can the Legislature thrust calomel and mercury down a man's throat while he wills to take only cayenne or lobelia. . . . Your committee thinks that justice should be done to the petitioners."[53] Legislation was passed repealing the medical licensing laws in 1844.

Elsewhere, public opinion also favored the Thomsonians. In South Carolina, a regular medical society brought suit against four Thomsonians in 1835 for illegal practice, but the grand jury refused to issue an indictment. The state legislature repealed all penalties for unlicensed practice three years later. In Ohio, the state legislature repealed the medical licensing laws a few days after the 1832 Thomsonian national convention in Columbus, Ohio. In these and the many other states in which licensing laws were repealed or their penalties

[51] *Ibid.*, p. 247.

[52] Charles J. Bartlett, "Medical Licensure in Connecticut," *Connecticut State Medical Journal* 6 (1942): 185.

[53] "Report of Minority of Select Committee," pp. 241, 243–44; "Report of the Select Committee . . . , Jan. 30, 1841," *Transactions of the Medical Society of the State of New York* (1841; reprint ed. Albany: 1868), pp. 265, 268.

eliminated, the Thomsonians were instrumental in securing the changes.[54]

The major fault with John Thomson's proposal for licensing botanical practitioners was that it was not radical enough. He merely wanted to revive the old apprenticeship system and apply it to botanical practitioners. What was needed if Thomson's system were to become a medical sect was a medical school. By understanding this, Alva Curtis, one of Samuel Thomson's lieutenants, had a much more profound impact on the movement. Curtis rose to the position of editor of a major Thomsonian journal and lobbied within the movement for a medical school. In 1836, he broke with Thomson over this issue and set up his own Botanico-Medical School and Infirmary in Columbus, Ohio; the school received a state charter to grant degrees in 1839. Curtis's successful efforts broke up the Thomsonian movement. After 1838, there were no more national conventions of the Friendly Botanical Societies. Instead, Thomson and Curtis organized separate societies, both using the word "Thomsonian" in the title. The movement rapidly fragmented thereafter, and Thomson's branch soon disintegrated altogether.[55]

During the period from 1827 to the Civil War, at least twenty-two botanical medical schools were founded, most of which were short-lived. The majority and the most stable of them were founded in the South and Midwest, frequently in small towns. Most of the schools were founded after 1845, a few years after the Thomsonian movement fragmented, and therefore were probably more closely associated with the long-run popularity of botanical medicine than with the Thomsonian movement specifically.[56]

THE THOMSONIAN MOVEMENT AND THE REGULAR PHYSICIANS

As Thomson's therapies became more widely used, regular physicians came to view them in a new light. With respect to lobelia, for example, articles by physicians in the *Boston Medical and Surgical*

[54] Joseph F. Kett, *The Formation of the American Medical Profession* (New Haven: Yale University Press, 1968), p. 23; Jonathan Forman, "Dr. Alva Curtis in Columbus: The Thomsonian Recorder and Columbus' First Medical School," *Ohio State Archaeological and Historical Quarterly* 51 (1942): 335; Berman, "Thomsonian Movement," p. 421.

[55] Berman, "Thomsonian Movement," pp. 425–27, 420–21.

[56] A detailed account of each school is provided in Waite, "American Sectarian Medical Colleges," pp. 150–62.

Journal in 1837, 1843, and 1844 all advised their colleagues that, as one said, "Were its medicinal properties well defined by observation and experiment, I think it would prove an auxiliary to our present means of cure." More generally, physicians began to turn from mineral to botanical remedies. C. G. Howard, who was quoted above as deploring the excessive use of calomel, suggested that many chronic diseases could be "relieved with more certainty and success, and with less risk, with vegetable, than with mineral medicines."[57] The major changes in regular therapeutics, however, were probably due to the influence of another sect, to be described in the next chapter.

Physicians had nothing but contempt for Thomson personally and for his system. They pointed out the errors in the idea that heat was life and cold death, and ridiculed his course of medicine. With respect to the latter, Thomson's basic approach was so similar to that of the regular physicians—to clean out the digestive system and restore the patient with tonics—that they might have been expected to see the parallel, but regular physicians were hardly interested in paralleling Thomson's system with their own.

Many physicians called Thomson a quack and stated that he did irreparable harm to medicine. Occasionally, a physician actually defended regular medicine against Thomsonism, as in this statement made in 1846:

. . . I have not the least doubt that bleeding, mercury, opium and antimony, separately or combined, save four times as many lives in these United States, every year, as are saved by all other medical means combined, and fifty times as many as would be saved if Thomsonism had the whole sway and practice. . . . I have in mind . . . our acute, internal inflammations, nine-tenths of which would most certainly terminate fatally, sooner or later, but for those remedies. I care not how much they might be steamed and dosed by all the means and appliances of pure Thomsonism, *they would die*.[58]

Other physicians were more cautious in attacking Thomsonism and defending regular medicine. Sumner Stebbins stated in 1837:

It cannot be denied that the pecularities of organization, the idiosyncracies of constitution, and the diversities of habit, and modes of living prevalent in civilized society, render the practice of medicine, in many instances, somewhat uncertain. This is admitted and lamented by all, but by none more so

[57] D. B. Slack, "The Extracts of Thoroughwort and Lobelia," *Boston Medical and Surgical Journal* 29 (1844): 279; also W. Procter, Jr. "Remarks on some Pharmaceutical Preparations of Lobelia Inflata," *Boston Medical and Surgical Journal* 27 (1843): 53–54; A., "Lobelia Inflata," *Boston Medical and Surgical Journal* 17 (1837): 329–32; Howard, "Calomel in Gangrenopsis," p. 413.

[58] C. Knowlton, "Quackery, etc." *Boston Medical and Surgical Journal* 34 (1846): 175.

than the enlightened physician. . . . there will always be diseases that will prove fatal. . . . But will the casting away the recorded experience—the well-attested facts—the collected wisdom of the ages—and launching, without compass or rudder, upon the ocean of empiricism, with no guide but blind and ignorant conjecture—have a tendency to improve the healing art? [59]

This is a powerful argument—the most powerful one available at the time, whether Stebbins knew it or not—and merits examination. Did Thomson advocate "casting away the recorded experience—the well-attested facts—the collected wisdom of the ages"? There is no evidence that he did.

Because of the limited amount of polemical writing by Thomson, it is necessary to draw on a paper by one of his trusted lieutenants, Thomas Hersey, to evaluate Stebbins's arguments. Although the use of such auxiliary sources must be approached with caution in a movement so heterogeneous and filled with internal dissension as Thomsonism, Hersey's paper coincides with Thomson's own arguments in so many respects and Hersey's role in the movement is so important that its use seems justified.

Hersey argued that regular medicine's claim to scientific and even professional status was a sham and pretense. He attempted to demonstrate this point by examining several major features of regular medical practice. First, he asked whether regular medicine was really responsible for the few medically valid therapies: "What great discoveries have been made by the schools of medicine, for the removal of disease, which is the great desideratum with the sick?" If regular medicine deserved the place it claimed for itself, its value could be demonstrated by its contribution to therapeutics. In fact, Hersey stated, "Many of the discoveries accounted most interesting in the healing art, can be traced to accident or a combination of incidents, that were independent of the efforts of deep, laborious, scientific research." At this point Hersey astutely turned to the two of the great contributions of pre-nineteenth-century medicine: cinchona bark and smallpox vaccination. With respect to the former, Hersey stated that it was discovered either by Jesuits or natives in South America and that the regular profession had nothing to do with its discovery. With respect to vaccination, while conceding that Jenner was "entitled for his ingenuous efforts to the gratitude of the world," Hersey stated that the value of cowpox in preventing smallpox was well known in dairy countries, and it also was not due to "the philosophical researches of medical professors." In addition, medical botany (which Thomsonians considered the only valuable part of the materia medica) was "de-

[59] Stebbins, *Refutation of the Thomsonian System*, pp. 37–39.

rived from savages, or from illiterate persons, urged by necessity to make experiments. The scientific faculty are more indebted to the illiterate for rudimental knowledge of the virtues of most of our simple remedies, than the illiterate are to all the learned labors of the world."[60]

Having demonstrated that regular medicine played only a minor role in developing the medically valid therapies of the time, Hersey turned to his second point: regular medicine did not even merit the professional status it claimed for itself. Regular physicians made a great pretense of their erudition and knowledge, and in this way sought justification for medical schools, licensing, and all the other exclusive arrangements which they designed to limit medical practitioners. Regular physicians claim that "diseases are so numerous; their symptoms so various in different diseases, and differ so widely at different stages of the same disease, and the remedies adapt to all these peculiar situations, so diversified and numerous, that none but an adept in medical science is competent to the task." Hersey's examination of the actual practices of regular physicians belied this argument. "Are the cardinal remedies on which the faculty rely, so numerous as pretended? Take from the faculty their emetic tartar, opium, calomel, nitre, cantharides, purgatives and the lancet, and you sweep from the arena of medical combat their main dependence." The "pompous display of remedies" in the materia medica of regular medicine only disguised the real paucity of therapies utilized by regular physicians.[61]

Furthermore, Hersey continued, regular medical schools were not even concerned with practical medical knowledge. "The attention of the student is diverted from the plain investigation of philosophical truth to an endless vocabulary of Greek and Latin names. Names, and the etymology of names, are a barren substitute for solid learning and philosophical research." We are not opposed to medical science, Hersey stated, but the regular medical schools do not provide practical, useful, clinical training in medicine:

We wish to know the situation and functional uses of the bones, sinews, muscles, joints, ligaments . . . et cetera, in plain English. Not that such a knowledge is indispensible or so materially necessary to enable a man to administer medicine to the sick, but because such knowledge is agreeable and sometimes useful when certain surgical operations become necessary, and because, . . . correct information, in the whole extent of this subject, serves to enlarge the boundaries of human thought, . . . and divest men's minds of that false confidence too often reposed in a merely scientific man, who has

60 T. Hersey, "Lecture, on the Thomsonian System of Medical Practice," *Thomsonian Recorder* 3 (1834): 36.
61 *Ibid.*, pp. 36–37.

but little experience or observation to direct him at the bed-side of the sick. Such men often know very little of disease, its nature, or its remedy. What little they do know, is what others have thought, and said, and done, and they rarely think and act for themselves.[62]

It is hardly insignificant that N. S. Davis made practically the same criticism of medical education a decade later.

Hersey's arguments do not give the impression of quackery, however much this may have been present in other elements of Thomson's movement. Both Thomson and Hersey maintained that regular medicine had become a sect: doctrinaire, unempirical, divorced from practical study and the concern with useful knowledge. Medical schools had separated medicine from the patient and made scholasticism an end in itself. Hersey and Thomson did not attack what was of proven value in medicine; they attacked the false erudition and unwavering dogmatic belief of physicians in "the life draining lancet, skin-rending cantharides, the salivating, bile-vitiating, bone-rotting mercury, and drastic purgatives."[63]

Stebbins made a second argument in his attack on Thomson; he stated that Thomson's system was based on conjecture, compared to regular "physicians whose practice is governed by scientific principles." While it hardly need be observed that regular medicine was not scientific, it was also true that Thomson's principles were not conjectural. Regardless of the intellectual window-dressing of his theory, Thomson based his remedies on his own experience and the experiences of the botanical practitioners who were his mentors. In his time, compared with the remedies of the regular profession, Thomson's system was no less scientific and considerably safer. The fact that Thomson was in error in his ideas must be compared to the even more dangerous errors of the regular profession. If Thomson, who accepted the valid therapeutics of his day, was a quack, then the great majority of the regular profession were likewise quacks.

CONCLUSION

In his own way, Thomson was the leader of a popular revolt against a new era. Shrewd and provincial, a man of the people, Thomson distrusted the new men of medicine, who depended on books and lectures for their learning rather than on clinical observation and practical botany. He saw these new men as the product of a system of education which moved continually in the direction of greater formalization of knowledge, greater specialization of activity, and an increased

[62] *Ibid.*, p. 35.
[63] *Ibid.*, p. 39.

breach between the knowledge of the physician and the knowledge of the people. In this tendency he saw not only the canonization of error, but also the inability of the people to judge for themselves the validity or invalidity of the doctrines on which they were asked to risk their lives through medical treatment.[64]

Thomson, however, was an anachronism in his own movement. He sought to lead his people away from a specialized society back to a wilderness where every man could be his own physician. But others in the heart of his own movement sought to establish infirmaries, found medical schools, and to make a professional medical sect out of his system. Many of Thomson's last writings were pleas against the transformation of his movement in the image of the regular profession:

Instructing the people is the only method to prevent the world from being thronged with cripples and invalids, as it is at the present day. Infirmaries, to cure the sick, is like working on the shadow, or the effects of disease, while the substance remains. There will be more sickness makers, and, of course, more sickness made, than we can provide Infirmaries to cure. Instruct the people, and the cause is removed. Let this point be attended to, and future generations will reap the reward of our labors. . . . For unless the cause is removed, the effect will not cease. All my discoveries will be bought up and kept from the people, and the whole system revert back into the fashionable mode of doctoring. "Is there no balm in Gilead? Is there no physician there?" No, no, there is no physician; but there are doctors without number! ! ! This is the reason why the sons and daughters of this boasted free country are not healed. . . .[65]

These pleas in 1836 harkened back to a by-gone age. A new era of medical practice was upon him, and he could not hold it back.

[64] Thomson, New Guide to Health, pp. 5–6.
[65] Thomson, "To the Public," p. 389.

CHAPTER 8 THE RISE OF HOMEOPATHY

JUST AS THE regular profession was recovering from its bout with Thomsonism, it suffered an attack from another quarter. While the Thomsonian practitioners were outside the ranks of the regular profession and their clients lived on the frontier and were usually poor, the practitioners of this new movement—homeopathy—were regular physicians and their clients were the urban wealthy. Thus, homeopathy posed a much greater threat to the regular profession than did Thomsonism, and the regular profession responded with more resolute and decisive countermeasures.

THE DISCOVERY OF THE HOMEOPATHIC LAW

Homeopathy[1] was the creation of Samuel Christian Friedrich Hahnemann (1755–1843), a German physician with a formal medical education and a marked proficiency in languages, of which he spoke at least nine. After his graduation from medical school, Hahnemann did not practice medicine regularly, but rather wandered about Europe, engaged in numerous activities. Lester King has observed that in these years Hahnemann "showed sound balance and good judgment" in such matters as his advocacy of proper diet, fresh air, and exercise as modes of treatment, his espousal of hygienic measures in epidemics, and his treatment of the insane.[2]

Early in his career, Hahnemann became a strong critic of regular medicine, particularly its "imaginary and supposed material cause of disease" as manifested in the therapies used by regular physicians. He attacked the belief in a "supposed plethora, or superabundance of

[1] Following the practice of other current writers, the spelling "homeopathy" will be used throughout, even though "homoeopathy" was the preferred spelling throughout the nineteenth century. References use the original spelling.

[2] Lester S. King, *The Medical World of the Eighteenth Century* (Chicago: University of Chicago Press, 1958), pp. 159–62.

blood" which required bleeding, when "the living human body may, perhaps, never have contained one drop too much." He criticized the practice of "drawing off the imaginary principle of the disease mechanically" through blisters and cathartics, all of which "were so many attempts to remove a hostile material principle which never did and never could have existed." He was especially critical of contemporary pharmacy and pharmacology, where he found drugs prescribed without an experimental knowledge of their effects and compounded by pharmacists haphazardly and often incorrectly.[3]

In order to increase his understanding of the effects of drugs, Hahnemann began his own experiments. In 1790, according to his account:

> For the sake of experiment I took for several days four drachms of good cinchona bark twice a day; my feet, finger-tips, etc. first grew cold. I became exhausted and sleepy; then my heart began to palpitate, my pulse became hard and rapid; I had intolerable anxiety, trembling (but no rigor), prostration in all my limbs, then throbbing in the head; flushing of the cheeks, thirst, and in short all the ordinary symptoms of intermittent fever appeared one after another, but without actual febrile rigor. . . . This paroxysm lasted two to three hours each time and returned when I repeated the dose, otherwise not. On leaving off the drug I was soon quite well.[4]

This description merits some elaboration. First, Hahnemann wisely chose the most important medically valid drug then available with which to experiment—cinchona bark. He took the drug when he was healthy to ascertain its effects on a healthy person, and he accurately described the effects of moderate doses of cinchona. Using the widely accepted theory that "the totality of the symptoms alone constitutes the disease," Hahnemann reasoned that because cinchona had given him all of the symptoms of malaria, it had given him, a healthy man, malaria. Then, using another widely accepted theory that "the physician has only to remove the totality of the symptoms, and he has cured the entire disease," he reached a logical conclusion.[5] It is a fact that cinchona cures malaria in a sick person (an error, as cinchona only relieves the symptoms of malaria), and it is also a fact that cinchona caused malaria in a healthy person, himself. Therefore, what causes an illness in a healthy person will cure the same illness in a sick person. He called this the "law" of *similia similibus curantur*—usually

[3] Samuel Hahnemann, *Organon of Homoeopathic Medicine* (New York: William Radde, 1849), 3rd American edition, pp. 29, 31, 38; King, *Medical World of the Eighteenth Century*, p. 162.
[4] *Ibid.*, p. 164.
[5] Hahnemann, *Organon*, p. 101.

translated like is cured by like—and the system based on that law as homeopathy.

Hahnemann believed that his discovery had major implications for medical practice. Physicians should test a large number of different drugs on healthy persons and have the subjects record their symptoms. Then, to treat a sick person, according to Hahnemann, "Of all those medicines, that one whose symptoms bear the greatest resemblance to the totality of those which characterize any particular natural disease, ought to be the most appropriate and certain homeopathic remedy that can be employed; it is the specific remedy in this case of disease."[6] Simply give the patient the medicine which, when tested in a healthy person, induces symptoms that resemble most closely the symptoms of the sick person.

Hahnemann also laid down two apparently arbitrary dicta regarding drug action. The first one was: "the symptoms, modifications, and changes of the health that are visible during the action of the medicine, depend upon that substance alone, and ought to be noted down as properly belonging to it, if even similar symptoms, occurring spontaneously, should have been experienced a *long time before* by the person on whom the experiment is made."[7] In other words, literally everything that happened to a person after he took a drug was due to the action of that drug alone. Hahnemann's second dictum concerned the length of time over which a single dose of a drug was effective:

One dose of a suitable homeopathic remedy, if its development be sufficiently subtle, gradually completes all the beneficial effects which, from its nature, it is capable of producing, and provided its operation be undisturbed, sometimes in the space of forty, fifty, to one hundred days. This, however, is seldom the case; and it depends upon the physician as well as upon the patient, whether these periods may not be abridged to the extent of one-half, one-fourth or to even a shorter time, and thus a more speedy cure effected.[8]

Thus it would appear that Hahnemann expected the action of a single dose of a drug to last from about ten to one hundred days.

The process of testing the effects of drugs, which came to be known as "provings," constituted one of the most debated points of homeopathic medicine. Each prover took designated doses of a drug, and recorded every symptom he thought interesting—twitches of the toe, feeling of sleepiness after dinner, eye blinks—in whatever fashion he desired and for as long as he thought useful—often as much as two

6 *Ibid.*, p. 171.
7 *Ibid.*, p. 166.
8 *Ibid.*, pp. 204–5.

months. These provings were frequently published in homeopathic journals and in a number of books. Because the provings were carried out in so unsystematic a manner, many homeopathic physicians were critical of them. One said of *Jahr's Manual*, the most famous of the books of provings, "Many symptoms are so trivial in their character, that they appear more like the imaginations of a healthy man expectantly watching his own organism, than the positive and uniform operations of a drug. Many of them were probably accidental."[9] Consequently, there were periodic calls for "reproving" all the homeopathic drugs.

After making one empirical finding, performing some deductions, and stating a number of wholly arbitrary rules about drug action, Hahnemann then attacked another question: what is the optimum homeopathic dose of any drug? Hahnemann's own experiments led him to some general conclusions. He soon discovered that large doses were very undesirable in ascertaining the effects of drugs: "If the dose be excessive, there will not only be several re-actions visible among the symptoms, but yet more, the primitive effects will manifest themselves in a manner so precipitate, violent, and confused, that it will be impossible to make any correct observation."[10] This overabundance of symptoms, as well as the severity of the symptoms, led him to believe that large doses disguised the true essence of the effects of any drug. If the dose were reduced, the superfluous symptoms would be eliminated. The more Hahnemann experimented with the proper homeopathic dose, the smaller the dose he recommended. By the time he was an old man, he believed that extremely small doses had to be used. He also discovered the principle of "dynamization"—shaking a solution of a drug increases its medicinal powers. He ultimately recommended the following means of making the optimum preparation of a drug, using very small doses and a certain number of shakes:

If two drops of a mixture of equal parts of alcohol and the recent juice of any medicinal plant . . . be diluted with ninety-eight drops of alcohol . . . and the whole twice shaken together, the medicine becomes exalted in energy . . . to the first development of power, or, as it may be denominated, the first potence. The process is to be continued through twenty-nine additional vials, each of equal capacity with the first, and each containing ninety-nine drops of spirits of wine; so that every successive vial, after the first, being furnished with one drop from the vial or dilution immediately preceding, (which had just been twice shaken,) is, in its turn, to be shaken twice. . . . These manipulations are to be conducted thus through all the vials, from the

9 William H. Holcombe, *The Scientific Basis of Homoeopathy* (Cincinnati: Derby, 1852), p. 75.

10 Hahnemann, *Organon*, p. 166.

first up to the thirtieth or decillionth development of power, . . . which is the one in most general use.[11]

It is important to realize that only one drop of the juice of the medicinal plant (in its original concentration) was used in this whole process. After the first dilution, the one drop of the plant was diluted to 1/100 of its original strength; after the second, to 1/10,000 of its original strength; after the third to 1/1,000,000 of its original strength. This constituted the *third* dilution; Hahnemann recommended the *thirtieth* dilution.

The resulting medicine could be administered in either of two ways, according to Hahnemann. A globule of sugar the size of a mustard seed could be moistened with the thirtieth dilution of the liquid and taken internally. Or, where the patient was "very weak and irritable, once smelling of [it] . . . is safer and more serviceable than when it is taken in substance." A globule used for smelling "retains its full power for this purpose undiminished for at least eighteen to twenty years (so far as goes my own experience), even though the vial should have been opened in the mean time a thousand times, provided it is only protected from heat and sunlight."[12]

These views on dosage were those of Hahnemann's later years. In his earlier years Hahnemann usually recommended doses of what came to be called the "low dilutions"—usually under the fifth, and often under the third. At all times in his career, he was extremely strict about not exceeding the dose, since "if *too strong* a dose of a remedy, that is even entirely homeopathic, be given, it will infallibly injure the patient."[13]

Hahnemann's more theoretical discussions are not of equivalent concern for this study for various reasons. He himself was unsure of the reason for the validity of the law of *similia similibus curantur*, and entitled his examination of this question: "Intimation how a homeopathic cure is probably effected." In his old age, Hahnemann developed a new theory in which he introduced the concept of "psora," a kind of itchy skin eruption, as the basic cause of all chronic diseases. Few of his followers accepted this theory, and it was in no way a part of his original system.[14]

Hahnemann's system extended beyond his theory of drug action.

[11] *Ibid.*, p. 217. Although Hahnemann here clearly defined a dilution as equivalent to a potence, elsewhere he defined a potence as every third dilution— twelve dilutions comprising only four degrees of potency.

[12] *Ibid.*, pp. 208–9; "Hahnemann," *Eclectic Medical Journal* 49 (1889): 236.

[13] Hahnemann, *Organon*, p. 219.

[14] *Ibid.*, p. 171; King, *Medical World of the Eighteenth Century*, pp. 184–85.

Because of his concern with the patient's symptoms, he insisted that physicians obtain an extremely detailed history of the patient's illness, not only from the patient himself, but from others who would be able to add information. He also taught that homeopaths should exercise extreme care in the purity and preparation of their drugs and avoid the use of compounds for single drugs given independently. These emphases were relatively novel at the time.[15]

Hahnemann expected that regular physicians would not greet his system enthusiastically. He called them the "allopathic" school because they used remedies whose action was opposite to the symptoms caused by the illness, and described their practice by the maxim *contraria contrariis*. In order to demonstrate the superiority of homeopathy over allopathy, Hahnemann pointed not only to his experiences with cinchona, but also to the efficacy of cowpox vaccine. He described numerous instances of medical treatment in classical literature to demonstrate that his discovery was known to writers of antiquity and was essentially rediscovered by him.[16] He also recognized that his doses would be considered ludicrous by physicians accustomed to heroic therapy and suggested:

If the allopathist, in essaying the homeopathic method, cannot resolve upon administering doses that are so feeble and attenuated, only let him ask himself what risk he ventures by doing so . . . a dose that appears to him like nothing, could have no worse results than that of producing no effect at all, which is at least far more innocent than the effects resulting from the strong doses of allopathic medicines.[17]

Basically, Hahnemann argued that skeptical regular physicians should not concern themselves with the logic of homeopathy, but rather look at the results. Homeopathic doses were effective in curing disease, he claimed, which was sufficient reason for their use.

Hahnemann's personal success as a practitioner came after 1835 when, at the age of 80, he married and moved to Paris. There he became fashionable among the upper class and acquired wealth and fame. He died in 1843.[18]

In his eccentric fashion, Hahnemann made one of the great discoveries of his time: he established that, given the existing state of medical knowledge, the absence of therapy was vastly superior to heroic therapy. The fundamental soundness of his perception is clearly manifested in the positive and negative hygienic and therapeutic measures

15 *Ibid.*, p. 189; Holcombe, *Scientific Basis of Homoeopathy*, p. 24.
16 Hahnemann, *Organon*, pp. 125, 119.
17 *Ibid.*, p. 222.
18 King, *Medical World of the Eighteenth Century*, pp. 177–78.

that he advocated: he accepted the medically valid therapies of his time, and he recommended the use of fresh air, bed rest, proper diet, sunshine, public hygiene, and numerous other beneficial measures at a time when many other physicians considered them of no value. He opposed bloodletting, blisters, large doses of drugs, and the whole host of heroic therapy. Unfortunately, Hahnemann misinterpreted his great discovery and attributed his success not to drugless therapy, but rather to his homeopathic doses. Nevertheless, Hahnemann's total therapeutic system was a marked advance over the heroic therapy of his contemporaries.

HOMEOPATHY IN AMERICAN MEDICAL PRACTICE

Homeopathy was brought to America about 1825 by a German physician, Hans Gram, who settled in New York City. The most important early American homeopath was Constantine Hering, a student of Hahnemann's who immigrated to America with a number of his colleagues a decade later.[19] By mid-century, homeopathy had become a significant part of American medicine.

Obviously, there was nothing in homeopathy to appeal directly to Americans the way Thomsonism did. Thomsonism had come directly and avowedly out of an American botanical tradition that was over two hundred years old by the middle of the nineteenth century and still viable and influential. Homeopathy, a rationalistic, dogmatic medical theory, had no roots in American medical practice, and therefore could hardly draw on American traditions. To understand the growth of homeopathy, one has to know something more about popular reaction to regular medicine in the second quarter of the nineteenth century.

THE STATE OF PUBLIC OPINION

It has already been observed that medical schools standardized regular medicine into a sect characterized by a system of distinctive but medically invalid therapy. The ensuing public dissatisfaction with this mode of therapy provided ample opportunity for its numerous critics to make themselves heard. Thomsonism was one major manifestation of public opposition to regular medicine, but other forms of protest also occurred.

The single most important long-run alternative to regular medicine was the patent-medicine industry. This industry grew rapidly in the early nineteenth century when inexpensive newspapers developed

---

[19] Thomas Lindsley Bradford, "Homoeopathy in New York," in William Harvey King, ed., *History of Homoeopathy* (New York: Lewis, 1905), 1: 44–45.

a mass circulation and provided a vehicle for the promulgation of patent medicines. Nostrum makers advertised that there was no mercury in their preparations and promised mild medication instead of the harsh therapies of the regular physicians. While the inexpensiveness of patent medicines was undoubtedly the major reason for their popularity, their therapeutic philosophy was a clear alternative to regular medicine.[20]

Hostility to regular medicine was also a characteristic of a number of social movements of the period that were less significant in terms of popular appeal than Thomsonism. One of the most popular of these was Sylvester Graham's popular health movement, which prospered in the 1830's. Graham opposed drugging generally and stressed exercise, frequent bathing, and temperance in food and drink. According to Shryock, he believed that "right living was a more certain means to health than was a resort to doctors and drugs." Graham's movement eventually merged with another movement of transient popular appeal, hydropathy (which, for a brief time, was thought to be a serious rival to Thomsonism), advocating water cures, Turkish baths, the use of wet sheets, etc. Shryock concluded from his study of these movements that their opposition to drugging and emphasis on personal hygiene and prevention of illness made a lasting contribution to medicine, which was ultimately accepted by the regular profession. Chronothermalism, another system which opposed bloodletting, became popular in the 1840's. A book describing its theory sold through thirteen editions, and a short-lived medical school was founded in Philadelphia to teach its doctrines.[21]

These and numerous other movements flourished and died, all different in doctrine and spirit, some organized and some unorganized, some ephemeral and some long-lived, all separate and usually unwilling to merge, all having only one thing in common—an unwavering hostility to the regular medical practice of the period.

THE APPEAL OF HOMEOPATHY

These social movements hostile to regular medicine all appealed primarily to the rural or lower-income segments of the population. Thomsonism attracted supporters primarily from rural and frontier

[20] James Harvey Young, "American Medical Quackery in the Age of the Common Man," *Mississippi Valley Historical Review* 47 (1961): 579–93; for a detailed history of the major nostrums, see James Harvey Young, *The Toadstool Millionaires* (Princeton, N.J.: Princeton University Press, 1961).

[21] Richard H. Shryock, "Sylvester Graham and the Popular Health Movement," *Mississippi Valley Historical Review* 18 (1931): 172–83; Charles S. Bryan, "Dr. Samuel Dickson and the Spirit of Chrono-Thermalism," *Bulletin of the History of Medicine* 42 (1968): 31–32.

areas. Grahamism and other comparable movements appealed to an urban working and lower-middle class population. None of these movements was able to attract many supporters from the urban middle or upper classes.

Homeopathy, on the other hand, appealed primarily to those urban middle and upper class persons who were seeking an alternative to regular medicine.[22] It was able to do so for two major reasons. First, unlike its competitors, homeopathy was extremely fashionable among the European nobility and upper classes, whose tastes were often copied by affluent Americans. Second, the leaders of Thomsonism and virtually all the other movements opposing regular medicine were often uneducated laymen. Patients who could afford to pay for the best in medical care would hardly be attracted to any movement with this kind of leadership. Homeopathy was devised by a physician and the early American homeopaths were all well educated and cultured physicians. The homeopathic physicians who wrote articles in the first important American homeopathic journal, the *Homeopathic Examiner*, were conversant with the writings of European homeopaths in the original French and German and manifested an erudition rarely found in the regular medical journals of the period. Many of them were also "persons of the highest respectability and moral worth," according to the editor of the *Boston Medical and Surgical Journal*.[23]

Conversely, the social position of homeopathy's clientele greatly influenced the kinds of American physicians who became homeopaths. The anonymous author of an article in the *Boston Medical and Surgical Journal* in 1844 suggested several of the reasons why American physicians adopted homeopathy. He placed great emphasis on the social class of its clientele:

Many of the learned, accomplished, and, what is more to the purpose, the *wealthy*, have an unconquerable aversion to taking nauseous and bitter medicines, such as the "regular physicians" employ in their pills, powders and potions; while such are very willing to place upon the tongue a pellet of sugar of milk every day, or smell a phial occasionally, containing these precious treasures. Hence a homeopathist is preferred by such, and by this craft has great gains. . . . the popular prejudice against bleeding, calomel, and mineral medicines generally, has become very prevalent and influential. It is in vain to say that it has originated in the abuse of these valuable remedies, for, whether well or ill founded, the prejudice exists. . . .[24]

22 "Hahnemann on Chronic Diseases," *New York Journal of Medicine* 6 (1846): 101.

23 "Homoeopathic Journal," *Boston Medical and Surgical Journal* 40 (1849): 266.

24 R., "Apology for Becoming an Homoeopathic Doctor," *Boston Medical and Surgical Journal* 30 (1844): 218.

He also observed that the relatively small number of homeopaths made it easier for a homeopath to achieve success:

In the "regular practice," a young doctor must often become gray-headed before he can attract attention, or inspire confidence in the public. . . . Not so, however, if he will only become a homeopathist, for however young and inexperienced, however obscure and unnoticed before, he will soon be summoned to "cure incurable cases," which have been justly decided to be such, by the regular fraternity, and he will find himself in families who else had never heard of him, and thus reap a golden harvest. And though the patient dies, because his potenzes come too late, yet his fame as a miracle-monger is not built upon his cures, but upon the mysticism of homeopathy.[25]

Last, he argued that a homeopath need not restrict himself to his new-found therapeutic system:

A young physician, or one without practice, has everything to gain, and nothing to lose, by turning homeopathist, for he will be careful not to take down his sign, much less substitute for his title "Doctor," that of a "practitioner of homeopathy." Hence strangers and casual patients are caught as before, while all he gains by his conversion is superadded to this emolument. Nor is he obliged to betray his art to everybody, and hence if he finds that his patient has been misled by his sign to mistake him for a "regular physician," he can fall back upon "allopathy," and treat him *secundum artem*.[26]

Other physicians became homeopaths because they shared the popular dissatisfaction with the state of regular medicine and sought an alternative. One Mississippi homeopath wrote that he began practice as a regular physician, and contracted yellow fever during the 1837 epidemic. He said, "I took a little calomel and quinine for two days, then abandoned medicines and let nature, untrammeled, do her own work. In a few days I was convalescent. Although I continued practice my faith in drugging was terribly shaken." In 1846 he became a homeopath. In New Orleans, homeopathy was popular among the many physicians descended from the early French population. These physicians had always avoided heroic therapy and found in homeopathy a theoretical justification for that practice.[27]

EARLY HOMEOPATHIC PHYSICIANS

The initial reaction of American physicians to homeopathy was skeptical, but not wholly unfavorable. The editors of the *Boston*

---

25 *Ibid.*, p. 217.

26 *Ibid.*

27 Thomas Lindsley Bradford, "Homoeopathy in Mississippi," in King, *History of Homoeopathy*, 1: 395; John Duffy, ed., *The Rudolph Matas History of Medicine in Louisiana* (n.p.: Louisiana State University Press, 1962), II: 36–37.

Medical and Surgical Journal stated in 1840, on receiving a copy of a homeopathic journal:

We are open to conviction, and to show that we entertain no hostility to homeopathia or the scientific followers of Hahnemann, every thing found in the [Homeopathic] Examiner, which can be of interest or utility to the profession at large, will be transferred to the pages of our Journal.[28]

Regular physicians in the large urban centers were the first American practitioners attracted to homeopathy. They organized themselves and attracted many other physicians to their ranks. For example, the Massachusetts Homeopathic Fraternity, established in 1839 with four members, had over twenty by 1843. All of the members were regularly educated physicians who were also members of the Massachusetts Medical Society. That they considered themselves regular physicians was made evident by one of their members in 1843:

In the pursuit of homeopathy . . . they fully and emphatically disclaim all fellowship or sympathy with those who are endeavoring to introduce or extend it by the tricks and arts of irregular practitioners or reckless imposters; and *particularly* such as have been, for the last year or more, advertising and puffing themselves in the newspapers, as "*Homeopathic Physicians*," offering for sale "homeopathic specifics" for all manner of diseases, and striving to impose on the uninformed and credulous, for homeopathy, that which is entirely adverse to its principles and practice.[29]

New York City was the major center of homeopathy in America. Some New York physicians became homeopaths in the 1830's, and in 1835, they and a number of regular physicians gained control of the Medical Society of the County of New York, the city's leading medical society, for a year. Many of the New York homeopaths were among the better-educated physicians of the city. Four of the original eighteen members of the New York Medical and Surgical Society, a small elite organization of young physicians, became homeopaths in the five years after its founding in 1836. The New York homeopaths, like those in Boston, considered themselves regular physicians. The president of the New York Homeopathic Physicians' Society stated in 1846 that every member of the society was a licensed physician and was required "to possess as thorough knowledge of every branch of medical science as the most respectable portion of his Allopathic brethren."[30]

[28] "The Homoeopathic Examiner," *Boston Medical and Surgical Journal* 22 (1840): 82.
[29] J. F. F., "Massachusetts Homoeopathic Fraternity," *Boston Medical and Surgical Journal* 29 (1843): 259.
[30] Daniel H. Calhoun, *Professional Lives in America* (Cambridge, Mass.: Harvard University Press, 1965), p. 39; Philip Van Ingen, *A Brief Account of the First One Hundred Years of the New York Medical and Surgical Society* (n.p., 1946), pp. 22–23; B. F. Joslin, "Address before the New York Homoeopathic Physician's Society," *American Journal of Homoeopathy* 1 (1846): 45.

American homeopaths rapidly developed a spectrum of divergent views on homeopathic therapeutics. A reviewer in the *New York Journal of Medicine*, a regular medical journal, observed in 1846 that "there are as wide differences of opinion among [homeopaths], both in relation to theory, and the *modus operandi* of remedial agents, as there is among allopathic physicians, and quite as great differences in modes of practice." On one side, many homeopaths did not consider homeopathy and regular medicine to be mutually exclusive, but rather believed them to be complementary. John F. Gray, one of the most eminent early American homeopaths, wrote in 1840 that in both homeopathy and regular medicine "there is certainly much error, but assuredly also a great deal of truth, and the sooner a catholic eclecticism inspires both parties, the better for mankind at large and for the true honor of the medical profession." On the other side, Hahnemann's dedicated supporters adopted his doctrines as articles of faith. One of these homeopaths stated that "those who undertake the study of homeopathy, must throw all their previous acquired knowledge overboard."[31]

The leaders of homeopathy were almost all arrayed on the more tolerant side of the question. They were often critical of Hahnemann himself, although they accepted the validity of the law of similars. One prominent homeopath said of Hahnemann's *Organon*, the veritable bible of homeopathy, "I was so dissatisfied with the loose statements, the hasty inferences, and the dogmatism . . . that I dropped it at about the 200th page, and have never finished its perusal."[32] Even Constantine Hering criticized Hahnemann openly. In his preface to an American edition of Hahnemann's works, he asserted that "Hahnemann's conception of the action of the homeopathic drug was altogether vague, incomplete and even erroneous." Elsewhere, in his preface to the *Organon*, he differentiated the law of similars from Hahnemann's theories and said, "since my first acquaintance with homeopathy, (in the year 1821), down to the present day, I have never yet accepted a single theory in the *Organon* as it is there promulgated. I feel no aversion to acknowledge this even to the venerable sage himself."[33] Hering also argued that a basic core of unity existed within the movement, regardless of controversy over what he considered details. He stated in his preface to the 1849 edition of the *Organon*:

[31] [John F. Gray], "Duty of Physicians of Either School to Study both Systems," *Homoeopathic Examiner* 1 (1840): 35 (the identity of the author is revealed in J. C. Peters, "To John F. Gray," *Homoeopathic Examiner* 3 (1843): 370); "Hahnemann on Chronic Diseases," p. 102.

[32] Holcombe, *Scientific Basis of Homoeopathy*, p. 269.

[33] "Hahnemann on Chronic Diseases," p. 104; Constantine Hering, "Preface to the First American Edition," in Hahnemann, *Organon*, p. 17.

[Among homeopaths] it is quite natural that different opinions should
be entertained and promulgated, and even that partisan conflicts should
arise. But against the stubborn adherents of the old-school doctrines, these
various parties stand united as the varied wings of one common army.

All Homeopathic physicians are united under the banner of the great
law of cure, *similia similibus curantur*, however they may differ in regard to
the theoretical explanation of that law, or the extent to which it may be
applied.

All Homeopathic physicians also acknowledge that provings upon the
healthy are indispensable in ascertaining the unknown curative powers of
drugs.

And finally: all Homeopaths concur in giving but one medicine at a
time, never mixing different drugs together under the absurd expectation
that each will act according to their dictum. This is the glorious tri-colour
of our school. . . .

The varied diversities among ourselves serve only to develop and advance our principles. What important influence can it exert, whether a
Homeopath adopts the theoretical opinions of Hahnemann or not, so long
as he holds fast the practical rules of the master, and the Materia Medica
of our school? What influence can it have, whether a physician adopt or
reject the Psora-theory, so long as he always selects the most similar medicine possible? Even in the larger or smaller doses, . . . allowing there is a
great difference between them according to the testimony of the friends of
each, yet all this difference dwindles into insignificance, when we compare
the results of Homeopathic with that of common Allopathic practice. . . .
There will always be a large number of [homeopathic] physicians who either
do not understand, or will not learn, how to select for each particular case
the one only proper medicine, and such will always find it most comfortable
to employ massive doses. . . .[34]

Despite Hering's attempt to minimize the differences over the size
of the dose to be used in homeopathic prescriptions, this question had
already become the great barrier to harmony among homeopaths, a
position it maintained throughout homeopathy's existence in America.
One group, the high-dilutionists, far exceeded Hahnemann's dilutions
and used doses of drugs in reductions up to the two-thousandth dilution. The other group, the low-dilutionists, used much less diluted
doses, and some even denied that homeopathy was "indissolubly bound
up in the doctrine of infinitesimal doses" at all. In a number of practical instances, however, the question of dosage was resolved empirically. In discussing the treatment of malaria, for example, one homeopath placed quinine as the most useful drug. He criticized the "massive doses" of the regular physicians as being too large (an accurate
observation), but said that European homeopaths had found that
homeopathic dilutions were too small, and he recommended a mod-

[34] Constantine Hering, "Some Remarks on the Third American Edition of
Hahnemann's Organon," in Hahnemann, *Organon*, pp. 3–4.

erate but non-homeopathic dose that was well suited to the needs of practicing physicians.[35]

The establishment of homeopathic medical schools and other institutions will be described in Chapter 12. Here it need only be observed that the wealth and influence of homeopathy's clientele assured it a degree of success and longevity unattainable by the other social movements, and made it a far greater threat to the regular profession.

THE REACTION OF REGULAR PHYSICIANS TO HOMEOPATHIC PHYSICIANS

Most regular physcans regarded their homeopathic colleagues first with skepticism, then with incredulity, and finally with bitter hostility. They considered many homeopaths to be opportunists who practiced both homeopathy and regular medicine, not from conviction, but "according to order, on the whims and caprice of their medical patrons."[36] They found the dedicated homeopaths wholly incomprehensible. The reviewer of Hahnemann's book maintained:

We hold that it is both difficult and useless to reason with the enthusiastic and credulous believers in any novel system, whether of medicine, politics, or religion . . . ; that those, who are, for the most part, ignorant of the ordinary laws which regulate the course of diseases, should mistake the recuperative efforts of nature, or the influence of a regulated diet, for the effect of their remedies, is what might naturally be expected; but the man who will entirely overlook these influences, and attribute to the 2000th potence of a drug, or the 30th, such favorable changes as may occur during its administration, is better fitted for a lunatic hospital than the practice of the healing art. It is a remarkable fact, that, so far as we know, no homeopathic writer or practitioner gives Nature any credit for cures effected under this system.[37]

This statement summarizes the regular physicians' two basic objections to homeopathy: (1) that the doses prescribed by homeopaths were too small to have any physiological effect whatever; and (2) that the cures which homeopaths attributed to their drugs were actually brought about by the "recuperative efforts of nature." The most interesting aspect of the criticism of the size of the dose was the almost complete absence of any reference to the law of similars on which it was based. Homeopaths themselves disputed the size of the dose and most regarded it as secondary. The primary characteristic of homeo-

35 H., "To the Sen'r Editor of the Homoeopathic Examiner," *Homoeopathic Examiner*, n.s. 1 (1845): 149; "Intermittent Fever," *Homoeopathic Examiner* 1 (1840): 416.

36 "Homoeopathy Considered Quackery in Philadelphia," *Boston Medical and Surgical Journal* 28 (1843): 303.

37 "Hahnemann on Chronic Diseases," p. 101.

pathic medicine was the law of *similia similibus curantur*, and if homeopathy was to be disproven, regular physicians had to demonstrate that this so-called law was invalid. Because regular physicians used the same clinical methodology of administering a therapy and watching for the effects on the patient as did the homeopaths, they were unable to verify or disprove it or any other scientific theory. Furthermore, regular physicians were the continual victims of their own clinical methodology to as great a degree as the homeopaths, and in such a situation neither system could attain scientific status. Regular physicians did admit that homeopathy had produced a surprisingly large number of successful treatments. They attributed this success to the effects of nature. Oliver Wendell Holmes, for example, said in 1861: "Homeopathy has taught us a lesson of the healing faculty of Nature which was needed." This criticism was two-edged, however. If nature cured the homeopath's patients, who cured the regular physician's patients? One homeopath said in reply to a regular physician, "if he says that our . . . cases got well without medicine, why may we not just as logically say that his . . . got well in spite of his medicine?"[38] These attacks on homeopathy were much like those on Thomsonism: they attacked the other sect, but were unable to defend their own.

To understand the actual validity of the regular physician's criticisms of homeopathic medicine, it is necessary to examine the relationship of homeopathic medicine to regular medicine. It has been shown above that both accepted cinchona bark and quinine in malaria, both accepted cowpox vaccination for smallpox, and both accepted surgery, for Hahnemann had declared that his system could cure all diseases "except such as require actual manual surgical interference."[39] Homeopaths and regular physicians alike accepted anatomy, physiology, and all of the other basic medical sciences, as evidenced by the similarities of the curricula of homeopathic and regular medical schools in this regard. The issue between the two rested solely with the materia medica. The homeopaths attacked the regular physicians' use of bloodletting, calomel, blisters, poisons, and the rest of heroic medicine as medically invalid, based on fallacious and speculative reasoning, and unsuccessful in treating disease. The regular physicians accused the

---

[38] Oliver Wendell Holmes, in his famous criticism of homeopathy, did attack the principle of *similia*, but the extent of his efforts was to argue that the principle was valid only in some situations and to show that some of the illustrations which Hahnemann drew from antiquity were erroneous and did not illustrate the principle. His major attack was on the size of the dose. Oliver Wendell Holmes, *Medical Essays, 1842–1882* (Boston: Houghton Mifflin, 1891), pp. 51–52, 64–65; Holcombe, *Scientific Basis of Homoeopathy*, p. 180.

[39] "Hahnemann," *Eclectic Medical Journal* 49 (1889): 236.

homeopaths of chicanery in administering drugs which could have no possible therapeutic effect of any kind. From the point of view of the patient's well-being, it is not difficult to conclude which was the superior system.

Jacob Bigelow, one of the truly great regular physicians of the early nineteenth century, recognized the real issue, although his comments have never received the attention they merited:

The broadest division which has been recognized for centuries in the treatment of disease, is that which resolves the whole subject into the active and the expectant modes of practice. The first employs various interfering agencies in the management of the sick,—the last waits more on the unassisted course of nature,—and both have long had their exclusive advocates.

To the last of these divisions Homeopathy really, though not avowedly belongs. Its character is, that while in reality it waits on the natural course of events, it commends itself to the ignorant and credulous by a professed introduction into the body of inappreciable quantities of medicinal substances. Now the nugatory effect of such quantities is demonstrated by the fact, that in civilized life every person is exposed to the daily reception, in the form of solution, dust or vapor, of homeopathic quantities of almost every common substance known in nature and art, without any appreciable consequences being found to follow. . . .

But it is not only to expectant medicine, in the form of its counterfeit, homeopathy, that the censure of prejudice and credulity is to be attached. The opposite system of active practice, carried to the extreme usually called heroic, is alike chargeable with evil to the patients, whenever it becomes the absorbing and exclusive course of the practitioner. Physicians are too often led to exaggerate the usefulness of the doctrines in which they have been educated, and especially of those by the exercise of which they obtain their daily bread. In such cases habit gets the ascendency over enlightened judgment, and the man of routine, or of narrow views, asks himself, from day to day, what drug or what appliance he shall next resort to, instead of asking the more important question, whether any drug or any appliance is called for, or is properly admissible in the case. . . .

I believe that much of the medical imposition of the present day is sustained in places where practice has previously been over-heroic, and because mankind are gratified to find that they and their families can get well without the lancet, the vomit and the blister, indiscriminantly applied; and because the adroit charlatan transfers the salutary influences of time and nature, to the credit of his own less disagreeable inflictions.[40]

Thus Bigelow—quite courageously—said there were two sects within medicine, the homeopathic and the regular, each with its dogmas, each with its fallacies, each placing doctrinal consistency over scientific considerations.

This is why the regular profession was forced to react so strongly

[40] Jacob Bigelow, *Nature in Disease* (Boston: Ticknor and Fields, 1854), pp. 103–6, 129.

to homeopathy, for homeopathy constituted the first attack on heroic therapy by physicians, rather than by outsiders. Regular physicians themselves recognized this. The reviewer of the Hahnemann book stated:

The mischief which has thus been done to our profession, by destroying the confidence once justly reposed in it by the public [because homeopaths attributed their failures to "former allopathic treatment"], and that, too, by men bound by the same code of honor, and of ethics (for, nominally, they are *of us*, if not *with us*), can neither be estimated nor repaired, at least in our generation. Can these men not see that this is a suicidal policy; that they are thus wielding a two-edged sword, which is as likely to wound them as us? We are told, on good authority, that "a house divided against itself, cannot stand;" neither can a profession. The warfare that has been waging by the two wings of the grand army has thrown the main body into confusion, and the public has sided with one or the other as humor, interest, chance, mental organization, or other circumstances dictated.[41]

Another physician, Charles B. Coventry, called by the editors of the *New York Journal of Medicine*, "one of the most distinguished professors and practitioners in our country," wrote:

Until within a few years, there was at least an apparent line of demarcation between the educated physician and the empiric; true, the quack denounced the regular profession, and the profession denounced the quack; but it was very rare indeed for a man who had been regularly educated in the profession and obtained license, however much quackery he might practice, to join the empiric in decrying the profession. But Hahnemann, an educated physician, came out and denounced the profession to which he belonged, and in which he had been educated, as knaves, as fools, and as murderers; his followers imitated his example, and whilst professing to be educated physicians (many of them having obtained licenses,) and members of medical societies, they were endorsing, retailing, and repeating all the abuse heaped upon the profession by their master. . . . Is it surprising that community should lose confidence in a profession so vilified and abused by its own members; and is it not certain that unless something can be done to arrest it, the profession will be irretrievably ruined.[42]

Regular physicians could have responded to this challenge from within their ranks in two ways. On the one hand, they could have tried to minimize the therapeutic differences between homeopathy and regular medicine by incorporating some elements of homeopathy into regular medicine. Apparently, many homeopaths hoped for this course of action, as exemplified by an editorial in the *American Journal of Homeopathy* in 1846 that criticized homeopaths who advertised them-

41 "Hahnemann on Chronic Diseases," p. 102.
42 C[harles] B. C[oventry], "Medical Convention," *New York Journal of Medicine* 8 (1847): 371–72.

selves in newspapers and on their signs as "homeopathic physicians." It considered the term to be a violation of medical ethics and looked "to the time when it will not be necessary to use the terms, homeopathy, or allopathy." On the other hand, regular physicians could have denounced homeopathy as a threat to the very existence of regular medicine and endeavored to destroy it by ostracism, legal action, and all other means available. The fact that the regular profession determined to pursue this latter course is further evidence of its basically sectarian nature. Homeopathy did not attack the science in regular medicine; it attacked only the sect in regular medicine. The regular profession could have tolerated an attack on medical science because it could demonstrate the validity of medical science. The sectarian aspects of regular medicine, however, had to be taken on faith, because there was no basic demonstrable validity to these practices. For this reason, the homeopathic heretics—like heretics of any religious sect—had to be cast out, if the sect's doctrinal purity was to be maintained.[43]

Thus, early in the 1840's, some regular physicians took the first steps to purge their ranks of homeopaths. In 1843, the Philadelphia Medical Society expelled all homeopathic physicians, a position with which the influential *Boston Medical and Surgical Journal* agreed. The *Journal*, however, criticized a case in which an upstate New York county medical society prosecuted a homeopath for illegal practice. The jury convicted the homeopath, fined him three-fourths of a cent, and contributed their own fees for jury duty to the Homeopathic Society. The *Journal* called the action of the regular society "the veriest piece of would-be despotism that has been exhibited for a long while," and observed that "the interference of a Medical Society, in the little business of silencing a single obscure dealer in pellicles will do much towards giving eclat to the system, ridiculous as it is."[44]

In New York City, regular physicians pursued a different course. Unable to throw the homeopaths out of the county society because of the provisions of its act of incorporation, they formed their own private medical society, the New York Academy of Medicine, in 1847. A leader of the academy asserted at one of its first meetings that the organization "would not admit irregular men. . . . Any swerving from the path of professional rectitude will not be recognized by us of the

[43] "Homoeopathy," *New York Journal of Medicine* 7 (1846): 264. Many homeopathic and botanical practitioners consistently used the analogy of religious sects in defending themselves. For example, see a history of the major botanical sects by one of their members: Alexander Wilder, *History of Medicine* (New Sharon, Me.: 1901).

[44] "Homoeopathy Considered Quackery," pp. 303–4; "Law vs. Homoeopathy," *Boston Medical and Surgical Journal* 29 (1843): 86.

old school." In a decade, the academy had become the largest medical society in the city, an achievement which one of its leaders attributed to its membership policy.[45]

In these and in other ways too numerous to mention, regular physicians drove homeopaths out of the regular societies, persecuted them in the courts, and otherwise endeavored to destroy homeopathy or at least separate it from regular medicine.

HOMEOPATHY AND THE AMERICAN MEDICAL ASSOCIATION

The problem of homeopathy was a major factor in the founding of the American Medical Association and was one reason for its survival and success. Coventry, like many other regular physicians, argued that a national medical society would aid in ostracizing homeopaths: "The first great step then should be to draw the line of demarcation between those who are of the profession and those who are not . . . [through] the formation of a national association. . . . Let a system of medical ethics be established by the national association, and signed by every member. . . ." This attitude complemented the motives of the physicians concerned with medical education. Men like Coventry, a medical school professor, who were opposed to any regulation of medical schools, were willing to join the AMA to rid the profession of homeopaths; others, like Davis, who never even referred to homeopaths in his arguments for the AMA, wanted the AMA to regulate medical schools and restore the medical societies. In this way, a coalition was formed between these two groups that was temporarily strong enough to overcome their mutual antagonism and permit the establishment of the AMA.[46]

HOMEOPATHY AND THE AMA CODE OF ETHICS

The major vehicle in the AMA for dealing with the homeopaths was the code of ethics established in 1847. This document devoted several important sections to relations with "irregular practitioners,"

45 "Proceedings of a Meeting for the Establishment of an Academy of Medicine and Surgery," *New York Journal of Medicine* 8 (1847): 125–26; "Abstracts of the Proceedings, Papers, etc. of Medical Societies of New York," *New York Journal of Medicine* 16 (1856): 257–58; for an analysis of the founding of the Academy from a different perspective, see Calhoun, *Professional Lives*, pp. 20–58.

46 Coventry, "Medical Convention," pp. 372–73. Some physicians argued that the problem of the excessive number of medical school graduates was related to the problem of homeopathic physicians. Because the graduates of the medical schools could not "all obtain a lucrative business (simply because there is not enough for them all) in an honorable way," they were forced to become homeopaths or adopt some other deviant form of medical practice: I. F. Galloupe, "One Cause of Empiricism," *Boston Medical and Surgical Journal* 41 (1849): 379–82.

as homeopaths and other non-regulars were called by the regular profession. The most important section concerned consultations, traditionally a major point of contention among physicians. By keeping irregular practitioners out of all consultations, the regular physicians hoped to destroy public confidence in them, deprive them of their clientele, and increase the gulf between them and the regular profession. The first section of the article on consultations read:

Section 1. A regular medical education furnishes the only presumptive evidence of professional abilities and acquirements, and ought to be the only acknowledged right of an individual to the exercise and honors of his profession. Nevertheless, as in consultation the good of the patient is the sole object in view, and this is often dependent on personal confidence, no intelligent regular practitioner, who has a license to practice from some medical board of known and acknowledged respectability, recognized by this association, and who is in good moral and professional standing in the place in which he resides, should be fastidiously excluded from fellowship, or his aid refused in consultation, when it is requested by the patient. But no one can be considered as a regular practitioner or a fit associate in consultation whose practice is based on an exclusive dogma, to the rejection of the accumulated experience of the profession, and of the aids actually furnished by anatomy, physiology, pathology, and organic chemistry.[47]

Related resolutions were passed in the same and in subsequent years to complement the above. A resolution in 1847 recommended to regular medical colleges "that the certificate of no preceptor shall be received, who is avowedly and notoriously an irregular practitioner, whether he shall possess the degree of M.D. or not." Another resolution in 1849 called for state societies "to recognize as regular practitioners, none who have not obtained a degree in medicine, or a license from some regular Medical body, obtained after due examination." Until 1855, the code and these interpretive resolutions were advisory. In that year, the AMA passed two resolutions which required all members to adopt the Code of Ethics as a condition of membership, and expelled any organization which "intentionally violated or disregarded any article or clause in the Code of Ethics."[48]

There are two major points of interest in these resolutions. The first is the definition of an irregular practitioner as one who (1) practiced using an "exclusive dogma," and (2) rejected "the accumulated experience of the profession, and . . . the aids furnished by anatomy, physiology, pathology and organic chemistry." A literal interpretation

---

[47] Austin Flint, "Medical Ethics and Etiquette," *New York Medical Journal* 37 (1883): 371–72.

[48] [Nathan S. Davis], "History of the American Medical Association," *New Jersey Medical Reporter* 7 (1854): 178, 346; "Minutes," *Transactions of the American Medical Association* 8 (1855): 56.

of these criteria would define most homeopaths as regular practitioners, because most of them did not practice homeopathy exclusively (as many regular physicians complained), and did not reject medical science. When the debate over the interpretation of these provisions became significant in the 1880's, supporters of the code stated that in fact this clause was not used to exclude homeopaths. Austin Flint, an eminent regular physician and a president of the AMA, made a detailed analysis and interpretation of the code in 1883 and asserted that "Any physician has a right either to originate or adopt an exclusive dogma, however irrational or absurd it may be." Furthermore, "opinions held by members of the regular profession, however at variance with those generally entertained, and however absurd, may fairly give rise to criticism and ridicule, but they can not be made occasion for professional discipline." He claimed that homeopaths were excluded from consultations not because of their dogma, but because they "adopt a distinctive title as a trade-mark, and . . . are banded in order to impair the confidence of the public in the medical profession."[49]

This interpretation does not correspond to the facts of the situation. It has been shown above that many homeopaths did not call themselves "homeopathic physicians" in the 1840's, and that regular physicians denounced them because they did not. Furthermore, homeopathic medical organizations which excluded laymen were not widespread until after the regular medical societies began to expel homeopaths or to refuse them admittance. Therefore, what Flint described as the cause of the professional ostracism of homeopaths was actually the effect of their ostracism. A regular physician who was critical of Flint's argument said in reply to him:

Surely the doctor is old enough to remember the persistent efforts made in the beginning by the homeopathists, when as yet they had no organization, to be admitted into our county medical societies, or in the case of members of the societies who adopted homeopathy, to resist expulsion. The numerous suits unsuccessfully brought before the courts to compel the societies to admit or retain them, sufficiently attest that if they now have a distinct organization, the fault is not on their side. We thrust them out-of-doors, and now it comes with a bad grace from us to give as a reason for refusing fellowship with them, that they are not in our house.[50]

The second point to be made about the code of ethics involves the provision that "the only presumptive evidence of professional abilities" was the student's preceptor and teachers. A literal interpretation of

49 Flint, "Medical Ethics," pp. 372–73.
50 Thomas Hun, "A Plea for Toleration," Alfred C. Post, ed., *An Ethical Symposium*, (New York: Putnam, 1883), p. 61.

this provision meant that a graduate of a homeopathic or other non-regular medical school would be denied access to the organized regular medical profession for his professional life, regardless of any subsequent conversion to regular medicine. Furthermore, any apprentice of a non-regular physician, regardless of his own intellectual orientations, would be denied admission to a regular medical school solely on the basis of the mode of practice of his preceptor. These provisions made it obvious that the intent of the resolutions was not to ostracize exponents of exclusive dogmas, but rather to make the penalties for any contact between a medical student and non-regular practitioners so severe as to make the persons rather than the dogmas of homeopathic physicians the object of the regulations.

OTHER ASPECTS OF THE AMA CODE OF ETHICS

The consultations provision exemplified the philosophy of the entire AMA code. Lester King called it a sense of *"noblesse oblige"* in his description of the code written by the English physician, Thomas Percival, which was the basis of the AMA code. It was reflected in the first paragraph of the AMA code which stated that physicians "should study, also, in their deportment, so to unite *tenderness* with *firmness*, and *condescension* with *authority*, as to inspire the minds of the patients with gratitude, respect, and confidence." The philosophy of the code was also manifested in its second article, entitled "Obligations of Patients to their Physicians." This article informed each patient of his obligation to select a physician who has a "regular professional education" and certain personal characteristics. The patient was instructed to confide in his physician freely without, however, wearying the physician "with a tedious detail of events or matters not appertaining to his disease" nor "the details of his business nor the history of his family concerns." Furthermore, the patient was warned that his "obedience . . . to the prescriptions of his physician should be prompt and implicit. He should never permit his own crude opinions as to their fitness to influence his attention to them" (this was adopted at the same time as the AMA's condemnation of medical schools for providing physicians with an inadequate education). The article concluded its proscriptions and warnings to patients: "A patient should, after his recovery, entertain a just and enduring sense of the value of the services rendered him by his physician; for these are of such a character that no mere pecuniary acknowledgment can repay or cancel them."[51]

It should not be thought that these provisions merely listed the

---

[51] King, *Medical World of the Eighteenth Century*, p. 255; Flint, "Medical Ethics," pp. 312, 342–43.

sentiments of the public toward the regular profession; far from it. The battles with the botanical practitioners and homeopaths had shown the AMA's members the precariousness of their support. The provisions expressed, rather, the ideals of the profession. The ideal physician was one who was viewed as infallible in his own realm; one who had the respect, deference, and undying trust of his patients; one whose patients expressed their gratitude with an open purse and a reverential heart. These were the ideals—so distant, so seemingly unattainable—expressed in the code.

Thus the fundamental motives of the founders of the AMA transcended the specific issues of the homeopaths and medical education. Their concern was the state of the profession: open to all who could afford a medical school education; unsure of its therapeutics and therefore the more determined to separate itself from its critics; distrusted and challenged by a much abused public; surrounded by non-regular practitioners who attacked it on every side. Yet 1847 was not the nadir of the profession; rather it was the beginning of a new era. The battles with the Thomsonians, and so far with the homeopaths, had shown the regulars that they had more strength and support than they must have thought possible. Medical societies continued to be formed on the frontier and most of the existing ones were surviving. Medical schools were being created at an unprecedented rate and displayed the prosperity and importance of the profession. It was a time of hope, of rebirth, of renewal. It was a time to gather the righteous under one banner, to seek out and destroy the foe.

PART IV THE INSTITUTIONALIZATION OF MEDICAL SECTS

THE OLD FASHIONED family physician and general practitioner was a splended figure and useful person in his day; but he was badly trained, he was often ignorant, he made many mistakes, for one cannot by force of character and geniality of person make a diagnosis of appendicitis, or recognize streptococcus infection.

CHARLES L. DANA

CHAPTER 9

THE THERAPEUTICS OF THE
REGULAR SECT AFTER
THE CIVIL WAR

As a result of the great conflicts among regular physicians, Thomsonians, and homeopaths, three major medical sects developed after
the Civil War. The regulars were the largest by far, the homeopaths
were influential and numerous in the northeast and in all the large
cities of the country, and the descendants of the Thomsonians, the
eclectics, practiced in the small towns and villages of the midwest.
Each sect had its own system of medically invalid therapeutics, each
had its own medical schools, each had its own professional societies,
each had its own pharmacies; the regulars and the homeopaths had
their own hospitals and dispensaries: in short, each sect constituted
an independent and autonomous system of medical practice. This
chapter will examine the therapeutics adopted by the regular sect in
the second half of the century.[1]

The Decline of Heroic Medicine

ATTACKS ON HEROIC THERAPY BY REGULAR PHYSICIANS

In the 1830's and 1840's, a few courageous regular physicians
began to criticize heroic therapy. Unfortunately, their circumspect
language and the restricted interpretations placed on their statements
by other physicians reduced or nullified their effectiveness. The most
famous of these critics was Jacob Bigelow, whose denunciation of
heroic therapeutics has already been mentioned. In his address on
"self-limited diseases," delivered in 1835, he argued that certain diseases ran a course to recovery or death that could not be altered significantly by the efforts of physicians:

By a self-limited disease, I would be understood to express one which
receives limits from its own nature, and not from foreign influences [i.e.,

[1] The epigraph for this part is from Charles L. Dana, "The Doctor's Future,"
New York Medical Journal 97 (1913): 3.

medical treatment]; one which, after it has obtained foothold in the system, cannot, in the present state of our knowledge, be eradicated, or abridged, by art—but to which there is due a certain succession of processes, to be completed in a certain time; which time and processes may vary with the constitution and condition of the patient, and may tend to death, or to recovery, but are not known to be shortened, or greatly changed, by medical treatment.[2]

Bigelow then drew the obvious implications for medical treatment:

. . . we should not allow [the patient] to be tormented with useless and annoying applications, in a disease of settled destiny. It should be remembered that all cases are susceptible of errors of commission, as well as of omission, and that by an excessive application of the means of art, we may frustrate the intentions of nature, when they are salutary, or embitter the approach of death when it is inevitable.[3]

Having opened the door to admit fresh light on the role of therapeutics in the treatment of the sick, Bigelow took advantage of the illumination to cast further doubt on the use of heroic therapeutics generally. He observed that the effects of treatments, such as the effects of mercury or bloodletting, had been confused with changes in the symptoms of the disease being treated, when in fact there was no relation between the two.[4] In this and other ways, Bigelow went far beyond self-limited diseases and questioned the role of heroic therapeutics in any situation.

Reviews of Bigelow's address in the medical journals, which employed some of the most enlightened members of the profession, were complimentary, although hardly ecstatic. The *Boston Medical and Surgical Journal,* for example, stated that "the best part of the dissertation" was the list of self-limited diseases, including whooping cough, measles, scarlet fever, smallpox, and other eruptive diseases.[5] Thus they emphasized the practical aspects of the discourse rather than its fundamental philosophy, which was designed to reorient medical therapeutics toward less heroic measures.

Oliver Wendell Holmes is also frequently considered an important contributor to the attack on heroic therapeutics, but his criticism was far more circumspect than is often alleged. He is most well known for having said in 1860 that "if the whole materia medica, *as now used,* could be sunk to the bottom of the sea, it would be all the better for mankind—and all the worse for the fishes." However, this statement was taken wholly out of context. Holmes advocated keeping on board

[2] Jacob Bigelow, *Nature in Disease* (Boston: Ticknor and Fields, 1854), p. 4.
[3] *Ibid.,* p. 35.
[4] *Ibid.,* p. 40.
[5] "Dr. Bigelow's Discourse," *Boston Medical and Surgical Journal* 12 (1835): 415.

a number of drugs, including opium, cinchona, mercury, arsenic, colchicum (a common treatment for gout with some extremely dangerous and toxic side effects), wine, and anesthetics. Although it is evident that the fishes got the worse of the bargain, the items left on board were sufficient to continue the slaughter unabated. Holmes himself complained about being misconstrued so as to overemphasize his therapeutic skepticism. He said in the 1891 preface to his volume of medical essays: "The sentence was misquoted, quoted without its qualifying conditions, and frightened some of my worthy professional brethren as much as if I had told them to throw all physic to the dogs." In the preface to the 1861 edition, he commented, "One thing is certain. A loud outcry on a slight touch reveals the weak spot in a profession, as well as in a patient."[6]

Criticisms of heroic therapeutics, no matter how tactfully stated, were strongly challenged by many regular physicians, including Bigelow's and Holmes's co-members of the Massachusetts Medical Society. In a well-received 1863 address before the society, Morrill Wyman called men like Bigelow and Holmes "nihilists" and "extromists." He questioned Bigelow's self-limited diseases on two counts. First of all, diseases like malaria, which had once been considered self-limited, were now treatable with quinine, so that the concept was historically determined. Second, he observed that "it would be a grave error to suppose that diseases cannot be abridged or mitigated by art, seeing that there are hardly any which cannot be prolonged or increased by imprudence." He also contended that the physician's actions bring "hope to the despairing, certainly to the doubting, calm to the alarmed," lessen pain and suffering, and ease death when that should occur.[7]

A more representative example of contemporary self-criticism than the writings of Bigelow and Holmes was a series of three articles on the effects of blisters, mercury, and bloodletting "on the young subject," written in 1847–48 by John B. Beck, a well-known physician of his day.[8] There is no reason to doubt the sincerity of his assertion

[6] Oliver Wendell Holmes, *Medical Essays, 1842–1882* (Boston, Mass.: Houghton Mifflin, 1891), pp. 203, xv, vii-viii.

[7] Merrill Wyman, "The Reality and Certainty of Medicine," *Medical Communications of the Massachusetts Medical Society* 10 (1863): 234, 237, 239, 250. For favorable comments about Wyman's article, see J. Mason Warren, "Recent Progress in Surgery," *ibid.* 10 (1864): 269–70; Henry Grafton Clark, "Medical Jurisprudence," *ibid.*, 11 (1868): 56; for comments similar to Wyman's, see George H. Lyman, "The Interests of the Public and the Medical Profession," *ibid.* 12 (1875): 9.

[8] John B. Beck, "On the Effects of Blisters on the Young Subject," *New York Journal of Medicine* 9 (1847): 7–14; "On the Effects of Mercury on the Young Subject," *ibid.* 9 (1847): 175–80; "On the Effects of Bloodletting on the Young Subject," *ibid.*, 10 (1848): 308–15.

that all three were useful and important therapeutic measures. None-theless, his findings led him to the conclusion that all three therapies were dangerous, sometimes lethal, abused beyond belief by reckless and foolhardy physicians, and—although this was never explicitly stated—of little demonstrable benefit in treating disease. Despite these findings, Beck was unwilling to draw the inescapable conclusion from his cata-logue of abusive overuse of these drugs. In the article on mercury, for example, he concluded by blaming homeopaths and patent medicines for its excessive use. In the last article, on bloodletting, he acknowl-edged that, whatever its merits, the public opposed bloodletting, homeopaths had taken advantage of this opposition, and the regular profession had to change its ways to induce the public to return to the fold:

A prejudice, if not general, at least very extensive, has been created against [bloodletting] itself; and empirics, always ready to play upon the weaknesses and prejudices of the community, have seized upon it for the mere purposes of traffic. Accordingly, the land is now filled with a set of men who pretend to practise medicine, without resorting not merely to bloodletting, but many of the other remedies sanctioned by long and tried experience. And what is melancholy, but true, they find a ready sympathy in a large portion of the community. . . . One thing, however, is very certain, and which we see illustrated every day. Whenever a person has been overtaxed with active medicine, he is apt to discard all belief in medicine generally, and he is then ready to fall into any absurdity [e.g., homeopathy]. . . . Calm reflection and rational inquiry are out of the question, and boasted independence [of the patient] speedily becomes the easy prey of the knave and the empiric.[9]

Thus, regular physicians' discussions of heroic therapeutics fre-quently turned from an analysis of the therapies' intrinsic properties to an examination of the preferences of the public and the behavior of their homeopathic and botanical competitors. Regular physicians proposed three alternative responses to the therapeutic challenges pre-sented by their competitors. One suggestion was that regular physicians should have no qualms about using the vegetable remedies of the Thomsonians or the infinitesimal doses of the homeopaths. A com-mencement speaker declared in 1848: "their remedies were yours, long before their systems originated."[10] This suggestion had little appeal because it made the regular physician merely a mime of his competitors and offered him no distinctive therapies which his competitors did not use. The second alternative advocated therapeutic nihilism, claiming that the role of the physician was to assist nature. The kinds of pro-

9 Beck, "Effects of Bloodletting," p. 315.
10 Josiah Gale Beckwith, *The Annual Address to the Candidates for Degrees and Licenses, in the Medical Institution of Yale College* (New Haven: 1848), p. 32.

fessional activities involved were described by Bigelow, who said, "he who turns a pillow, or administers a seasonable draught of water to a patient, palliates his sufferings."[11] Physicians realized that professional training was not required in these tasks and that the average patient would hardly pay good money simply to receive a drink of water from the hand of a physician. Furthermore, nature effected her cures without any expense to the patient, but physicians were compelled by economic necessity to demand fees for their treatments. Competition from homeopaths was tolerable, for at least they charged fees, but competition from nature was asking too much. The inevitable consequence was that regular physicians succumbed to public and competitive pressures, reluctantly abandoned heroic therapy, and adopted a distinctive new set of sectarian therapies.

THE DEMISE OF HEROIC THERAPEUTICS

Most recent studies have found that the decline in the use of bloodletting, calomel, and other elements of heroic therapy occurred in the second half of the nineteenth century. Bonner's history of medicine in Chicago found that heroic therapy declined in the 1860's. Rosenberg's study of medical practice in New York City in the 1860's found a decrease at that time in the extensive use of bloodletting, emetics, and cathartics. The same author's study of the cholera epidemics of 1832, 1849, and 1866 found a decline in the use of bloodletting and calomel only in the 1866 epidemic. Ackerknecht's study of malaria in the midwest found a decline in heroic treatment of that disease after 1850.[12]

These dates appear to be representative for both bloodletting and calomel. With respect to the former, Cowen's history of medicine in New Jersey found that bloodletting was common until the Civil War, and retained its popularity in many places for two decades thereafter. Bonner's history of medicine in Kansas found a gradual decline in bloodletting in the 1860's, and little use of it in the 1870's. A study of bloodletting as described in therapeutics textbooks found that their authors restricted the therapeutic use of bloodletting in the 1860's and 1870's. Last, a lecture on trends in therapeutics in 1870 by William

[11] Bigelow, *Nature in Disease*, p. 4.
[12] Thomas Neville Bonner, *Medicine in Chicago 1850–1950* (Madison, Wis.: American History Research Center, 1957), p. 31; Charles Rosenberg, "The Practice of Medicine in New York A Century Ago," *Bulletin of the History of Medicine* 41 (1967): 244; Charles E. Rosenberg, *The Cholera Years* (Chicago: University of Chicago Press, 1962), pp. 151–53, 222–23; Erwin H. Ackerknecht, *Malaria in the Upper Mississippi Valley 1760–1900* (Baltimore: Johns Hopkins Press, 1945), p. 118.

Wellington stated that bloodletting was becoming "one of the lost arts."[13]

Bloodletting continued to be recommended in specific illnesses for decades. William Osler, one of the most eminent of all American physicians, advocated bloodletting in pneumonia as late as the turn of the twentieth century. In 1893, he said: "Pneumonia is one of the diseases in which timely venesection saves life." By 1912, he modified this to the following: "To bleed at the very outset [in pneumonia] in robust, healthy individuals, in whom the disease sets in with great intensity and high fever, is, I believe, a good practice," adding that "small amounts are often sufficient." In 1913, Fielding Garrison wrote in his history of bloodletting, "there is hardly a physician with a good practice who may not suddenly encounter some circumstances in his experience in which venesection would turn out to be his sheet anchor and his patient's salvation."[14]

The decline in the use of calomel also occurred during the middle of the century. An Indiana physician observed in 1849 that "its use is much less now than it was a few years since." Bellevue Hospital in New York City purchased no calomel and only five pounds of jalap in 1866. Nevertheless, its use was sufficiently widespread during the Civil War to cause a major alteraction between the Surgeon General and many physicians. Joseph Woodward stated in his 1879 medical history of the Civil War that military physicians used calomel in numerous diseases during the war. William Hammond, the Surgeon General of the United States Army at the time, became so disturbed over what he believed to be the excessive use of calomel and tartar emetic by army physicians that he removed both drugs from the supply table of the army in 1863. This action created such a furor in regular medical societies and medical journals that, although never revoked, the order was never enforced and the drugs remained in use throughout the war.[15]

13 David L. Cowen, *Medicine and Health in New Jersey* (Princeton, N. J.: Van Nostrand, 1964, p. 35; Thomas Neville Bonner, *The Kansas Doctor* (Lawrence: University of Kansas Press, 1959), p. 20; Leon S. Bryan, Jr., "Blood-Letting in American Medicine, 1830–1892," *Bulletin of the History of Medicine* 38 (1964): 520; William W. Wellington, "Modern Medicine," *Medical Communications of the Massachusetts Medical Society* 11 (1870): 159.

14 B. M. Randolph, "The Blood Letting Controversy in the Nineteenth Century," *Annals of Medical History*, n.s., 7 (1935): 181–82; Fielding H. Garrison, "The History of Bloodletting," *New York Medical Journal* 97 (1913): 501.

15 A. B. Shipman, "Treatment of Malarious Diseases at the West," *Boston Medical and Surgical Journal* 40 (1849): 239; Rosenberg, "Practice of Medicine," pp. 243–44; Joseph Janvier Woodward, *The Medical and Surgical History of the War of the Rebellion*, Pt. II, vol. 1: Medical History, Second Issue (Washington:

Calomel survived in the therapeutic arsenal for many years. As late as 1937, a Louisiana physician complained that calomel was "a close second" to quinine as "the most used and abused remedy" among many physicians in the South. He stated that "there are those who believe that every treatment should begin with calomel or other drastic purgative. I have seen it given in large doses to babies with dysentery."[16]

Another way of examining the decline of heroic therapy is found in a detailed study of every case of acute lobar pneumonia—one thousand in all—treated in the Massachusetts General Hospital in Boston from 1822 to 1889. Prior to 1850, almost two-thirds of the patients were bled, and "almost every case was vomited and purged, given mercury to salivation and sore gums, [and] blistered with cantharides." The period from 1850 to 1860 was transitional: bleeding was used in less than one third of the cases, "and the other heroic measures were proportionately decreased." After 1860, heroic therapy was almost never used, and only 6 of 741 cases in this period were bled.[17]

THERAPEUTIC NIHILISM

A few physicians who abandoned heroic therapy took refuge in a cynical nihilism. For example, H. C. Wood wrote in the 1875 edition of his *Therapeutics*:

The old and tried method in therapeutics is that of empiricism, or, if the term sounds harsh, that of clinical experience. . . . the best possible development of this plan of investigation is to be found in a close and careful analysis of cases before and after the administration of a remedy, and if the results be feasible, the continued use of the drug in similar cases. It is evident that this is not a new path, but a highway already worn with the eager but weary feet of the profession for 2,000 years. . . . What has clinical therapeutics established permanently and indisputably? Scarcely anything beyond the primary facts that quinine will arrest an intermittent, salts will purge and that opium will quiet pain and lull to sleep. The history of medical progress is a history of men groping in the darkness, finding seeming gems of truth one after another, only in a few minutes to cast each back into the

---

1879), pp. 718–22. In addition to Woodward's account, a description of the incident can be found in Gert H. Brieger, "Therapeutic Conflicts and the American Medical Profession in the 1860's," *Bulletin of the History of Medicine* 41 (1967): 215–22. For a short biography of Hammond, see Albert F. Heck, "William Alexander Hammond—1828–1900." *JAMA* 183 (1963): 466–68.

16 S. W. Douglas, "Medical Fads and Fallacies," *New Orleans Medical and Surgical Journal* 90 (1938): 610.

17 C. W. Townsend and A. Coolidge, Jr., "The Mortality of Acute Lobar Pneumonia," *Transactions of the American Climatological Association* 6 (1889): 41–43.

vast heap of forgotten baubles that in their day had also been mistaken for verities. In the past there has scarcely been a conceivable absurdity that men have not tested by experience and found for a time to be the thing desired. . . . Looking at the revolutions and contradictions of the past, is it a wonder that men should take refuge in nihilism?[18]

This cynicism was stimulated by comparisons of trends in therapeutics with developments in other areas of medical science—surgery, pathology, anatomy, etc. Therapeutics, Wellington stated in 1870, "have not kept pace with other departments of medicine" and constituted "the weak spot in our profession, against which the arrows of the adversary are aimed with most effect." Twenty-one years later in 1891, another physician could make precisely the same complaint: "While hygiene, pathology, and clinical research in the natural history of diseases have made great advances during the past three decades, therapeutics has remained tentative and empirical." Therapeutics, which Wellington conceded to be the major justification for the role of the physician in the community, continued to suffer from a lack of medical validity.[19]

The cynicism of these physicians was a luxury which most of their colleagues could not afford. Physicians who had to contend with a world of patients seeking relief from their ills could hardly solace anxious patients with cynical disclaimers about the historical futility of therapeutics.[20] As physicians themselves observed, patients demanded that physicians use active therapy in treating their illnesses. A regular physician, Maurice Clarke, complained of the "popular clamor for dosage" in these words in 1889:

How often . . . after having inquired as to the patient's bodily functions, regulated the diet, made suggestions as to bed and bedding, urged the importance of fresh air, and carefully attended to all the minute details for the patient's comfort, how often has it fallen to the lot of all of us to be confronted by the anxious friends with the inquiry, "But aren't you going to do something for him, Doctor?"[21]

18 Quoted in W. H. Witt, "The Progress of Internal Medicine since 1830," in Philip M. Hamer, ed., *The Centennial History of the Tennessee State Medical Association 1830–1930* (Nashville, Tenn.: 1930), p. 268.
19 Wellington, "Modern Medicine," pp. 141–42, 148; A. S. Coe, "Therapeutics," *New York Medical Journal* 54 (1891): 239.
20 Rosenberg has made this same observation with respect to medical treatment during cholera epidemics in the middle of the nineteenth century. Rosenberg, *Cholera Years*, p. 154.
21 Maurice D. Clarke, "Therapeutic Nihilism," *Medical Communications of the Massachusetts Medical Society* 14 (1888): 221; see also Wellington, "Modern Medicine," p. 152.

Moreover, a patient did not request a dose of medicine for its own sake: he wanted relief from his pain and discomfort. A homeopath observed in 1912:

None of us like to suffer pain, yet, as physicians, we are somewhat inclined to be philosophical about it when treating a patient; but the latter wants relief and quickly, and if he or she does not get it in what is considered a reasonable time, criticism will probably develop. We all know that the proper remedy will relieve pain and quickly because we have seen it do so, but we do not always know what is the proper remedy, so the physician succumbs to temptation because of his uncertainty and prescribes something which will have an anodyne effect; the patient is satisfied with the relief and with the doctor, and the latter justifies his procedure on the ground that the temporary relief has probably done the patient good rather than harm, and that time has been gained for finding the proper remedy without destroying the patient's confidence and prolonging his or her suffering.[22]

Physicians did not merely acquiesce grudgingly in these requests for palliative relief. According to Clarke, most of them shared the belief of their patients "that he fails of his duty and his privilege who neglects to do something for the patient."[23] As another physician complained, practicing therapeutic nihilism required courage and self-restraint in the face of the demands of patients for active therapy:

How many physicians know anything of the natural course of most diseases, except by hearsay? How many have had the courage to observe for themselves, while sternly combatting the seductive opportunity of prescribing a variety of unnecessary medicines? Most diseases, as they are met in practice, are so overlaid, disguised, and their symptoms colored and mingled with the effects of drugs that have been administered, that only a mongrel type is known to the profession. . . .

It is a convenient mask to a perplexed spirit to be industriously giving something when the case is not understood. The doctor's dignity of knowledge is not questioned—he is hard at work dosing the obstinate sick man, all must be right![24]

Surely it comes as no surprise that therapeutic nihilists were rarely to be found among practicing physicians.

In their search for new therapies to replace those rejected by patients, physicians were still in the grips of nineteenth-century clinical methodology. The lack of any scientific knowledge of etiology meant a continued emphasis on symptomatic treatment. Bacteriology contributed nothing to therapeutics until 1894.[25] Histology was equally

[22] James W. Fox, "The Practice of Homoeopathy," *The Chironion* 29 (1912): 29.

[23] Clarke, "Therapeutic Nihilism," pp. 221–22.

[24] George T. Welch, "Therapeutic Superstitions," *Medical Record* 44 (1893): 37.

[25] This question will be examined in detail in Chapter 14.

unproductive: Henry J. Bigelow, one of the leaders of the profession, complained in 1871 that theories of diseased tissues were "as change- able and uncertain as groups in clouds" and that every decade brought "a new crop." The indifference to the more basic medical sciences characterized medical education as well as medical practice. Bigelow expressed the opinion of most physicians when he objected to medical school curricula which sent students "wool-gathering among the abstract and collateral sciences" like chemistry, and comparative anatomy and physiology, instead of emphasizing the core of the cur- riculum—therapeutics, pathology, anatomy, and general physiology.[26]

THE NEW VIGOROUS THERAPY

Taking advantage of numerous developments in pharmacology through- out the second half of the century, physicians continued to use therapies to "make an impression on the patient"—to use the words of their forebears. New antipyretics continued to reduce fever at any cost. Analgesics and anodynes continued to relieve pain and hypnotics to induce sleep despite their addictive properties and other undesirable side effects. Stimulants were widely employed to strengthen the pulse and improve appetite and digestion, when their long run effects were deleterious in the extreme. Throughout the period, harmful drugs made the presence of the physician a dubious advantage in much medical care. Wellington stated in 1870 that "over-medication has been the besetting sin of the medical profession"; another physician ob- served in 1894 that "one of the most pernicious practices of the regular profession is excessive medication."[27] Some physicians even doubted whether the doses were smaller than those used in the first half of the century. D. W. Cathell, the author of a widely-read handbook for physicians, wrote that "in serious illness it is doubtful whether we have lessened our doses of standard reliable remedies half as much as some imagine," although he felt that there was less heroic treatment in

[26] Henry J. Bigelow, "Medical Education in America," *Medical Communica- tions of the Massachusetts Medical Society* 11 (1871): 190, 203–4, 232; Henry Bigelow was the son of Jacob Bigelow.

[27] Wellington, "Modern Medicine," p. 151; Edwin J. Kuh, "Sectarianism in Medicine," *Journal of the American Medical Association* 23 (1894): 907; see also Augustus Caille, "The Relation of the Family Doctor to Recent Progress in Medical Science," *American Monthly Review of Reviews* 23 (1901): 462. For a detailed critique of late nineteenth-century drug abuse by physicians, see John T. G. Nichols, "The Misuse of Drugs in Modern Practice," *Boston Medical and Sur- gical Journal* 129 (1893): 239–42, 261–64, 292–94.

"trifling, obscure or undeveloped" cases.[28] Drugging continued to be the watchword of American medicine in the second half of the century.

ANTIPYRETICS

If the public would no longer tolerate bloodletting, the resourceful American physician could turn to other antipyretics, but the objective remained the same: in the words of a well-known physician, "the one idea of the modern therapist being to reduce temperature at all hazards."[29] The second half of the nineteenth century witnessed a succession of antipyretics, each having such severe side effects that it was rapidly cast aside for another development of contemporary pharmacology.

Among the first were aconite and *Veratrum viride*, two vegetable poisons which acted as "cardiac sedatives," reducing fever by their direct effect on the heart's action. Aconite, one of the most powerful known poisons, remained popular with physicians for decades. Veratrum was so popular for a while that it was called the "vegetable lancet" because of its antipyretic properties. The harshness of its effects made it controversial before 1880, although it was still being used a decade later.[30]

The discovery of alkaloids led to the development of a more important antipyretic—quinine, which was isolated from cinchona bark in 1820. The much greater potency of quinine made it a considerable improvement over cinchona, but its substantially higher cost for several

28 D. W. Cathell and William T. Cathell, *Book on the Physician Himself, and Things that Concern His Reputation and Success* (Philadelphia: Davis, 1902), 11th ed. p. 275. Because Cathell will be referred to with some frequency in the remainder of the study, a brief description of his book is warranted. It was an extremely popular *vade mecum* for physicians on how to be successful in medical practice. The author dedicated the book to the "younger men of our profession"—it must have been a popular graduation gift to new physicians—"and also to the older ones who have paused at less than the average degree of success in life." The book was first published in 1882 and went through nine editions by 1889, and three more from that date to 1922. Obviously, it was a very popular book in its day. Cathell was quite conscientious in his revisions, and incorporated his views on the major issues of the day, which adds to the book's usefulness to the historian.

29 Alfred L. Loomis, "Anniversary Address," *Transactions of the Medical Society of the State of New York* 1888: 69.

30 Henry Morris, *Essentials of Materia Medica, Therapeutics and Prescription Writing* (Philadelphia: Saunders, 1912), 7th ed., pp. 163–66; *American Cyclopedia* (New York: Appleton, 1881), s.v. "Aconite"; Witt, "Progress of Internal Medicine," pp. 263–64; Cowen, *Medicine in New Jersey*, pp. 48–49; G. F. Cooper, "Veratrum Viride . . . ," *Transactions of the American Medical Association* 30 (1879): 213; Aaron C. Ward, "Veratrum Viride," *Medical and Surgical Reporter* 64 (1891): 297–302. Samuel Thomson had denounced veratrum decades earlier: Samuel Thomson, *New Guide to Health* (Boston: 1831), p. 32.

decades after its development delayed its replacement of the bark. As it became cheaper and more widely used, physicians recognized that large doses tended to reduce fever in most diseases consistently and demonstrably, by depressing the heart's action. Thus it was usable not only in malaria, where its value was widely recognized, but also in most other fevers, such as pneumonia, typhoid, yellow fever, etc. Reasoning backward from quinine's therapeutic uses, physicians assumed that these other diseases could be classed as malarial. One physician said that malaria "became a component part of almost every other ailment such as malarial-neuralgia, malarial-headache, malarial-pneumonia, malarial-rheumatism, etc., . . . when a trouble was obscure, physicians were wont to call it malarial—malaria *latent* in form. Much too often malaria served as a kind of blanket to cover up the diagnostician's ignorance."[31]

Thus quinine became a panacea for all ills in the 1870's and 1880's. The physician who said in 1884 that he considered quinine second only to opium "in our armamentarium of drugs" spoke for a large part of the profession. When confronted with fevers of all kinds, according to one physician, quinine was "firmly fixed in the minds of many practitioners as the one means of treatment to be at once seized upon." It was also used as a general tonic to improve the appetite and digestion, and as such it became so popular that a committee of the AMA stated, "with this in their hands, [many physicians] do not need or desire any other articles of this class." Quinine's combined antipyretic and tonic qualities undoubtedly made many physicians believe that it could be used in virtually any illness. One physician complained: "It is the custom with most physicians of this country, to give quinine during some stage of every disease that flesh is heir to. Some give it for one purpose and some for another; many because they don't know what else to do." The consumption of quinine in the United States was so large that in the decade after the Civil War, the AMA sought unsuccessfully to induce the federal government to cultivate the tree in the United States for medicinal purposes. By 1888, the United States was using about forty percent of the total world consumption. Indeed, for over two decades after the Civil War, quinine

---

[31] Erwin H. Ackerknecht, *A Short History of Medicine* (New York: Ronald Press, 1955), p. 155; Tom Kirkwood, "The General Practitioner . . . ," in David J. Davis, ed., *History of Medical Practice in Illinois, Vol. II: 1850–1900* (Chicago: Illinois State Medical Society, 1955), p. 99; Ackerknecht, *Malaria in Mississippi Valley*, pp. 113–4; Charles B. Johnson, *Sixty Years in Medical Harness . . . 1865–1925* (New York: Medical Life Press, 1926), p. 96.

replaced calomel in the materia medica as the standard medication in fevers and other acute diseases.[32]

Like calomel, quinine had some deleterious side effects. In moderate doses it weakened the heart and pulse, caused gastro-intestinal irritation, and produced nervousness and giddiness. These side effects were accentuated by repeated doses of the drug. In large doses—and physicians were often extraordinarily liberal in their dosage of quinine —it produced a set of symptoms which became so common that they were given a name—cinchonism. This was characterized by the symptoms described above and by ringing of the ears and, in severe instances, deafness, blindness, and other toxic effects.[33]

This abuse of quinine led patients to rebel against it; as early as 1849, one midwestern physician spoke of the "universal antipathy which the great mass of the inhabitants of the West have against sulphate of quinine." This antagonism continued for some time, because another physician spoke of a "popular prejudice against quinine" in 1884. Strangely enough, many physicians believed that the side effects of quinine rarely occurred, undoubtedly because there were no visible physiological manifestations comparable to calomel's effect on the teeth. Cathell observed that many people believed that "quinine gets into the bones, affects sight and hearing, causes dropsy, etc. So firmly do some people believe these things that you will at times have to humor their prejudices, and change to sulphate of cinchona . . . or some other preparation of bark, when bark is indicated."[34]

In the 1880's, research with coal-tars led to the development of synthetic antipyretics which rapidly replaced quinine. The first of these was antipyrine, about which one physician said in 1886: "antipyrine, in sufficiently large doses, is the most powerful, the most certain, and

[32] A. A. Smith, "The Danger of Large Doses of Quinine," *New York Medical Journal* 39 (1884): 115; D. B. St. John Roosa, "On the Injudicious Use of the Sulphate of Quinine," *Medical Record* 23 (1883): 145; Lemuel J. Deal and Thomas M. Logan, "Report of the Committee to Memorialize Congress on the Cultivation of the Cinchona Tree in the United States," *Transactions of the American Medical Association* 21 (1870): 154; George M. Dewey, "Sulphate of Quinine—its Use and Abuse," *Eclectic Medical Journal* 47 (1887): 176–77; Erwin H. Ackerknecht, "The American Medical Association and the Cultivation of the Cinchona Tree in the United States," *Journal of the American Medical Association* 123 (1943): 375; Ackerknecht, *Malaria in Mississippi Valley*, p. 115.

[33] Otis Frederick Manson, *A Treatise on the Physiological and Therapeutic Action of the Sulphate of Quinine* (Philadelphia: Lippincott, 1882), pp. 97–101; Dewey, "Sulphate of Quinine," pp. 177–79; Kaspar Pischl, "Quinine-Blindness," *Medical News* 63 (1893): 122–25.

[34] A. B. Shipman, "Professional Matters at the West—Malarious Fever," *Boston Medical and Surgical Journal* 40 (1849): 73; Smith, "Large Doses of Quinine," p. 116: Cathell, *Physician Himself*, 10th ed. (Philadelphia: 1895), p. 196.

the safest anti-febrile drug that we have in our materia medica." It rapidly became a panacea because of its analgesic as well as antipyretic effects. One prominent physician claimed in 1893 that there was "certainly no drug ever discovered which is so universally applicable as antipyrine, the powers of which are almost as diverse as disease itself." Almost immediately after its introduction, however, antipyrine was found to produce many undesirable side effects, including profuse perspiration, nausea, and irregular heart action. These and other even more toxic side effects frequently occurred after the administration of average doses, making antipyrine dangerous and inconsistent under most circumstances.[35]

For these reasons, many physicians welcomed antipyrine's synthetic successor, acetanilid (introduced as antifebrin) as a demonstrably superior antipyretic. However, when this drug was used habitually, it produced serious cardiac symptoms and other toxic effects, so that it did not prove a panacea either, although it was demonstrably superior to its predecessor. Ultimately, acetylsalicylic acid (aspirin) was developed as a successor to these drugs, but during the nineteenth century, according to Walsh, synthetic drugs "proved each in succession to have certain serious very lasting effects that made them eminently undesirable when used over long periods."[36]

ANALGESICS

The relief of pain has always been one of the major symptomatic treatments used by physicians. During the second half of the century, developments in analgesics added considerably to their importance in the physician's armamentarium. Many physicians felt that analgesics were the *sine qua non* of medical practice. Henry J. Bigelow said in 1870 that the physician's "sheet-anchor, whether in life or at the hour of death, is narcotism in some degree or form, and without which his profession, if not his prescriptions, would be comparatively a farce."[37]

[35] E. P. Lacey, "The Effect of High Temperature in Continued Fevers . . . ," *Virginia Medical Monthly* 17 (1890): 10–12; J. H. Frankenberg, "Antipyrine," *Medical Record* 29 (1886): 591; H. A. Hare, "The Present State of Therapeutics," *International Medical Annual* (1893), p. 4. For a description of the variety of uses to which antipyrine was put, see John Aulde, "Studies in Therapeutics—Antipyrin," *Medical Record* 39 (1891): 195–98; William H. Draper, "Antipyrine and its Effects," *New York Medical Journal* 41 (1885): 429–31; Morris, *Essentials of Materia Medica*, pp. 78–79.

[36] William Osler, "Antifebrin," *Therapeutic Gazette* 11 (1887): 163–67; *New International Encyclopedia*, (New York: Dodd, Mead, 1914), 2nd ed., s.v. "Acetanilid"; James J. Walsh, *History of Medicine in New York* (New York: National Americana Society, 1919), 1: 262.

[37] Bigelow, "Medical Education in America," p. 214.

The most important analgesics during the last half of the nineteenth century were opium and its alkaloid, morphine. One physician said in 1889: "Opium is the most conspicuous article in the pharmacopeia. Its extraordinary efficacy in relieving pain, the versatility of its powers, and its reliability in emergencies, give it a preeminent standing." Opium was used by physicians in every conceivable illness. Another physician said: "Modifying the several processes by which life is maintained, secretion, ennervation, respiration and circulation, its broad application and various uses in disease commend it to the medical philosopher as the best adaptation of means to ends that comes within the scope of his knowledge." Physicians used it in fevers, inflammations, and aches and pains of all kinds. It was probably the most common treatment for diarrhea. In 1888, Virgil Eaton, a nonmedical writer, surveyed over ten thousand prescriptions by visiting numerous pharmacies and examining 300 prescriptions at each. He found that 14 percent of all prescriptions involved some preparation of opium, and that the percentage increased considerably among refilled prescriptions. He concluded that opium was "the great panacea and cure-all." Eight years later, a physician inquired among pharmacists and wholesalers who sold directly to physicians, and found that the therapeutic use of opium was increasing at that time.[38]

Because opium was such a successful painkiller, physicians even invented a new disease for it to treat, called neuralgia (a term still in use today, but in a more restricted sense). An English encyclopedia defined neuralgia succintly as a "term which is frequently employed, both technically and popularly in a somewhat loose manner, to describe pains the origin of which is not clearly traceable."[39] Obviously, opium was just the thing to treat this sort of disease.

The extraordinary aspect of the therapeutic use of opium was the complete indifference of many physicians to its addictive properties. Cathell advised physicians to "carry a supply of morphia granules or tablets with you constantly, and give a proper number of them in an ounce or two of hot water as soon as you reach one of the thousand cases in which great pain is a symptom." He recommended that physicians use morphine "to give any jaded sufferer an occasional night of

38 J. F. A. Adams, "Substitutes for Opium in Chronic Diseases," *Boston Medical and Surgical Journal* 121 (1889): 351; L. L. Todd, "The Therapeutic Properties of Opium," *Transactions of the Indiana State Medical Society* 20 (1877): 79–80; Virgil G. Eaton, "How the Opium-Habit is Acquired," *Popular Science Monthly* 33 (1888): 665; G. Walter Barr, "The Therapeutic Abuse of Opium," *Journal of the American Medical Association* 26 (1896): 162.

39 *Encyclopedia Britannica* (New York: Scribner's, 1884), 9th ed., s.v. "Neuralgia."

delicious visions, or of placid slumber." The problems of addiction increased considerably when the hypodermic injection of morphine became popular during and after the Civil War. This development was particularly welcome to physicians because the oral administration of opium produced "unpleasant gastric effects and cerebral disturbance" and was less powerful in its effects. For the same reasons, hypodermic injections were much more likely to lead to addiction.[40] Many physicians exhibited only casual concern with this new and intensified problem. Cathell, for example, wrote:

> Among the lesser evils connected with [hypodermic medication] is that those who are soothed and temporarily comforted by it, or have become habituated to it, are apt to harass and worry you for its application at all hours, day and night; and you will often find it a real hardship, after doing your day's work, to be obliged to go and administer a hypodermic (night-cap) of morphia to the Rev. Mr. Cantsleep at eight o'clock P.M., to Mrs. Allnerves at nine, to Colonel Bigdrinks at ten, and to Miss Narywink at eleven o'clock, and probably be called from bed again to insert the sleep-giving needle for one or all of them before morning.
>
> Much of such work is not only a hardship but a nuisance. Far better is it for both the patient and yourself that anodynes be administered by the mouth or rectum in such cases, than for you to . . . expose him to what may prove, to him, a fatal charm, and, to you, a sorrowful lesson.[41]

Even the medical schools did not instruct their students about the addiction problem in any detail during this period. In their comprehensive study of opium addiction, Terry and Pellens found that the authors of the "great majority of textbooks on the practice of medicine, materia medica, and therapeutics failed to issue any warning of the dangers" involved in the hypodermic use of morphine.[42]

Those concerned with addiction frequently blamed physicians as a major cause of the problem. Some physicians criticized their colleagues for starting patients on the road to addiction by administering morphine hypodermically too often and by teaching patients how to use the hypodermic syringe themselves. A committee of the American Pharmaceutical Association reported in 1903 that physicians were to blame for much addition. Eaton stated: "The parties who are responsible for the increase of the habit are the physicians who give the

---

40 Cathell, *Physician Himself*, pp. 241–42; J. B. Mattison, "The Responsibility of the Profession in the Production of Opium Inebriety," *Medical and Surgical Reporter* 38 (1878): 101–4.

41 Cathell, *Physician Himself*, p. 207.

42 Charles E. Terry and Mildred Pellens, *The Opium Problem* (New York: 1928), p. 72.

prescriptions."[43] Physicians defending the profession argued that the increase in addiction was due, instead, largely to the lack of any effective legal regulations governing the sale of opium in most states and to the widespread use of patent medicines with opium as their only or major therapeutic ingredient.[44] The consensus of most writers on the subject was that all these factors aggravated the addiction problem.

Addiction became a major social issue by the end of the nineteenth century. The amount of opium imported into the United States was enormous. About 1910, the United States imported over 20 times as much opium per capita as such countries as Germany, Italy, and Austria-Hungary. In the years from 1860 to 1910, the amount of opium imported into the United States increased almost three times as fast as the population. The number of addicts in the United States at this time was the subject of considerable debate, and Terry and Pellens have shown that the empirical evidence on the subject is extremely unreliable. Nonetheless, there was widespread agreement that addiction was a rapidly growing problem which affected a surprisingly large proportion of the population.[45]

The desire of a number of physicians "to be emancipated" from opium as an analgesic led to the rapid acceptance of newly developed alternative drugs. One of the most popular of these was cocaine, which physicians felt could be administered with "comparative impunity." It also was found that, when sprayed in the nose, cocaine contracted the mucous membranes and was therefore useful for rhinitis, which led one physician to state that there was "no longer any excuse for any one suffering from a cold in the head." This use of cocaine became so popular that it contributed to the rapid development of the nose and throat specialty. A considerable debate developed in the profession

43 *Ibid.*, pp. 94–135. See also Mattison, "Responsibility of the Profession," p. 102; J. C. Wilson, "The Causes and Prevention of the Opium Habit and Kindred Affections," *Boston Medical and Surgical Journal* 119 (1888): 505–6; F. W. Comings, "Opium. Its Uses and Abuses," *Transactions of the Vermont State Medical Society*, 83d meeting (1896), pp. 365–66; Frederick T. Gordon and E. G. Eberle, "Report of Committee on the Acquirement of Drug Habits," *Proceedings of the American Pharmaceutical Association* 51 (1903): 472; Eaton, "Opium Habit," p. 666.

44 "How the Opium Habit is Acquired," *Journal of the American Medical Association* 11 (1888): 419–20; Adams, "Substitutes for Opium," p. 352; Terry and Pellens, *Opium Problem*, pp. 74–75.

45 Martin I. Wilbert and Murray Galt Motter, "Digest of Laws and Regulations in force in the United States Relating to the Possession, Use, Sale and Manufacture of Poisons and Habit-Forming Drugs," *Public Health Bulletin*, No. 56 (1912), pp. 14–15; Terry and Pellens, *Opium Problem*, pp. 1–52.

over whether cocaine was addictive, and many physicians felt that it was not.[46]

A number of hypnotics, or sleep-inducing drugs, were also developed during this period and partly replaced opium in this regard. One of the most popular was chloral hydrate, which produced a more natural sleep than opium. It was widely recommended for infants and children. Chloral was toxic in large doses and had serious side effects when used over any length of time. Another popular hypnotic was sulphonal, which also had toxic side effects.[47]

TONICS

Tonics or stimulants, the third major category of late nineteenth-century drugs, were loosely defined terms, referring to drugs which produced demonstrable and beneficial changes in pulse, respiration, appetite, digestion, and skin color. Arsenic had been a popular tonic in the pre-Civil War period. After the war, it was replaced first by quinine and later by strychnine. Strychnine, a poison which is now considered to have little or no therapeutic value, was employed by many physicians "day after day for considerable periods of time for the purpose of stimulating the heart."[48]

The most important tonic and probably the most important medicinal agent of the second half of the century was beverage alcohol, almost always in the form of whiskey or brandy. Alcohol had always been popular as a therapy because of its low cost and accessibility, but after the Civil War its use increased considerably. Alcohol was believed to produce an amazing variety of beneficial effects. One physician observed: "It is a generally accepted doctrine that alcohol is a stimulant to the digestion, a cardiac tonic, a conservator of tissue, capable

46 Adams, "Substitutes for Opium," p. 352; John A. Wessinger, "The Untoward Effects of Cocaine," *New York Medical Journal* 51 (1890): 70; F. H. Bosworth, "An Additional Note on the Therapeutic Action of Cocaine," *New York Medical Journal* 43 (1886): 324; for an account of a physician who took cocaine for several months for rhinitis, see Frank W. Ring, "Cocaine and its Fascinations, from a Personal Experience," *Medical Record* 32 (1887): 274–76; Caille, "Family Doctor," p. 459. For a debate on cocaine addiction, see "New York Neurological Society," *New York Medical Journal* 44 (1886): 637–39.

47 For a detailed description of chloral, see H. H. Kane, "Chloral Hydrate," *Medical Record* 18 (1880): 702–5; 19 (1881): 4–7, 32–37, 60–65, 284–88, 310–13, 460–63, 482–84; Adams, "Substitutes for Opium," p. 355; Morris, *Essentials of Materia Medica*, pp. 100–102.

48 Arthur Osol, Robertson Pratt, Mark D. Altschule, *The United States Dispensatory* (Philadelphia: Lippincott, 1967), 26th ed., p. 1100; "The Abuse of Strychnine as a Stimulant," *Therapeutic Gazette* 22 (1898): 307; see also Thomas J. Mays, "Is the Continual Use of Strychnine Unwise?" *New York Medical Journal* 68 (1898): 525–26.

of increasing and sustaining the vital energy, and therefore indispensable in the treatment of all low grades of disease, shock, collapse, etc." The authors of most leading textbooks recommended it unhesitatingly: one said that the early use of beverage alcohol "furnishes our best means of counteracting the depressing action of disease in general."[49]

Alcohol was used in both acute and chronic diseases. Foremost among the former were typhoid and pneumonia. In the treatment of typhoid one extremely popular textbook advised: "Alcohol in some form should be used in *every* case of typhoid *from the beginning,* unless there is some very strong reason for refusing it, as where there is a distinct heredity toward drunkenness." In the treatment of cases of pneumonia, the Massachusetts General Hospital study found that, after 1860, one half the cases were given alcohol, including nearly all the severe and fatal cases. This ratio was conservative compared to the practices of physicians elsewhere: one physician complained that the effects of alcohol in treating pneumonia were not well understood because there were so few cases where it was not used. The dosage of beverage alcohol in acute disease was so large that continual inebriation must have been the state of many patients. The most common dose for adults was one half to one ounce of whiskey or brandy every two or three hours. One physician said that he would not hesitate to give children ill with diphtheria ten to twelve ounces of whiskey a day if necessary, but the more usual dose was from one-half to two teaspoons every three hours for infants and young children. In chronic diseases, most notably tuberculosis, beverage alcohol was highly recommended for continued use over long periods of time because of the widespread belief that alcohol had actual food value in addition to its other desirable properties.[50]

The discoveries in bacteriology tended to increase the use of alcohol. It was discovered that alcohol acted as a germicide when

[49] John Duffy, ed., *The Rudolph Matas History of Medicine in Louisiana* (n.p.: Louisiana State University Press, 1962), II: 30; Walsh, *History of Medicine in New York,* p. 262; Rosenberg, "Practice of Medicine in New York," pp. 243–44, n. 45; A. A. Kent, "The Abuse of Alcoholic Stimulants in Practice," *Medical and Surgical Reporter* 74 (1896): 72; J. M. Farrington, "The Use of Alcohol in Medicine," *New York Medical Journal* 50 (1889): 352. This article examines a number of textbooks to show their enthusiasm for beverage alcohol.

[50] Quoted in Richard C. Cabot, "Alcoholic Stimulants in Continued Fevers," *Boston Medical and Surgical Journal* 137 (1897): 573; Towsend and Coolidge, "Mortality of Pneumonia," pp. 43–44; Kent, "Alcoholic Stimulants," p. 73; Edward Field Parsons, "Alcohol in Therapeutics," *Proceedings of the Connecticut Medical Society,* n.s. vol. 4 (1888): 65–66; Robert Bartholow, "Alcohol: Its Therapeutic Uses, Internally and Externally," *Philadelphia Medical Times* 11 (1881): 649; H. C. Wood, "Is Alcohol a Food?" *Philadelphia Medical Times* 11 (1881): 656.

placed in contact with bacteria, and it was deduced from this that alcohol would kill bacteria when administered internally. Primary among the bacterial diseases in which alcohol was used was diphtheria, where, as one physician said, it was believed that "heroic doses are not only justifiable but almost omnipotent in rescuing the patient from the jaws of death." The more scientifically inclined physicians recognized the error in this reasoning; Hermann M. Biggs, for example, advised his colleagues in 1889 that the administration of alcohol as a germicide through sprays, inhalations, injections, or enamata in cases of tuberculosis was useless: "They have not one single physiological or pathological fact for their basis, and are founded on a kind of a sentimental system of bacteriological empiricism."[51]

Beverage alcohol was obviously popular with many patients, and some physicians complained that this was why it was prescribed so frequently. One physician observed that a prescription of alcohol "needs no thought, is easy to be made, and agreeable to the patient. The prescription costs nothing, and is quite sure to institute friendly relations." Another physician stated that in a country with taverns everywhere, physicians either had to prescribe alcohol or lose their patients.[52]

On the other side of the coin, the temperance movement and the medical profession carried on a running dispute about the therapeutic use of beverage alcohol through the last two decades of the century. Some physicians considered the temperance movement a threat to medical therapeutics. On one occasion, the Women's Christian Temperance Union addressed a questionnaire to the Michigan State Medical Society, containing complaints about the "free and sometimes reckless prescription of alcoholic liquors." A committee of the society, formed to respond to the WCTU, strongly defended the use of alcohol in therapeutics: "The cause of temperance cannot be promoted by ignoring or denying the often proved and constantly recurring benefits obtained from the use of alcohol liquors as a therapeutic agent."[53]

Thus physicians in the period after the Civil War were still limited

[51] Parsons, "Alcohol in Therapeutics," p. 65; H. D. Didama, "Should Alcohol be Used in the Treatment of Disease?" *Journal of the American Medical Association* 25 (1895): 493; Hermann M. Biggs, "The Principles of Treatment in Pulmonary Tuberculosis . . . ," *Buffalo Medical and Surgical Journal* 28 (1889): 645; G. H. Chapman, "Diphtheria; the Germ Theory and the Alcohol Treatment," *New York Medical Journal* 41 (1885): 74–76.

[52] Benoni Carpenter, "Quackery in the Regular Profession," *Boston Medical and Surgical Journal* 84 (1871): 312; "Medical Societies," *Medical and Surgical Reporter* 49 (1883): 543.

[53] Parsons, "Alcohol in Therapeutics," pp. 67–68; G. W. Toppings, "Report," *Transactions of the Michigan State Medical Society* 8 (1881): 32.

in their use of drug therapy by their almost complete ignorance of the etiology of disease, and by their consequent dependence on symptomatic treatment alone. For this reason, regularly educated physicians were not necessarily better therapists than their untrained competitors. Charles L. Dana observed in 1902: "the limit of actual medical knowledge and its inefficiency in practice made distinction between the learned and pompous physician and the unlearned vendor of drugs one of little moment at the bedside. Experience and good sense belonged to the charlatan perhaps even to a greater extent than to the erudite product of the school."[54] Nevertheless, despite the lack of progress in drug therapy, other advances in medical science during this period had profound effects on the structure of the medical profession and medical practice.

[54] Bernhard J. Stern, *American Medical Practice* (New York: Commonwealth Fund, 1945), p. 27.

CHAPTER 10 STRATIFICATION
AND SPECIALIZATION IN
THE REGULAR MEDICAL
PROFESSION AFTER
THE CIVIL WAR

AFTER THE CIVIL WAR the activities of medical societies shifted from licensing and membership restriction to a more open membership policy and a greater concern with regulation of the conduct of their members. The medical profession also became more stratified internally, as the number of wealthy physicians increased and as medical specialties developed. The wealthy physicians and the specialists formed elite medical societies to serve their own interests, which established new divisions within the profession.

DEVELOPMENTS IN MEDICAL SOCIETIES

The physicians who populated the growing number of cities and states organized many new medical societies. The estimated 125 medical societies in 1846 expanded to over 1200 in 1874, so that virtually every state then in the union had at least one medical society.[1] The increasing preponderance of medical-school graduates in the profession led medical societies to deemphasize licensing and exclusiveness and to place greater stress on the regulation of the conduct of their members. These changes were illustrated by the activities of the AMA, which was founded at the beginning of this new period in the history of medical societies.

THE AMERICAN MEDICAL ASSOCIATION

The AMA was formed in part to separate regular physicians from non-regulars, but this was virtually the only restriction in its membership policies. This decision was reached after considerable debate at its first convention. One group, including N. S. Davis, wanted the associa-

[1] Joseph M. Toner, "Address," *Transactions of the American Medical Association* 25 (1874): 71–72, n. 2; for a tabulation of state medical societies, see Stanford E. Chaille, "State Medicine and State Medical Societies," *Transactions of the American Medical Association* 30 (1879): facing p. 320.

tion to be a representative body composed of delegates chosen by medical societies, medical schools, hospitals, asylums, and other medical institutions. After a physician served as a delegate, he would become a "permanent member" of the association. Davis argued that this membership policy would give the association "a legitimate claim to the character of a true representative of the whole profession. . . . [It] would have more influence both with the profession and public, than one organized on any other plan." It would also "constantly hold a strong inducement to form and sustain in active operation, state, county, and city Associations in every state in the Union." Another group of founders wanted to make the AMA an exclusive organization. They argued that a body which elected its own members and was independent of the state and local organizations would be more stable and more effective as a scientific body. The convention's acceptance of the proposal advocated by Davis was symptomatic of the changing concerns of the profession of that time: the founders were willing to sacrifice exclusiveness to obtain greater influence with the public and greater control over the behavior of the members of the constituent societies.[2]

The AMA's adoption of the delegate system did limit its scientific activities. J. Collins Warren, a well-known surgeon, wrote in 1881 that the AMA's delegate system offered "but little inducement for membership" for physicians interested in scientific work. John S. Billings, the distinguished medical librarian, wrote in 1876 that the AMA appealed primarily to physicians who did not play a conspicuous role "as sources of addition to the science and literature of medicine." He also said that no "effectual supervision" was exercised over the content of papers read at the AMA meetings and printed in the transactions. Proposals to improve the quality of the papers by referring them to an editorial board for criticism were rejected in 1856 and 1878 on the ground that this would discourage the contributions of ordinary physicians.[3]

The major issues debated at the AMA's meetings concerned violations of the code of ethics by individual members or member societies. Charges of improprieties were often subject to disputation, and the early meetings sometimes became rancorous. Henry I. Bowditch, an eminent physician of his time and a secretary of the association during

[2] [N. S. Davis], "History of the American Medical Association," *New Jersey Medical Reporter* 7 (1854): 183–84.

[3] J. Collins Warren, "Medical Societies: their Organization and the Nature of their Work," *Medical Communications of the Massachusetts Medical Society* 12 (1881): 503; John S. Billings, "Literature and Institutions," in Edward H. Clarke *et al., A Century of American Medicine* (Philadelphia: Lea, 1876), p. 347; Donald E. Konold, *A History of American Medical Ethics 1847–1912* (Madison, Wis.: State Historical Society of Wisconsin, 1962), p. 34.

its first years, spoke of the "wild tumults which often pervaded [the early] meetings. The sessions resembled nothing, except perhaps some of the riotous displays witnessed during the closing scenes of our national congress, when both parties are very nearly balanced and party feeling runs high." The displays of temper were more muted in later years, but the issues remained the same: economic competition had to be regulated, physicians who consulted with homeopaths had to be rooted out and exposed for their doctrinal shortcomings; users of patent medicines had to be censured; in short, violators of the code of ethics had to be brought forth and exposed. Indeed, the code of ethics became so important in the organization that J. Marion Sims said of it in his AMA presidential address in 1876: "I know that there are many, indeed a large majority, of this Association who believe it to be as perfect as the Decalogue, and as incapable of improvement. It is looked up by some of its High Priests as the Holy of Holies, and not to be desecrated by the touch of vulgar hands."[4]

While the AMA's activities were meaningful and important to its members, they were insufficient to make the organization large and influential. The AMA led a sporadic, haphazard, conflict-ridden existence during its first several decades. Warren stated that between the annual meetings "the association is a blank; beyond the feeble efforts of a few committees, its work seems to have come to a stand-still." Another physician complained in 1879 that the AMA did not know the correct titles, addresses, or membership of its component state societies, and had made no effort to secure the information.[5] Even the annual meetings themselves were more social than professional gatherings. Henry Bigelow observed in 1871:

> The American Medical Association is a body of medical gentlemen, practically volunteer delegates, having primarily in view the agreeable and commendable object of a journey to break the monotony of medical practice and give them an apology for leaving their homes and their patients at a pleasant season of the year. They assemble to revive old friendships, to form new acquaintances, to make excursions, and to settle down into relations of good fellowship, after a healthy difference of opinion over current medical topics and parliamentary forms.[6]

4 "Minutes," *Transactions of the American Medical Association* 28 (1877): 54; J. Marion Sims, "Address," *Transactions of the American Medical Association* 27 (1876): 96.
5 Warren, "Medical Societies," p. 505; Chaille, "State Medicine," pp. 310–11.
6 Henry J. Bigelow, "Medical Education in America," *Medical Communications of the Massachusetts Medical Society* 11 (1871): 234. Billings shared Bigelow's view of the delegates to the AMA convention: Billings, "Literature and Institutions," p. 347.

By the early 1870's, the AMA's debates had become so notorious that many leaders of the profession seriously questioned the association's usefulness. The *Boston Medical and Surgical Journal* spoke of its "downward progress to disgraceful imbecility," and the *Medical Record* of New York City suggested that the association required wholesale reorganization. These and other criticisms led to the first major change in the AMA's structure. In 1874, the association created a judicial council which was empowered to decide all code violations in private, away from the floor of the convention. Although this served to restrain the excesses of previous meetings, it did not alter the organization fundamentally. In 1877, Bowditch observed that the organization's prestige among the prominent men of the profession was still low and that they did not participate in its activities.[7]

STATE AND LOCAL MEDICAL SOCIETIES

The activities of state and local societies were basically the same as those of the AMA. The local societies met more regularly and were composed of individual members rather than delegates, but their activities also consisted largely of regulating the professional behavior of their members. Local societies were more successful than the AMA in maintaining their standing in the profession, because they were more significant to their members. Membership in the AMA provided some prestige, but membership in a local society was, according to Austin Flint, "essential to an unequivocal professional status." It demonstrated that the member was orthodox in his sectarianism, and gave him access to consultations and opportunities for appointments to dispensaries, clinics, hospitals, medical school faculties, etc.[8]

ELITE MEDICAL SOCIETIES

The regional medical societies were advantageous to those physicians who wanted to regulate the economic conditions of the profession. Some physicians, however, were not interested in these activities. The best educated, wealthiest, and most successful physicians did not suffer extensive competition from their colleagues and therefore were not likely to be concerned with codes of ethics and fee bills. Neither were they concerned with consultations with irregular practitioners,

---

[7] "The American Medical Association," *Boston Medical and Surgical Journal* 87 (1872): 69; "Shall We Have Another American Medical Association," *Medical Record* 8 (1873): 205–6; "Minutes," *Transactions of the American Medical Association* 24 (1873): 35–36; Henry I. Bowditch, "Address," *Transactions of the American Medical Association* 28 (1877): 99.

[8] Austin Flint, "The First Century of the Republic: Medical and Sanitary Progress," *Harper's New Monthly Magazine* 53 (1876): 72.

nor with licensing legislation to control entry into the profession. John S. Billings commented:

These physicians, whose positions are fairly assured, and who, as a rule, have all the practice they desire, are not usually active leaders in movements to secure medical legislation, although they passively assent to such efforts, or at least do not oppose them; and their names may sometimes be found appended to memorials urging such legislation. They are clear-headed, shrewd, "practical" men, who know that their business interests are not specially injured by quacks and ignoramuses, rather the contrary in fact, for they are called on to repair the damage done by the quack to people who have more money than brains; and they are not inclined to risk [their positions on] other people's troubles.[9]

It is, he continued, rather the "young men who have not yet acquired local fame" who "feel the competition of the local herb-doctor or of the traveling quack more keenly, and have more decided views about the importance of diplomas." These physicians are "apt to become very indignant over the doings of some charlatan in the neighbourhood, or of some druggist who prescribes over the counter" and "are usually quite clear in their minds that the State ought to interfere and prevent injury to the health of the people." Thus, for example, N. S. Davis observed that one feature of the early meetings of the AMA was "the absence of those to whom the profession had long been accustomed to look as leaders in all important professional matters. . . . it may be said with propriety, that the Convention was composed of the younger, more active, and perhaps, more ambitious members of the profession." The elite of the profession was simply unconcerned with those facets of medical practice of greatest concern to the AMA—reducing the number of physicians by raising the standards of medical education and regulating professional behavior through a code of ethics.[10]

The concerns of the elite physicians had not changed since the beginning of the century: they still wanted to separate themselves from the rank-and-file of the profession and to develop some mechanism for sharing prestige and the emoluments to be gained from interaction among themselves. Indeed, such organizations were even more important than in the past as the ranks of the profession multiplied. The estimated 36,000 regular physicians in 1850 grew to over 110,000 by 1900.[11] Thus once again elite physicians formed small, select organizations for prestige and mutual economic benefits.

The nominal basis of these elite societies was scientific. In most

9 John Shaw Billings, *Selected Papers* (n.p.: Medical Library Association, 1965), p. 191.

10 *Ibid.*; Davis, "History of the American Medical Association," p. 48.

11 See Appendix IV.

large cities the elite of the profession formed local societies with the stated objective of scientific inquiry. However, Billings claimed that these societies seldom brought out "the best work of their members," and their work very rarely compared with that of the London and Paris societies. Their success was actually due to the prestige and power of their members. In New York, for example, 17 of the 34 members of the Medical and Surgical Society held teaching positions in the three medical schools in the city in 1866 and constituted a large majority of their total faculties. Members of the same society held about half of the consulting and attending appointments at the city's hospitals and dispensaries. The New York Academy of Medicine was a larger elite organization in the same city, and the members of the Medical and Surgical Society were active in its leadership. Other prestigious organizations appealed to other groups of physicians in the city. At the bottom of the hierarchy was the county medical society, which was open to all regular physicians. The members of the Medical and Surgical Society were not active in this organization.[12]

Most of the elite societies had some informal connection with a medical school or a hospital. In Cincinnati, for example, the Academy of Medicine, founded in 1857, was the open membership society. The Cincinnati Medical Society, founded in 1874, was the elite organization whose members were affiliated with a local medical school.[13] A close relationship with a medical school provided the maximum amount of mutual self-interest for a professional clique, according to the editor of the *Medical Record*:

There are always several so-called professional rings which exist in large towns and cities. The principal ones are those which revolve around a particular college, and are almost absolute in their exclusiveness. The members of the faculties and the lesser lights are bound by an honorable understanding to look after each other on any and every occasion. . . .

The college ring is usually a perfect one, and contains all those elements of self-interest which give it its greatest strength. It is well understood that no case for consultation goes begging outside the circle. The professor of medicine always sends his surgical cases for opinion to the professor of surgery, and so on to the end of the chapter.[14]

These elite societies excluded many physicians who would have liked to participate in them. The wealthier outsiders therefore tended

[12] Billings, "Literature and Institutions," p. 349; Charles Rosenberg, "The Practice of Medicine in New York a Century Ago," *Bulletin of the History of Medicine* 41 (1967): 227–28.

[13] Otto Juettner, *Daniel Drake and His Followers* (Cincinnati: Harvey, 1909), pp. 446, 454–56. The two organizations merged in 1893.

[14] "Medical Cliquism," *Medical Record* 12 (1877): 521.

to form competing elite societies. For example, the Boston Society for Medical Improvement was founded in 1828 as an elite organization which soon became a major influence in the local profession. Some younger physicians who were excluded from membership formed a competing society in 1835, the Boston Society for Medical Observation. The two organizations were both important in the local profession until their merger in 1894.[15]

In this way, elite and not-so-elite societies proliferated in large cities, and any well-informed local physician of the time could have ranked them according to wealth, power, and prestige. A list of the local regular medical societies in New York City in the years between 1870 and 1874 would have included the following, gathered from lists of delegates at AMA conventions during that period and from the study by Rosenberg:

> East River Medical Association of the City of New York
> New York Academy of Medicine
> New York County Medical Society
> New York Medical Union
> New York Dermatological Society
> New York Medical Association
> New York Medical Library and Journal Association
> New York Medical and Surgical Society
> New York Medico-Legal Society
> New York Obstetrical Society
> New York Pathological Society
> Order of Aesculapius (New York)
> Roman Medical Society of New York
> Society of German Physicians[16]

This incomplete list had to be supplemented at least by the alumni associations of the local medical colleges and probably by other associations of physicians with the same ethnic background. While New York City medical societies were undoubtedly more numerous than those in other communities, multiple societies were common in virtually every large city in the country.

SOCIAL STRATIFICATION IN THE MEDICAL PROFESSION

Elite societies were manifestations of increasingly important distinctions among the physicians of large cities—gross differentials in wealth, social position, and influence. Young physicians beginning practice in

15 J. G. Mumford, "The Story of the Boston Society for Medical Improvement," *Boston Medical and Surgical Journal* 144 (1901): 247–53.

16 *Transactions of the American Medical Association* 21–25 (1870–74); Rosenberg, "Medicine in New York," pp. 227–28.

New York City after the Civil War earned about $400 a year. A very eminent surgeon who died in New York City in 1865 left an estate of almost a million dollars. The young physicians obviously did not travel in the same professional or social circles as the surgeon. Income was not the only basis of stratification within the profession. Ethnic background constituted a source of professional distinction. No immigrants were members of the New York Medical and Surgical Society, even though some of the city's leading medical scholars were immigrants. Ostentatious display also became common. Wealthy San Francisco physicians, for example, often owned foreign-made gold-plated instruments and rode to work "behind spick and span horses drawing costly landaus or victorias, with liveried drivers, shiny harnesses and fashionable coach dogs."[17]

The differences in wealth and status were manifestations of more fundamental differences within the profession. John S. Billings wrote the following discerning description of the major social strata in the medical profession in 1875:

We have had, and still have, a very few men who love science for its own sake, whose chief pleasure is in original investigations, and to whom the practice of their profession is mainly, or only, of interest as furnishing material for observation and comparison. . . . The work of our physicians of this class has been for the most part fragmentary, and is found in scattered papers and essays . . . ; but buds and flowers, rather than ripened fruit, are what we have to offer. Of the highest grade of this class we have thus far produced no specimens; the John Hunter, or Virchow, of the United States, has not yet given any sign of existence.

We have in our cities, great and small, a much larger class of physicians whose principal object is to obtain money, or rather the social position, pleasures, and power, which money only can bestow. They are clear-headed, shrewd, practical men, well educated, because "it pays," and for the same reason they take good care to be supplied with the best instruments, and the latest literature. Many of them take up specialties because the work is easier, and the hours of labour are more under their control than in general practice. They strive to become connected with hospitals and medical schools, not for love of mental exertion, or of science for its own sake, but as a respectable means of advertising, and of obtaining consultations. They write and lecture to keep their names before the public, and they must do both well, or fall behind in the race. They have the greater part of the valuable practice, and their writings, which constitute the greater part of our medical literature, are respectable in quality, and eminently useful.

They are the patrons of medical literature, the active working members of municipal medical societies, the men who are usually accepted as the representatives of the profession, not only here, but in all civilized countries; they

[17] *Ibid.*, pp. 228–29; Henry Harris, *California's Medical Story* (San Francisco: Stacey, 1932), pp. 261–62.

may be famous physicians and great surgeons in the usual sense of the words, and as such, and only as such, should they receive the honour which is justly their due. They work for the present, and they have their reward in their own generation.

There is another large class, whose defects in general culture and in knowledge of the latest improvements in medicine, have been much dwelt upon by those disposed to take gloomy views of the condition of medical education in this country. The preliminary education of these physicians was defective, in some cases from lack of desire for it, but in the great majority from lack of opportunity, and their work in the medical school was confined to so much memorizing of text-books as was necessary to secure a diploma. In the course of practice they gradually obtain from personal experience, sometimes of a disagreeable kind, a knowledge of therapeutics, which enables them to treat the majority of their cases as successfully, perhaps, as their brethren more learned in theory. Occasionally they contribute a paper to a journal, or a report to a medical society; but they would rather talk than write, and find it very difficult to explain how or why they have succeeded, being like many excellent cooks in this respect. They are honest, conscientious, hard-working men, who are inclined to place great weight on their experience, and to be rather contemptuous of what they call "book learning and theories." To them our medical literature is indebted for a few interesting observations, and valuable suggestions in therapeutics, but for the most part, their experience, being unrecorded, has but a local usefulness.

These three classes have been referred to simply for the purpose of calling attention to the fact that, in speaking of "the physicians of the United States," it is necessary to be careful. There are many other classes, and they shade into each other and into empiricism in many ways.[18]

Billings argued that physicians were readily differentiated into several social strata, varying in degrees of wealth, fame, social position, power within the profession, and influence in the community. He traced all these differences to one fundamental factor: the professional knowledge of the physician. Physicians who were well-educated, aware of the latest scientific developments, equipped with and competent to use the finest instruments and facilities were the men who held appointments in medical schools and hospitals, wrote articles for medical journals, obtained frequent consultations, and were the most successful members of the profession. Thus he found a direct relationship between professional competence and social status in the profession.[19] To be sure, other elements did enter into the picture. Family background and wealth, social standing, and friendships were paramount in gaining admission to a medical school, setting up a practice, obtain-

18 Billings, "Literature and Institutions," pp. 363–65.

19 It should not be thought that differentials in professional skill are the result of intelligence alone or even primarily. Differences in social class enable some medical students to attend better schools, obtain post-graduate education, and purchase more and better equipment.

ing appointments to hospitals, medical schools, and elite medical societies, and attracting a wealthy clientele. Billings did not necessarily neglect these; rather, even these upper-class physicians had to maintain a superior level of competence or else "fall behind in the race."

If professional competence was the primary source of success in medical practice, and if a superior medical education was the major vehicle for attaining greater competence, then the route to professional distinction was obvious. Aspiring physicians should obtain as much education in the best medical schools as possible. Because both lengthy education and high-quality education were expensive, this alone would force many physicians out of the race. However, the number of competitors eliminated in this manner was inadequate to assure success to the survivors. The physician seeking the highest distinction had to go one step further. He had to specialize, to differentiate himself from his competitors not only in the amount of his knowledge, but also in the character of that knowledge. Specialization could maximize a physician's chances for success by minimizing his potential competition. Therefore, as Billings observed, most of the more successful and important members of the profession in the last half of the century were specialists.

SPECIALIZATION IN THE MEDICAL PROFESSION

THE DEVELOPMENT OF MEDICAL SPECIALTIES[20]

Specialization could not develop in medicine until a number of conditions were fulfilled: (1) a medically valid body of medical knowledge and techniques had to develop in a given specialty; (2) urban population aggregates had to become sufficiently large to support a specialist in the practice of his specialty; and (3) institutions and arrangements within the profession had to make it financially rewarding for a physician to restrict his practice to a specialty.

A medically valid body of knowledge developed in certain specialties during the middle of the nineteenth century. The division of labor in the medical schools gave impetus to specialization in medicine. Even more important were several major discoveries and inventions which had immediate practical consequences for medicine. The discovery of anesthetics in the late 1840's made surgery painless and enabled physicians to place less emphasis on speed and more on precision. The ophthalmoscope was invented in 1851 and the laryngoscope in 1855. These instruments enabled physicians to examine the eye,

[20] This account relies heavily on George Rosen, *The Specialization of Medicine* (New York: Froben Press, 1944).

larynx, and ear with much greater precision and to refine and develop their knowledge of those organs.[21]

The invention of an instrument like the ophthalmoscope was not in itself sufficient to cause an increase in the body of knowledge about the eye. It was also necessary to observe numerous cases of various kinds of eye diseases and to obtain first-hand knowledge of the effects of various treatments on large numbers of cases. A large population of patients with eye diseases was needed to provide cases for accurate description, analysis, and treatment. Such a situation exists only in a large city, where a sufficient number of residents suffering from disorders of specific organs can be found. Specialization, therefore, depended upon urbanization for its development, and urbanization in America was a nineteenth-century phenomenon.

Furthermore, institutions had to be devised to bring numerous cases to the specialist and to permit him to treat them under controlled conditions. One such institution was the specialty hospital, whose visibility and accessibility attracted many patients with relevant disorders. For example, an eye infirmary which opened in New York City in 1818 to treat poor patients gratuitously soon became sufficiently well known to provide the staff of physicians with an ample supply of patients.

Another institution was the medical society, which provided specialists with a means of notifying their colleagues of their special interests and persuading general practitioners to refer cases to them. Specialty medical societies enabled specialists to communicate their knowledge to each other in meetings and through professional journals (the latter serving as a vehicle for the international as well as the national promulgation of knowledge), and in this way contributed to the expansion of knowledge in the specialty.

One more factor was required, however, to induce physicians to limit their practice to a specialty. It was one thing to study a specialty and to use that knowledge in one's medical practice; it was quite another to limit one's entire practice to a specialty and to refuse all unrelated cases. Specialization had to be profitable, and it became profitable only when specialists had sufficient medically valid knowledge to attract patients whom general practitioners were unable to treat. This situation developed in America in the 1870's and 1880's.

---

21 A. C. Furstenberg, "A Chronicle of 100 Years of Otolaryngology," *Laryngoscope* 57 (1947): 599; Thomas J. Harris, "The Early Years of the American Otological Society . . . ," *Annals of Otology, Rhinology, and Laryngology* 35 (1926): 459; Arthur J. Bedell, "The First Ten Years of Ophthalmoscopy, 1851–1861," *Transactions of the American Ophthalmological Society*, 1951, 86th meeting, p. 38.

In 1886, William Brodie, president of the AMA, said that physicians had begun "to realize that by devoting themselves to one branch instead of working up a general practice, they could often do more good, earn more money, and have less arduous work to perform."[22]

Specialists and specialties multiplied during the last decades of the century. Ophthalmology was the first major specialty, but surgery soon overtook it in scientific precision and importance, and numerous others assumed stature in the profession. Training programs for specialists developed in Europe more rapidly than in America, and thousands of wealthy American physicians found it worthwhile to travel to Vienna, Berlin, and other European centers to obtain post-graduate instruction in medical specialties.[23] Specialization also fragmented the curriculum of American medical colleges. One physician said of changes in one academic area in 1880:

> Thirty years ago the Chair of Obstetrics included the Diseases of Women and Children, and embraced some forty lectures, in which the forceps . . . were shown to the class by a professor who perhaps had applied them half a dozen times in his life . . . , while the vaginal speculum, if known to the professor, was hardly exhibited. . . . Now there are delivered during each regular session some thirty or forty didactic lectures on Obstetrics, and some thirty or forty more on the Diseases of Women, while the Clinical Professor of Gynecology delivers some fifty lectures with an almost unlimited amount of clinical material . . . ; moreover the subject of the diseases of Children is turned over to another professor.[24]

Thus specialization rapidly became a major influence on all aspects of medicine and medical practice.

REACTIONS OF GENERAL PRACTITIONERS TO SPECIALIZATION

Fundamentally, specialization was no different than the use of secret nostrums: in both instances, physicians claimed to offer services unavailable from their competitors. It was therefore hardly surprising that general practitioners reacted to specialization much as they had responded to sales of secret nostrums by physicians. When specialization was just beginning to develop in the 1850's, some general practitioners suggested that specialists be ostracized from the profession and denied representation in the AMA. The editor of the *Medical Record*

---

[22] George Rosen, "Changing Attitudes of the Medical Profession to Specialization," *Bulletin of the History of Medicine* 12 (1942): 352.

[23] S. Weir Mitchell, "The History of Instrumental Precision in Medicine," *University Medical Magazine* 4 (1891): 2; Thomas Neville Bonner, *American Doctors and German Universities* (Lincoln, Neb.: University of Nebraska Press, 1963), pp. 73–78.

[24] G. M. B. Maughs, "Medical Ultraisms," *Transactions of the Missouri State Medical Association*, 23d session, 1880, p. 21.

later recalled that any practitioner who defended specialization at that time "risked his reputation for respectability and invited aspersions on his professional integrity."[25] As late as 1866, the president of the AMA, Humphreys Storer, bluntly warned specialists in his presidential address:

A growing disposition is apparent in a portion of the profession to direct their individual attention to some one department, to the exclusion of others; to confine their researches to the derangements of one organ or system of organs, to stand aloof from the rest of their brethren; to disclaim the title of general practitioner, and to assume that of specialist. . . .

It is not surprising that much diversity of opinion should exist as to the expedience or propriety of a step which in this country is comparatively new, and which may be considered as an inroad, an interference, something subversive of old and cherished opinions. Our brethren . . . look with suspicion upon any act which implies important changes, which would tend to affect its conservatism.[26]

General practitioners justified their hostility to specialization by claiming that it led to a "heedless neglect of general medicine," according to an 1875 report of a committee of the Medical Society of the State of New York. The committee deplored the tendency of physicians to specialize before they became competent general practitioners, and claimed that younger physicians specialized only because they saw the financial and professional success of some older specialists.[27]

However, the advance of specialization could not be stopped. Even the New York medical society committee conceded that "the progress of medicine depends on the continual efforts of specialists."[28] By 1880, as one physician observed, specialists dominated urban medical practice:

Within the last thirty years departments of the healing art that were embraced within the narrowest limits have widened into vast fields that engage the labors of the most intelligent and industrious to comprehend them. This has been accomplished by the division of labor whereby men of talent by devoting themselves to a single branch of medicine have been enabled to develop it to an extent otherwise impossible. But while by this division of labor an infinite amount of good has been accomplished, which would have been impossible had all been general practitioners, there is now danger lest, all being specialists, none shall be general practitioners. Indeed in some of our large cities specialism is now carried to such an extreme, and the human body is so nicely mapped out and divided, that there is only left

25 "Specialism as a Practice," *Medical Record* 10 (1875): 489.

26 D. Humphreys Storer, "Address," *Transactions of the American Medical Association* 17 (1866): 56.

27 "Specialties in Medicine," *Medical Record* 10 (1875): 158.

28 *Ibid.*

to the general practitioner or family physician the umbilicus. In country districts where from necessity the physician has to treat all diseases, and consequently where specialism is an impossibility, the family doctor still holds his own; but in all our large cities and densely populated districts specialism revels in tropical luxuriance.[29]

RELATIONS BETWEEN GENERAL PRACTITIONERS AND SPECIALISTS

The proliferation of specialists adversely affected the economic well-being of many general practitioners, who were now confronted with the dilemma of treating patients themselves or referring them to specialists. Cathell had only contempt for the weak-willed general practitioner who chose the latter course:

Never turn your cases over to *"specialists,"* but keep them under your own watchful supervision, unless they present features which render it an actual duty to do so. If you distrust your own capacities, shrink and shirk and timidly refer your cases [to specialists] . . . , you will soon lose all familiarity with the diseases that specialists treat, they will be "out of my line," and you will dwindle and degenerate into a mere distributor of cases . . . advancing everybody's professional and pecuniary interest except your own, aiding them to gain the admiration of the community, and to make reputation and fees out of that which sinks your own individuality, robs your own purse, and throws (little) you into the shade. . . . Timidity, from a want of confidence in one's own merits, and rashness are both bad traits in a physician, but the former is the greater drawback, since every physician's success must be within himself and must come out of himself. . . .[30]

General practitioners also complained that specialists engaged in a number of unethical practices. According to Storer, specialists were often self-proclaimed without any formal training for their specialty; they sometimes treated cases outside their specialty; they obtained higher fees than did general practitioners; and they tended to "ridicule the course pursued by the older men of the profession," who were general practitioners. The greatest problem was advertising, according to an AMA committee. Specialists advertised their specialties in medical and public journals, and sent handbills to their colleagues notifying them of their specialties.[31]

Eventually the AMA, as the ultimate source of the codes of medical ethics, was forced to rule on the legitimacy of specialization. A committee of the Association which reported in 1866 was divided on the

[29] Maughs, "Medical Ultraisms," pp. 23–24.

[30] D. W. Cathell, *Book on the Physician Himself* (Philadelphia: Davis, 1895), 10th edition, pp. 208–9.

[31] Storer, "Address," pp. 57–60; Worthington Hooker and James Kennedy, "Report of the Committee of Medical Ethics on Specialties," and Henry J. Bowditch, "Minority Report," *Transactions of the American Medical Association* 17 (1866): 503–12.

issue, but in 1869 the delegates passed a number of resolutions defining relations between general practitioners and specialists. The resolutions recognized specialties, but bound specialists to the code of ethics and banned advertising by specialists. Exclusive practitioners of specialties were permitted to notify the public in limited ways, but not through handbills or the mass media.[32]

Considering the hostility of so many general practitioners to specialists, these resolutions were surprisingly mild and even sympathetic to specialization. This occurred because specialists had become very powerful men in the profession. Specialists controlled the elite medical societies, dominated the faculties of the medical colleges and the staffs of the hospitals, clinics and dispensaries, and many had wealthy and powerful clients. Specialists soon assumed a dominant position in the AMA itself, as shown by an analysis of the type of practice of AMA presidents from 1850 to 1899 (Table X.1). Surgeons dominated the presidency after 1880 and often assumed the position even before that time.[33]

SPECIALTY MEDICAL SOCIETIES

While general practitioners eventually resigned themselves to the presence of specialists in their societies, specialists found the general medical societies ineffective for the promotion of their interests.

TABLE X.1
PRESIDENTS OF THE AMERICAN MEDICAL ASSOCIATION BY TYPE OF PRACTICE, 1850–99

Years	General Practitioners*	Surgeons	Other Specialists
1850–1859	6	3	1
1860–1869**	4	2	1
1870–1879	5	3	2
1880–1889	4	5	1
1890–1899	2	7	1

* Including physicians not in private practice.
** No meetings held in 1861 and 1862; the same president served in 1864 and 1865.

SOURCE: Morris Fishbein, *A History of the American Medical Association 1847 to 1947* (Philadelphia: W. B. Saunders, 1947), pp. 579–678.

[32] "Minutes," *Transactions of the American Medical Association* 20 (1869): 28–29.
[33] Fishbein's data did not reveal whether the AMA presidents described here as specialists limited their practices to specialties or simply devoted special attention to them. Given the historical development of specialties in the United States, it is improbable that most of the specialists listed before 1880 actually limited their practices to the specialties described in Fishbein's history.

Local specialty societies were formed in many large cities and replaced the scientific medical societies as the elite societies of the profession. Numerous national specialty societies were also founded during this period (Table X.2). Many national specialty societies had extremely restrictive membership policies which limited their total membership to fifty or one hundred members and required new members to be elected by an almost unanimous vote of the membership.[34]

N. S. Davis, the leading figure in the AMA of the time, stated that specialty societies were formed because the AMA refused to grant specialists concessions on advertising. He believed that specialty societies fragmented the profession:

> In proportion as it became evident that no concessions [toward permitting advertising by specialists] could be obtained through the national organization, it also became apparent that these restless classes were taking less interest in the general organization, and inclining to the formation of societies of their own. This disintegrating influence has continued to increase until we have general and local organizations, distinct from either the State or national societies, representing not only every specialty worthy of mention, but also some having no well defined purpose. . . . We have thus lost in some measure the unity of our professional organization, and in the same proportion we have come to perceive clearly the existence of diverse, if not directly antagonistic interests. So much so, indeed, that it has become quite

TABLE X.2
DATE OF FOUNDING OF NATIONAL SPECIALTY MEDICAL SOCIETIES, 1864–1902

Date of Founding	Organization
1864	American Ophthalmological Society
1868	American Otological Society
1875	American Neurological Association
1876	American Dermatological Association
	American Gynecological Society
1879	American Laryngological Association
1880	American Surgical Association
1886	American Association of Genito-Urinary Surgeons
1887	American Orthopedic Association
1888	American Pediatric Society
1895	American Laryngological, Rhinological and Otological Society
1896	American Academy of Ophthalmology and Otolaryngology
1897	American Gastroenterological Association
1899	American Proctological Society
1902	American Urological Association

SOURCE: Margaret Fisk, ed., *Encyclopedia of Associations*, 6th ed., vol. 1, (Detroit: Gale Research Co.: 1970).

[34] [N. S. Davis], "An Important Question," *Journal of the American Medical Association* 11 (1888): 741–42.

common to hear the interests of the general practitioner and the wants of the specialist spoken of as essentially distinct.[35]

Specialists, however, claimed that the ineptitude of the AMA forced them to turn to independent societies. The eminent surgeon, Samuel D. Gross, said in his presidential address to the American Surgical Association in 1883: "If it be said that we are striking a blow at the American Medical Association, we deny this soft impeachment. On the contrary we shall strengthen that body by rousing it from its 'Rip Van Winkle slumbers' and infusing new life into it." Abraham Jacobi, one of the outstanding physicians of his time and a president of the AMA, stated that the national specialty societies were founded by physicians "who had no time to spare for entertainment, excursions, medico-political wrangling and other pastimes" of the AMA. Even Davis was forced to concede that "the absence of clear, definite, well-considered plans or lines of inquiry and schemes of original investigation" was a major defect of the AMA.[36]

Overall, several factors contributed to the formation of specialty medical societies. First of all, specialty organizations provided a valuable service for their members by promulgating recent advances in the specialty, which had never been a major activity of the AMA. Second, the AMA was a large and relatively open organization, and specialists tended to form small exclusive organizations which provided prestige and other economic advantages. Third, specialists did have interests distinct from those of general practitioners: specialists used clinics and hospitals more extensively, and were much more concerned with becoming well known in the professional community. The AMA and the general medical societies failed to satisfy these and other needs of specialists, who therefore formed their own societies.

THE CONGRESS OF AMERICAN PHYSICIANS AND SURGEONS

In 1888, a Congress of American Physicians and Surgeons was formed as a federation of the most prominent national specialty societies. Each member national society held separate annual meetings for two years, and on the third year all the societies held their meetings simultaneously in Washington, D.C., when the congress held its triennial meeting. Several reasons were advanced for the formation of

35 N. S. Davis, "Address on the Present Status and Future Tendencies of the Medical Profession in the United States . . . ," *Journal of the American Medical Association* 1 (1883): 37–38.

36 J. Englebert Dunphy, "Medical Care, Education and Research," *New England Journal of Medicine* 271 (1964): 1245; A. Jacobi, "Medicine and Medical Men in the United States," *Journal of the American Medical Association* 35 (1900): 430; Davis, "Present Status of Medical Profession," p. 38.

the Congress. Jacobi stated that "the fear of unchecked specialism" was a major reason. Other founders wished to provide a mechanism whereby members of more than one specialty society could attend the meetings of all their societies with a minimum amount of inconvenience and expense. Probably the most significant reasons for the formation of the congress were to maintain the elite membership standards of the member societies and to prevent the establishment of duplicate societies in any one specialty. The congress took several steps to insure this. Additional societies could become members of the congress only with unanimous approval of all eleven member societies. Because the member societies represented practically all of the existing specialties, they would oppose the admission of new organizations duplicating their areas of interest. According to the chairman of the executive committee of the congress, this would prevent the "needless increase of societies devoted to minute fragments of medical science [that] would have a disintegrating and injurious result." Furthermore, participation in the meetings of the congress was limited to a small number of members chosen by each of the member societies as their "guests," although any physician could listen to a session of the congress. This was done, according to the chairman, to encourage the same men to attend successive meetings "in order to produce the best scientific results. . . ."[37] He stated further that these policies would insure the continued exclusiveness of the member specialty societies:

Each society participating will be stimulated to continuous and lofty endeavors. Membership in any of these bodies will come to be regarded as more and more an honor; and in time the scientific qualifications of candidates will be more and more strictly scrutinized. . . .

If it is to remain a high and coveted honor to be a member of the Congress of American Physicians and Surgeons, it will be because each special society guards its portals even more and more strictly: makes genuine ability and solid work the indispensable qualifications for admission; and continued scientific activity the recognized duty of membership.[38]

The leaders of the AMA were critical of the congress. N. S. Davis accused the directors of the congress of being "actuated by the desire that the [congress] should ultimately displace and supersede the American Medical Association." On its side, the congress initially attempted

[37] Jacobi, "Medicine and Medical Men," p. 430; "Historical Introduction," *Transactions of the Congress of American Physicians and Surgeons* 1 (1888): xiv; "Minutes," *Transactions of the Congress of American Physicians and Surgeons* 1 (1888): xxvi, xxiv; "The Congress of American Physicians and Surgeons," *New York Medical Journal* 48 (1888): 250.

[38] "Minutes," *Transactions of the Congress of American Physicians and Surgeons* 1 (1888): xxv, xxxvi.

to placate the AMA. The chairman of the executive committee said at its first meeting that the directors of the congress were "warmly attached" to the American Medical Association and "determined to exert their influence to maintain and promote" its success. They believed that the plan of their organization "would prevent even the least interference" with the AMA. At the congress's second meeting in 1891, the chairman went somewhat further in defining its role. He stated that the national specialty societies and the congress formed a structure parallel to that of the AMA and "doubted if further steps are needed in the organization of the medical professional in this country."[39]

Davis, however, had dismissed the congress in 1888 as no real threat to the AMA. He said at that time:

Instead of . . . having any serious tendency to supersede the American Medical Association, it will only serve as a convenient and really useful place in which the small but respectable class of exclusionists can work and dine without personal contact with the sunburned and weatherbeaten general practitioners of the healing art.[40]

Davis was an astute observer of medical politics, and he was correct in his assessment. The congress had fewer than 500 members in its constituent societies combined, no effective policy-making body, infrequent meetings, and little interest in medical politics. More basically, specialists obtained nothing from the congress which could not be obtained from other societies. The specialty societies offered their members all the prestige and technical information they desired, and the general societies were the only societies large and powerful enough to affect the economic position of the profession. For these reasons the congress never became an important influence in the profession.

Whatever their differences, all regular medical societies maintained a policy of rigidly excluding physicians who used the therapies of other sects. Homeopaths and other non-regular physicians were therefore compelled to develop independent institutional structures, which paralleled those of the regular sect.

---

[39] Davis, "An Important Question," p. 741; "Minutes," *Transactions of the Congress of American Physicians and Surgeons* 1 (1888): xxiv; 2 (1891): xiv–xv.
[40] Davis, "An Important Question," p. 742.

CHAPTER 11 THE ECLECTIC SECT:
SUCCESSOR TO
BOTANICAL MEDICINE

ECLECTIC MEDICINE was the only botanical movement to become a major force in American medical practice after the Civil War. Eclectic physicians differed from most other botanical practitioners in that they did not limit their practice to botanical remedies. The intellectual fountainhead of the eclectic movement and its major medical school was the Eclectic Medical Institute in Cincinnati. The practices espoused by this school after the Civil War paralleled those of the regular profession in most important respects.

The professional Thomsonian and other botanical practitioners who sought to turn Thomsonism into a medical sect succeeded only in fragmenting it into a number of factions. Alva Curtis, alone among Thomsonian leaders, was able to develop a reasonably stable institutional structure. He and his supporters held a national convention, formed a few regional medical societies, and chartered eight medical colleges—four in the South, two in Ohio, one in New York City, and one in Massachusetts. Although Curtis's faction survived until the twentieth century in the form of "physio-medicalism," it never became a prominent part of American medical practice. The other Thomsonian factions lost their popularity after the Civil War and dwindled away.[1]

THE ORIGINS OF ECLECTICISM

One group emerged out of this melange as a successful and influential medical sect in the nineteenth century. Its founder was Wooster Beach (1794–1868), a medical school graduate who also studied with botanical practitioners. Beach became a critic of heroic therapy and turned to

[1] Alex Berman, "Neo-Thomsonianism in the United States," *Journal of the History of Medicine and Allied Sciences* 11 (1956): 133–55; Alex Berman, "The Impact of the Nineteenth Century Botanico-Medical Movement on American Pharmacy and Medicine" (Ph.D. Dissertation: University of Wisconsin, 1954), pp. 133–44.

Thomsonians, Indian doctors, herb doctors, and others for ideas on medical practice. Because he drew his ideas from all these sources, he decided to call himself an eclectic. This was an apt description, because Beach never did develop any systematic or sectarian dogma and did not limit his practice to botanical medicines.[2]

Beach founded the United States Infirmary in New York City in 1827 and turned it into the Reformed Medical Academy two years later. He was unable to secure a charter from the state to confer degrees, and the school languished. Thomson's movement was demonstrating its great appeal to the midwestern population about this same time and Beach decided to establish a branch of his school in the midwest. He managed to locate a defunct liberal-arts college in Worthington, Ohio, with a charter from the state to issue degrees. Using the charter of this institution, a number of Beach's colleagues opened a medical school in 1830. The school was quite popular with the local population, and its faculty members supplanted the regular physician in the community. Part of the reason for the early success of the school was that a number of the faculty members adopted Thomson's system. Thomson himself complained in his *Narrative* that the faculty used all his medicines "in manner and form, as I had laid down in my books," and that, if these medicines were taken from them, "their Institution would not be worth one cent." He added that they did not even purchase a right from him: that "would have been too much for such dignitaries; but, to steal it from a *quack*, was, perhaps, in their estimation, much more honorable!!!" Ideological quarrels soon developed among the faculty and were intensified by the inadequate financing of the school. In 1839, the local population attacked the school in an anti-dissection riot following the disappearance of the corpse of a deceased resident, and the school closed the next year.[3]

A few of the faculty moved to Cincinnati, and although their charter had been revoked by the legislature, they began a series of lectures on medicine in 1842. The legislature granted them a charter in 1845 after receiving a petition signed by "1,100 of the foremost citizens, including the mayor and members of the City Council," according to Felter's history of the school. Beach himself joined the faculty in that year, and the Eclectic Medical Institute of Cincinnati began a long career which ended in 1939.[4]

[2] Jonathan Forman, "The Worthington Medical College," *Ohio State Archaeological and Historical Quarterly* 50 (1941): 376.

[3] *Ibid.*, pp. 375–79; Samuel Thomson, *Narrative of the Life and Medical Discoveries of the Author* (Boston: 1832), p. 182; Harvey Wickes Felter, *History of the Eclectic Medical Institute, Cincinnati, Ohio, 1845–1902* (Cincinnati, Ohio: 1902), pp. 15–17.

[4] *Ibid.*, pp. 19–24.

In the next decade, the institute underwent what must have been the most extraordinary period in the history of any American medical school. In 1846 Joseph Rhodes Buchanan was appointed to the faculty. "Though having but little medical knowledge," Felter wrote, he was a fluent speaker and writer, and had given public lectures on phrenology, anthropology, and kindred topics. Many years later, Buchanan sold hundreds of bogus diplomas using the names of defunct medical schools whose charters he had purchased. Many of the diplomas were sold to Europeans, and the matter became an international scandal. For the time being, however, Buchanan was content to teach physiology and medical jurisprudence.[5] In 1850, he was chosen dean of the institute. However, his "peculiar theories" and "domineering course" caused dissension among the faculty and led to the resignation of Wooster Beach and some others. The dissension was abetted by Buchanan's great innovation in medical education: although the school's only source of income was students' fees, Buchanan convinced the faculty in 1852 to eliminate tuition charges altogether. The matriculation, graduation, and laboratory fees were retained, but the tuition fees which constituted faculty salaries were abolished. Buchanan's hope was that the faculty would earn even more than they did in the past through the sale of their textbooks and their employment as preceptors to increased numbers of students. Needless to say, this new policy led to further resignations.[6]

To replace these faculty members, Buchanan hired, among others, a regular physician who denounced eclectic remedies in his classes, as well as George W. L. Brickley (1823–67) who, alone among the faculty, was a fit companion for Buchanan. Felter described him as a brilliant man, an eloquent speaker, and an "inveterate worker." In the four months after he joined the faculty, he wrote a book on "physiological botany," 2,700 pages of manuscript lectures, hundreds of pages of newspaper correspondence, and a 300-page novel (which was translated into French and German). During and after his years at the institute, which he left in 1859, Buchanan engaged in numerous activities, such as organizing the Knights of the Golden Circle, which had 17,000 members at one time. He hoped to use the Knights to invade Mexico and set up a military government with himself as emperor. Benito Juarez, then in exile in America and later president of Mexico, offered him

[5] For a biography of Buchanan, see *ibid.*, pp. 98–100; for an account of his later activities, see Harold J. Abrahams, *Extinct Medical Schools of Nineteenth-Century Philadelphia* (Philadelphia: University of Pennsylvania Press, 1966), pp. 436–55; for a description of his system of phrenology, see Madge E. Pickard and R. Carlyle Buley, *The Midwest Pioneer* (New York: Henry Schuman, 1946), pp. 227–38.

[6] Felter, *Eclectic Medical Institute*, pp. 98–99, 25–33.

"grants of land, and other great advantages" for his support. The United States government opposed Brickley's efforts, and the organization was eventually suppressed by President Lincoln as being pro-Southern.[7]

Under the leadership of this stalwart band, the institute careened toward bankruptcy. In 1855, the free tuition venture was abandoned, although the school's leadership was not altered. Meanwhile, a dispute had been developing between two factions of the faculty over the actual ownership of the stock of the school. Buchanan and his followers were on one side, another group of faculty and their supporters were on the other. The latter group seized the school building, and Buchanan's faction endeavored to wrest it away from them. Brickley wrote the following account of the skirmish:

While [the anti-Buchanan] party stood on the steps . . . , the opposite party thronged the entrance, and in threatening attitude, endeavored to overawe the little Spartan band who had taken possession and bid defiance to their foes. Knives, pistols, chisels, bludgeons, blunderbusses, etc., were freely displayed, and the usually staid Professor Buchanan urged his troops to enter. . . . [but] the brave outsiders could not be persuaded, coaxed, nor driven upon those murderous weapons, which grinned solemn death from hand to pocket, and rendered terrific the bare thought of carrying the stairway by storm. "On, on! my lads," shouted Professor Buchanan, but no commander— even had he been one who would lead—could remove the belief which the outsiders entertained of the character of Colt's pistol in a storm. The night and the day passed, and the night again witnessed renewed efforts to get the outsiders in, when finally a six-pound cannon was procured to sweep the passage if a rush should be made by the outsiders. The sight of this gun was enough, and the besiegers retired in utter disgust with the attempts to storm medical colleges.[8]

The police intervened at this point and ended the battle. Buchanan and his faction, unable to gain control of the institute, formed a rival school in the city in 1856. Buchanan left the new school shortly thereafter, and the two schools merged in 1859.[9]

Despite the machinations of the faculty, the institute actually grew during this hectic decade. When the free tuition plan was announced, the enrollment increased from about two hundred to about three hundred students annually. Even the reinstatement of tuition and the establishment of the rival school failed to depress the enrollment seriously. Furthermore, students came to the institute from surround-

[7] *Ibid.*, pp. 33, 37, 110–113.
[8] *Ibid.*, pp. 41–42.
[9] *Ibid.*, pp. 43–44; Frederick C. Waite, "American Sectarian Medical Colleges before the Civil War," *Bulletin of the History of Medicine* 19 (1946): 157.

ing states and even from the South and the East in these years.[10] In this extraordinary manner, a foundation was laid for the subsequent development of the eclectic sect.

THE DEVELOPMENT OF ECLECTIC THERAPEUTICS

During the period before the Civil War, eclectic physicians were unable to agree on a body of therapeutics. The problem was: how could eclecticism be eclectic in a distinctive way? The regulars had their bloodletting and calomel, the homeopaths their dilutions and little pills, and the Thomsonians their lobelia, steam, and cayenne. The eclectics needed something which would give them a distinctive place in the therapeutic spectrum, and yet take advantage of the public's hostility toward regular medicine and sympathy for botanical drugs.

In its early years, the eclectic sect was distinguished by neither the calibre of its practitioners nor the character of their medical practices. An eclectic historian, Alexander Wilder, wrote that, before the 1850's, "most of the teachers and others who were prominent in [eclecticism] were men little versed in classic and general literature, and many were hardly redeemed from actual illiteracy." These early practitioners used a heroic botanical therapy. They dosed the patient with nauseating botanical drugs in enormous doses, and administered vegetable cathartics and emetics with the same conviction with which their regular counterparts used mineral ones.[11] This form of eclecticism had little popular appeal, according to Wilder:

It could not be denied that the agents employed from the vegetable kingdom, while superior to the others in use, were crude and bulky, as well as often distasteful and repulsive beyond the power of sensitive patients to endure.

Under this condition of facts, it was morally certain that the New Practice of Medicine, notwithstanding its many merits, would hardly become general or popular. It was likely to be circumscribed to the rural and humbler population, to the "plain people," and to be virtually precluded from a standing with the cultured, the wealthy and fashionable. Indeed, Homeopathy coming from Europe with practitioners liberally educated, with a milder dosage and ready flexibility in remedial properties, was in better plight to earn favor in those circles, debarring its American competitor from that opportunity so essential to its prosperity.[12]

10 Felter, *Eclectic Medical Institute*, pp. 38, 146, 170–77.

11 Alexander Wilder, *History of Medicine* (New Sharon, Me.: 1901), p. 609; J. U. Lloyd and G. C. Lloyd, "The Eclectic Alkaloids, Resins, Resinoids, Oleo-Resins and Concentrated Principles," *Bulletin of the Lloyd Library of Botany, Pharmacy and Materia Medica*, Bulletin No. 12, Pharmacy Series No. 2 (1910): 4–5.

12 Wilder, *History of Medicine*, p. 656.

In the early 1850's, John M. King, an eclectic physician and a member of the faculty of the Eclectic Medical Institute, discovered a new type of drug preparation. King was a thoroughly qualified physician whose interest in Virchow's work led him to publish in 1859 a *Manual of Practical Microscopy*, intended for both medical and botanical use. According to a medical historian, this was "quite an ambitious undertaking considering the time in which the book was written."[13] Some years earlier, King worked on the problem of reducing the bulk of botanical drugs. He added alcohol to the powdered root of podophyllum, an emetic, added water, and let the solution stand. The next day, King later recalled, he discovered "numerous pieces of a dark somewhat porous and rather brittle body" floating in the fluid:

Many were the surmises as to what they were, and the query arose as to their value, if any, as a medicinal agent.

In the midst of these speculations, a young lady, about seventeen years of age, who was present, complained of feeling ill. Having no idea of the intense activity of the article just discovered, I administered twelve or fifteen grains. Nothing further was thought of the matter until about an hour afterward, when my attention was called to her condition. She was in severe pain and distress, cramps in the stomach and extremeties, pulse small and feeble, extremities cold, excessive vomiting and hypercatharsis, and apparently sinking rapidly. . . . To say that I was greatly alarmed would but feebly describe my mental condition. I ran to secure the aid of two or three professional friends, but could find none of them in their offices. Then I ran back again, trembling over what might be the consequences, and thinking out a course of treatment to pursue. A princely fortune could not induce me to undergo a repetition of such a condition. . . . the patient recovered in six or seven days, but unfortunately, with some chronic gastro-enteritic abnormal condition that remained for many years. From this experience I was so influenced that I feared to use any of the remainder of the resin until at least eighteen months had passed, when I ventured a repetition of its use, but in much smaller quantities, and with most excellent results.[14]

Podophyllin (the name given to the drug) soon became extremely popular. Eclectic physicians had been seeking distinctive therapies, and podophyllin was a palatable cathartic which was ideal as competition for calomel and lobelia and, indeed, became known as the "eclectic calomel." Podophyllin was prescribed by many regular physicians also, and was listed in the U.S. Pharmacopoeia in 1860 under the name of *Resina Podophylli*.[15]

A fad developed, and dozens of other resinoids and alkaloids de-

---

[13] Otto Juettner, *Daniel Drake and His Followers* (Cincinnati: Harvey, 1909), pp. 374–75.
[14] Lloyd and Lloyd, "Eclectic Alkaloids," pp. 8–9.
[15] *Ibid.*, pp. 11–12.

rived from botanical drugs were placed on the market. Most of these were therapeutically useless. The bubble soon burst, and by 1855, King was calling the manufacture of these resinoids a "most stupendous fraud." Another eclectic claimed that manufacturers were selling fraudulent and adulterated products, and that most of the resinoids "contain but little, if any, of the medicinal value of the substances they may be obtained from, being far more inferior than a common extract." The craze lasted through the 1860's and probably as many regular physicians as eclectic ones succumbed to the blandishments of the resinoids.[16]

The residue of all this gave the eclectics a body of therapies that paralleled, in many ways, the worst of the regular practice. John M. Scudder, the most eminent of all eclectic physicians, wrote:

The older eclectics had not a single *principle* to guide them in therapeutics. They *objected* to, and *discarded* the four "regular" agencies—blood-letting. mercury, antimony, arsenic—because they were *injurious* to the sick, and left behind them various diseases, and not because they were anti-phlogistic or depressant. For each and every one they proposed a substitute, claiming that they could obtain with it *all* the good results, without any of the bad. When I attended lectures, the professors labored to show the advantages of Eclectic blood-letting over the lancet, by free catharsis, and hemostasis; the advantages of Podophyllin, Leptandrin, and other agents to "tap the liver," and produce the cholagogue effects of the common preparations of mercury, without the unpleasant results; the advantages of [other] compounds . . . to produce the nausea, relaxation and sedation of Tartrate of Antimony. . . .

Remedies were given in large doses, and for their crude and poisonous influence, cathartics were freely and continually used; emetics played an important part in many acute diseases; diaphoretics were given in large doses and for their *sudorific* effect; nauseants were in common use to produce sedation, and it was not thought possible to treat diseases of the respiratory apparatus without them. . . .

Perpetual blisters, and prolonged supperation, counter-irritation with the irritating plaster, were freely used in chronic diseases, and they would not object to a pea under the skin as an issue, or the seton. . . .[17]

Thus, eclectic practitioners, unlike homeopaths, merely aped regular heroic medicine, replacing regular drugs with others which produced similar physiological effects.

It is hardly surprising that this system did not flourish in the period before the Civil War. The public was not seeking a botanical heroic practice; they were rebelling against the principles of heroic medicine, and any system which persisted in using those principles was

16 *Ibid.*, pp. 24, 33–39.
17 [John M. Scudder], "The Philosophy of Modern Eclecticism," *Eclectic Medical Journal* 39 (1879): 144–45.

hardly likely to succeed. After the first flush of the resinoids, the sect deteriorated steadily. Eclecticism reached its lowest ebb during the depression of the late 1850's and early 1860's. The National Eclectic Medical Association, founded in 1848 as a response to the formation of the AMA, suspended its activities after 1857. The eclectic medical schools, with the exception of those in Cincinnati and Philadelphia, all discontinued their activities. Many eclectic physicians abandoned eclecticism for regular medicine or homeopathy. Scudder stated: "We were overweighted with . . . a lot of miserable 'concentrated medicines,' with a poor pharmacy, and druggists that sought to make things cheap rather than good, and with a constituency that, using a western expression, were 'down at the heel.' "[18]

The eclectic sect appears to have split into several groups at this point. Some eclectics became disreputable charlatans. Others continued as nondescript physicians, with no distinctive therapies. The largest and most important single faction developed along more respectable lines under the leadership of Scudder and the Eclectic Medical Institute in Cincinnati. After his graduation from the Institute in 1856, John M. Scudder (1829–94) became an extremely successful practitioner in Cincinnati. During the Civil War, when the school reached its nadir in terms of enrollment and solvency, he assumed the position of dean, and through astute management restored it to a sound financial and intellectual basis. He resumed publication of the *Eclectic Medical Journal*, which became a successful and influential medical journal under his editorial leadership.[19]

In addition to his extraordinary entrepreneurial and managerial talents, Scudder developed in 1869 a new system of eclectic therapeutics which became the basis of the eclectic practice. He called this system "specific medication." Scudder's system paralleled homeopathy in a number of important respects. Like Hahnemann, Scudder was concerned solely with pathological symptoms. The physician looked for a "constantly occurring symptom or symptoms," and treated the patient on the basis of a specific remedy for a specific symptom.[20] Whereas the homeopath's treatments were based on *similia similibus curantur*, Scudder was far more pragmatic. He developed botanical remedies empirically, and subsequently bottled and sold them as com-

[18] J. M. Scudder, "A Brief History of Eclectic Medicine," *Eclectic Medical Journal* 39 (1879): 305; Wilder, *History of Medicine*, pp. 618–619, 653.

[19] A biography of Scudder can be found in Felter, *Eclectic Medical Institute*, pp. 118–20.

[20] [John M. Scudder], "Is Specific Medication Practical?" *Eclectic Medical Journal* 39 (1879): 193; Alex Berman, "Wooster Beach and the Early Eclectics," *University of Michigan Medical Bulletin* 24 (1958): 282.

mercial preparations, although the latter was not part of his original system. Had his system been extended to its logical extreme, it could easily have reverted to heroic therapy. Scudder's real contribution was his philosophy of therapeutics, which closely resembled that of Jacob Bigelow. He wrote:

> The necessity for small doses of pleasant medicines for direct action became greater each year. Our fathers had used infusions, decoctions, and weak tinctures of our indigenous remedies with marked success, and our earlier journals were filled with information regarding them. They had fallen into disuse on account of their form, but principally from inefficient teaching of materia medica and practice. A series of experiments found that they could be put in the form of a very strong tincture, and dispensed in water, and could then be easily carried, and would not offend the palate or stomach of our patients. It was also found that quality in a medicine was far more important than quantity, indeed that the dose might be very minute as compared with the drugging of the olden time. . . .
>
> Of necessity the old antiphlogistic treatment must be discarded, as it had been discarded in the past; of necessity much of the harsh medication that had held its ground even with Eclectics must go with it. The free purgation, harsh purgation, alterative purgation, nauseants . . . blisters, and a host of associated means were to be laid aside and replaced with simpler and better means. The old dose of medicine and its *poisonous* action must be replaced with the small dose and its medicinal action. The stomach was to be kept in comfortable condition for the reception of food and the bowels in such restful condition that they would not disturb the patient. "Rest for the weary," "cleanliness which was better than godliness," kindliness which bound up the wounds and said, "take care of him," became important elements in the modern practice of medicine.[21]

Scudder's system attracted much attention among both eclectic physicians and members of the other sects; Felter said that Scudder's book on the subject had a "remarkably large sale." Although specific medication soon became the nominal therapeutic hallmark of eclectic medicine, it was probably more honored in the breach than by observance. Eclectic physicians continued using heroic therapies—like emetics, cathartics, and blisters—well into the 1870's.[22]

INSTITUTIONAL DEVELOPMENTS IN THE ECLECTIC SECT

The Eclectic Medical Institute prospered under Scudder's leadership, particularly from the late 1870's to the mid-1890's. The school had a distinguished faculty: in addition to Scudder, it included John King,

[21] Scudder, "History of Eclectic Medicine," p. 306.

[22] Felter, *Eclectic Medical Institute*, p. 50; [John M. Scudder], "Be Kind to the Sick," *Eclectic Medical Journal* 37 (1877): 281–82; Scudder, "History of Eclectic Medicine," p. 307.

A. J. Howe, a successful surgeon and author of medical textbooks, and John Uri Lloyd, a nationally known and highly respected (by members of all sects) pharmacist and chemist. The student enrollment was also large. During the mid-1880's, the institute was the largest of the six medical schools of all sects in Cincinnati. It was also the largest and most influential eclectic medical school: in 1894, it had about 44 percent of the students in the eight eclectic medical schools approved by the national association. Although the institute was never a leader in medical education, it compared favorably with the better medical schools of all sects.[23]

The eclectics were the smallest and weakest of the three major medical sects in the last half of the nineteenth century. In 1900, there were approximately 4,000 eclectic physicians, compared with 10,000 homeopaths and over 110,000 regular physicians. Most eclectics practiced in midwestern states. In Kansas, for example, there were 729 regular physicians, 515 eclectics, and only 104 homeopaths in 1883. In Missouri about the same time, there were an estimated 3,453 regular physicians, 581 eclectics, 217 homeopaths, and 583 practitioners classified as nondescript. In New York, on the other hand, there were only an estimated 100 eclectics practicing in the whole state in 1890. Furthermore, 538 of the 743 students in eclectic medical schools in the same year were from the midwest. The National Eclectic Medical Association was revived in 1870, and it grew slowly until it included 32 state societies by 1900. The state societies were usually small, as evidence by the existence of additional local societies in only 12 of the states. Most of the state societies were also in the midwest. Surprisingly, eclecticism was weak in the South, where Thomsonism had been strong.[24]

The scientific and intellectual content of eclecticism was inferior to that of homeopathy and regular medicine. Most eclectic medical colleges were undistinguished and unsuccessful. Up to 1892, 32 eclectic medical colleges had been founded; of the ten surviving at that time, only three or four were in a "flourishing condition," according to an eclectic physician. Nonetheless, eclectic medical education did not have

[23] Ralph Taylor, "The Formation of the Eclectic School in Cincinnati," *Ohio State Archaeological and Historical Quarterly* 51 (1942): 286; Felter, *Eclectic Medical Institute*, p. 55, 59, 61, 69–71; Juettner, *Daniel Drake*, p. 377.
[24] See Appendix IV; Thomas Neville Bonner, *The Kansas Doctor* (Lawrence: University of Kansas Press, 1959), pp. 72–73; Willis P. King, "Quacks and Quackery in Missouri," *Transactions of the Missouri State Medical Association*, 25th session, 1882, p. 33; "The Eclectics," *Medical Record* 38 (1890): 212; Wilder, *History of Medicine*, pp. 672–76, 695, 726; J. A. Harrison, "Mr. Editor," *Eclectic Medical Journal* 45 (1885): 471–72.

a wholly undistinguished history. The Eclectic Medical Institute did much useful work in medicinal botany. Furthermore, the Penn Medical University, an eclectic school founded in 1853 in Philadelphia, was probably the first medical school in the United States to offer graded courses, using a novel and carefully considered curriculum in which the two six-month terms were divided into four graded semesters. It was also the first American medical school to provide coeducational instruction to large numbers of men and women in the same classes, a policy it adopted about 1857. Although the school declined steadily after the Civil War until it discontinued operations in 1881, it was one of the very few impressive innovations in American medical education before the Civil War.[25]

Some eclectic physicians had reputations as violators of professional ethics. A Massachusetts eclectic disclosed in 1880 that many eclectics in Boston practiced "under illicit diplomas" and were "so discreditable in their professional ways that they cannot join our local or state associations."[26] Scudder's colleague, A. J. Howe, attributed this behavior to regular physicians' ostracism of eclectics:

Not infrequently an Eclectic practitioner does business in a community where he has no brethren, yet in company with a horde of "regulars" who treat him like an outlaw, and thus convert him into a profession freebooter. After they have striven to deprive him of a livelihood in a free country, ought they to complain that the "irregular" disregards all ethics and professional rules?

But too many of our men, in the struggle for existence under disadvantages, have become callous to the decencies which belong to medical men of the same school or organization. They have been freebooters so long that they seem to have forgotten that such a thing as professional etiquette anywhere exists.[27]

Scudder and the Eclectic Medical Institute remained aloof from developments elsewhere in the eclectic sect. An examination of the *Eclectic Medical Journal* from 1876 to 1891 revealed few references to professional eclectic activities. On some occasions, Scudder seemed to go out of his way to dissociate himself from the rest of the sect. He said of the National Eclectic Medical Association in 1886: "as an expounder of doctrine, a means of improving the practice of medi-

---

[25] E. Melvin McPheron, "Does Denver Need an Eclectic Medical College?" *Eclectic Medical Journal* 52 (1892): 66; Abrahams, *Extinct Medical Schools*, pp. 176–203.

[26] "A Letter and a Reply," *Eclectic Medical Journal* 40 (1880): 168.

[27] [A. J. Howe], "Professional Etiquette," *Eclectic Medical Journal* 39 (1879): 48.

cine, or of developing our knowledge of the materia medica, it is a failure."[28]

THE DISTINCTIVENESS OF THE ECLECTIC SECT IN THE MEDICAL PROFESSION

The problem of therapeutic distinctiveness haunted eclectic physicians throughout the nineteenth century. Scudder himself declared that "in many things the three schools of medicine agree. The anatomy, the physiology, the chemistry, the art of obstetrics, the art of surgery, the preventive medicine, are the same in all. . . . The points of differences, then, are in materia medica, and the administration of remedies for cure." Even here, however, Scudder was hard pressed to find a clear-cut distinction between regular and eclectic medicine. He conceded that many eclectic physicians were "a very poor species of old school medicine," but held that "your sound Eclectic to-day believes in small doses of pleasant medicines for direct effect. He takes his remedies from every source."[29] Of course, the latter group hardly qualified as a distinctive sect. The many eclectic physicians who wrote to the *Eclectic Medical Journal* on this topic were equally unable to define eclectic medicine satisfactorily. One of them suggested the following:

There are many honest and sincere men calling themselves Eclectic, who can not give a plain distinction between their practices and that of the other schools . . . .
    The difference is not great, but it is enough to ostracise the eclectic from the regular ranks. If I were asked in a court . . . . "What is an eclectic physician?" I would answer, a regularly (in the sense of school training) educated, legally qualified practitioner, who has not subscribed to the Hippocratic oath, and who owes no allegiance to the time honored code of ethics.[30]

Several important differences between eclectic and regular physicians had nothing to do with therapeutics. One was the size of the communities in which they practiced. An examination of the residences of the contributors to the *Eclectic Medical Journal* showed that most of the physicians practiced in midwestern villages or very small towns. Howe observed that "one reason why eclectics settled in villages and small towns was that their personal accomplishments were not of

28 [John M. Scudder], "A Brief History of Eclecticism," *Eclectic Medical Journal* 46 (1886): 92.
    29 [John M. Scudder], "The Essential Differences between the Three Schools of Medicine . . . ," *Eclectic Medical Journal* 52 (1892): 346; [John M. Scudder], "What is Eclecticism in Medicine?" *Eclectic Medical Journal* 43 (1883): 399–400.
    30 A. H. Hattan, "What is Eclecticism in Medicine?" *Eclectic Medical Journal* 43 (1883): 467, 469.

sufficiently high order to win a way into the elegant families of large towns and cities." He believed that, by 1878, eclectic physicians were "making headway in county seats, and even in the largest cities."[31] The eclectics' small-town practices probably enhanced their influence and political power, because eclectic physicians were often the only physicians in their communities. This gave them the enthusiastic support of the local residents in any state-wide battle with the regular physicians.

Eclectic physicians differed from regular physicians in another major respect. They probably came from poorer families than the regular physicians did and, for this reason, were more poorly educated than many regular physicians. For example, when several regular medical schools raised their entrance requirements and changed their degree requirements from a two-year repeated course to a three-year graded course, Scudder commented that there were "enough students who can see the value of such thorough instruction to give them a good support. In the Eclectic branch of the profession a college adopting an exclusive graded course would starve."[32]

From the patient's perspective, there was little to choose between eclectic physicians and their competitors in the other sects. The therapeutic differences among the sects did not give the patient a choice between medically valid and invalid treatments: what was valid in medicine was shared by all sects; where physicians in one sect groped in ignorance, physicians in the other sects were equally unenlightened. To be sure, few eclectics were specialists, but in the small communities where eclectics practiced, equally few regular physicians specialized. The continuing lack of medically valid therapeutics that sustained sectarianism also made differences among sects of little significance for the well-being of the patient.

31 [A. J. Howe], "Are We Moving in the Right Direction?" *Eclectic Medical Journal* 38 (1878): 430.
32 [John M. Scudder], "Medical Education," *Eclectic Medical Journal* 38 (1878): 531.

CHAPTER 12 THE HOMEOPATHIC SECT

AFTER THE homeopathic physicians had separated themselves from the homeopathic quacks and were driven out of regular medical institutions, they developed homeopathy into a prosperous and progressive medical sect with an affluent clientele. The increasing interest of the main body of homeopaths in palliative therapy, clinical specialties, and medical science caused considerable conflict with the small number of dogmatic homeopaths throughout the century.[1]

THE STRUGGLE WITH THE HOMEOPATHIC QUACKS

Because Hahnemann altered his views during his lifetime from a less to a more doctrinaire belief in the therapeutic value of the homeopathic law, his teachings could be approached from either of the two perspectives. On the one hand, homeopathy could be considered as superseding both the scientific and sectarian elements of regular medicine, rejecting its valid as well as its invalid components. On the other hand, homeopaths could accept the medical sciences and the medically valid clinical specialties like surgery and ophthalmology, and reject the medically invalid therapeutics of the regular sect, replacing the latter with therapies derived from Hahnemann's law.

Those homeopaths who had been educated as regular physicians did not forsake medical science when they became homeopaths; they abandoned only the regular medical sect. One homeopath said in 1854:

Is it as necessary that the homeopath should be a man of *learning*, as the allopath? . . . many suppose that the homeopathic system can be successfully sustained and practiced by those who are not learned, but on the contrary,

[1] A history of American homeopathy has been published too late for inclusion in this study. In addition to its discussion of many issues confronting nineteenth-century homeopaths, it also examines homeopathy's twentieth-century history: Martin Kaufman, *Homeopathy in America* (Baltimore: Johns Hopkins Press, 1971).

are almost destitute of medical education. This, however, is a very erroneous conception of our system. Because we see quacks and empirics administering the small doses, we must not suppose that the merit of the system is in harmony with the attainments of such individuals. . . .

Homeopathy . . . does not discard any of the branches of medicine. . . . we discard many fashions [and] obsolete methods of relieving diseases by the old school [e.g. bloodletting and cathartics]. . . . Reasoning upon the indispensability of blood-letting in fever, and cathartics in constipation, [people] very naturally conclude, no doubt, that if we should discard these, we would certainly not hesitate to discard even anatomy, or some other branch of as much importance.[2]

These educated homeopaths strongly defended the valid aspects of medicine. One of them wrote in 1846 that "the merits of surgery are so true, certain and undeniable, and so conformable to the great object of all medical art, that it deserves to be placed in rank far above physic in its ordinary form." Another said that the homeopaths who "exclaim with vehemence" against the recently developed use of auscultation and percussion "must grope in doubt and ignorance."[3]

The educated homeopaths separated themselves from the homeopathic quacks by forming exclusive professional societies. The most important of these was the American Institute of Homeopathy (AIH), founded in 1844. A resolution passed at the first meeting of the AIH stated two reasons for organizing the institute. One was to improve knowledge of the homeopathic materia medica, which could "only be obtained by associated action." The second was the "restraining of Physicians from pretending to be competent to practice Homeopathy who have not studied it in a careful and skilful manner." According to a history of homeopathy in America, the organization sought to protect educated homeopaths against "quacks, charletans and medical pirates, who without the warrant of medical training sought to prey upon the credulous public at the expense of the new school."[4]

[2] Dr. Rowland, "What is Homoeopathy?" *Philadelphia Journal of Homoeopathy* 3 (1854): 294, 298–99. See also "Educational Requirements of the Homoeopathic Physician," *Homoeopathic Examiner* 2 (1841): 17–22.

[3] C. V., "Homoeopathy Supersedes the Necessity of a Great Number of Surgical Operations," *American Journal of Homoeopathy* 1 (1846): 144. (The title refers to those operations which do not lead to cures, but palliative relief.) Homeopaths later stated that before the 1850's very few homeopaths practiced surgery: I. T. Talbot, "Address on the Recent History of the Institute, . . ." *Transactions of the American Institute of Homoeopathy*, 47th session (1894): 65; N. F. Cooke, "Advantages of Physical Diagnosis to the Homoeopathic Physician," *Philadelphia Journal of Homoeopathy* 3 (1854): 1, 3.

[4] "Minutes of the Sessions of 1844 and 1845," *Transactions of the American Institute of Homoeopathy* 1, (1846): 3; Thomas Lindsley Bradford, "Homoeopathic Societies," in William Harvey King, ed., *History of Homoeopathy* (New York: Lewis, 1905) III: 255.

HOMEOPATHY'S BREAK WITH REGULAR MEDICINE

In the late 1840's, regular physicians undertook a series of measures to ostracize homeopaths from the major regular medical institutions. The most important of these steps concerned medical education. In 1847, the AMA passed a resolution urging medical colleges not to accept the certificate of any preceptor who was "avowedly and notoriously an irregular practitioner." Many medical colleges endorsed this resolution. In 1850, a student asked the faculty of Rush Medical College in Chicago whether they would grant him a degree if he fulfilled the graduation requirements, even though he was "a homeopathist from a conviction of the truth of the principles and the efficacy of the practice of homeopathia." N. S. Davis, who was then on the faculty, was no man to temporize over matters of principle. He wrote back to the homeopath: "I am directed to inform you that the faculty of Rush Medical College will not recommend you to the trustees for a degree so long as they have any reason to suppose that you entertain the doctrines, and intend to trifle with human life on the principles that you avow in your letter." Apparently, the faculty of Rush Medical College was not satisfied to have a student fulfill the graduation requirements in order to receive a degree. The intention to practice as a homeopath was sufficient reason to deny the application.[5]

Homeopaths were therefore forced to open their own medical colleges. The Homeopathic Medical College of Pennsylvania was established in Philadelphia in 1848 as the first chartered homeopathic medical school in America. Homeopaths and sympathetic laymen, the most prominent of whom was William Cullen Bryant, founded the Homeopathic Medical College of New York in 1860. Homeopathic medical schools were also established in Cleveland in 1850 and in Chicago in 1860.[6]

Regular physicians took equally vigorous efforts to bar homeopaths

[5] Lucius H. Zeuch, *History of Medical Practice in Illinois*, vol. I (Chicago: 1927), pp. 239–40, 243.

[6] Frederick C. Waite, "American Sectarian Medical Colleges Before the Civil War," *Bulletin of the History of Medicine* 19 (1946): 162–65; Thomas Lindsley Bradford, *History of the Homoeopathic Medical College of Pennsylvania* (Philadelphia: Boericke and Tafel, 1898), p. 9; Leonard Paul Wershub, *One Hundred Years of Medical Progress: A History of the New York Medical College* . . . (Springfield, Ill.: Thomas, 1967), pp. 14–19, 31. The first homeopathic medical school, the Allentown (Penn.), Academy, was established in 1836 by Constantine Hering and other German immigrants. Instruction was in the German language and the school gave no degrees. It ceased operation in 1841, due to the failure of the bank in which its funds were invested. Its faculty was active in founding the Homeopathic Medical College of Pennsylvania.

from treating patients at public hospitals. In Chicago, a number of homeopaths and their supporters sought in 1857 to obtain facilities to treat patients in the Cook County Hospital then under construction. The board of health acceded to their request and allocated one-quarter of the hospital to the patients of homeopathic physicians. The regular physicians thereupon refused to serve in the hospital under those conditions. The hospital's opening was delayed for many months because of this conflict, but eventually it was opened only to the patients of regular physicians. The New York homeopaths were more successful when they sought hospital privileges during the 1866 cholera epidemic. There, the intervention of prominent lay supporters of homeopathy enabled homeopaths to overcome the opposition of the New York Academy of Medicine, and the Metropolitan Board of Health permitted homeopaths to staff wards at two city hospitals.[7]

In these and other ways, regular physicians systematically endeavored to exclude homeopaths from their institutions: homeopaths were barred from regular medical societies, denied hospital privileges at regular hospitals, excluded from many boards of health, forbidden to serve on the faculties of regular medical schools, and blacklisted from consultations and any professional association with regular physicians. Even their apprentices were denied certification of preceptorship at regular medical schools.

The expulsion of homeopaths from the ranks of the regular profession did not proceed with equal celerity or thoroughness in all communities. The battle began early in New York and Chicago. It progressed more slowly in Boston. The Massachusetts Medical Society was practically overrun with homeopaths by the standards of other regular medical societies. A few members had converted to homeopathy in the early 1840's without being expelled. An acknowledged homeopath was admitted to membership in 1846. In 1850, the society defeated a motion to exclude all homeopaths, but passed another motion banning them from the position of Fellow of the society. At the same time, it disallowed any education at a homeopathic medical school from fulfilling that part of the entrance requirement. Finally, in 1859, the society resolved to exclude all non-regular physicians from membership. For some reason, this new policy was not strictly enforced, because at the 1870 AMA meeting, representatives from the Boston Gynecological Society claimed that some members of the Massachusetts Medical Society were homeopaths, and successfully demanded that the society's

[7] Zeuch, *Medical Practice in Illinois*, pp. 241–42; Charles E. Rosenberg, *The Cholera Years* (Chicago: University of Chicago Press, 1962), pp. 223–24.

membership in the AMA be discontinued if the homeopaths were not expelled. This action did lead to a purge of the homeopathic members of the society, at least nine of whom were expelled in the years between 1873 and 1877.[8]

Regular medical schools also often disregarded the ban on apprentices of sectarian physicians. They were proprietary institutions and not all of them could be expected to refuse a paying student simply because of his preceptor's medical philosophy. Not only did many students of homeopathic physicians attend regular medical schools, but students of eclectic physicians were also accepted. Scudder reported that a student of an eclectic physician applied to the University of Michigan about 1882 and received the following letter in reply: "Dear Sir:—By the rule of the Department, we can not accept time from an Eclectic preceptor. But you can without trouble make affidavit that you have been studying medicine for three years and that will answer every purpose."[9]

THE SUCCESS OF HOMEOPATHY

For the reasons discussed in Chapter 8, homeopathy rapidly became extremely popular among the wealthy in many communities throughout the country. By 1883 the president of the American Institute of Homeopathy claimed that "it is accurately safe to say that in the aggregate at the lowest calculation fully one-third of the taxable property is held by the people who employ homeopathic treatment."[10] While this was undoubtedly one of the flights of campaign oratory common among the medical sects of the period, homeopathy did maintain its popularity among the upper classes for many years. A homeopathic historian described the situation in Chicago in 1871 in this way:

From Michigan avenue to State street, the choice residential portion of the city, it was acknowledged that more than one-half of the families preferred

8 Reginald H. Fitz, "The Rise and Fall of the Licensed Physician in Massachusetts, 1781–1860," *Transactions of the Association of American Physicians* 9 (1894): 14–17; Walter L. Burrage, *A History of the Massachusetts Medical Society* (n.p., 1923), pp. 127–31. According to a homeopath, the expulsion was carried out without any regard for the rules of the society, and the homeopaths were denied all procedural rights: I. T. Talbot, "A Telegram from Boston . . . ," *Transactions of the American Institute of Homoeopathy*, 26th session (1873): 90–96. For statements by the accused homeopaths during the trial, see *Trial of William Bushnell, et al, for Practising Homoeopathy* (Boston, 1873). For a description of cooperation between homeopaths and regular physicians in a Michigan community, see C. B. Burr, ed., *Medical History of Michigan* (Minneapolis: Bruce, 1930) II: 3–4.

9 [John M. Scudder], "Let Them Rub It In," *Eclectic Medical Journal* 42 (1882): 477; Bradford, *History of the Homoeopathic Medical College*, p. 137.

10 W. James Bushrod, "Annual Address," *Transactions of the American Institute of Homoeopathy*, 36th session (1883): 33.

and used the homeopathic practice. From State to Clark street, only about one-fourth, while from Clark street to the river, among the lower classes, and the disreputable portions of the city, the allopaths had full sway, and the homeopaths were scarcely represented. One member [of the regular medical society] suggested that the newspapers should be induced to take the matter up, but on investigation this was found to be impracticable as the newspapers were owned and edited largely by men employing the homeopathic practice in their own families. . . .[11]

In New York City in 1875, a petition requesting that a public hospital be set aside for the use of homeopathic physicians was signed by 655 citizens, who represented more than half of the estimated wealth of the city. Medical histories of Cleveland and Detroit also found that many of the wealthy families in those cities employed homeopathic physicians.[12]

The success of homeopathy among these families enabled the movement to grow steadily. By the end of the century, approximately 10,000 homeopaths—about eight percent of all practitioners—practiced throughout the nation. The homeopaths were concentrated in the urban states like Massachusetts, New Jersey, and Illinois, where they comprised between 13 and 15 percent of all practitioners, and were virtually nonexistent in the southern states like Mississippi, North Carolina, and South Carolina, where they constituted less than one-half of one percent of all practitioners.[13]

Homeopathy continued to attract physicians who had been educated in regular medical schools and who had apparently practiced for some time as regular physicians. Of the 141 physicians admitted to the AIH in 1872 and 1873, 17 percent were educated in regular medical schools. Almost 80 percent of the regularly educated physicians had received their degrees before 1870 (compared to 59 percent of the physicians educated in homeopathic schools), and 62 percent had received their degrees before 1865 (compared to 29 percent of the physicians educated in homeopathic schools).[14] Thus the regularly educated

[11] John E. Gilman, "History of the Medical Profession and Medical Institutions of Chicago: Homoeopathy in Chicago," *Magazine of Western History* 12 (1890): 544–45.

[12] Wershub, *New York Medical College*, pp. 110–11; Frederick Clayton Waite, *Western Reserve University Centennial History of the School of Medicine* (Cleveland, Ohio: Western Reserve University Press, 1946), p. 321; Burr, *Medical History of Michigan* I: 541.

[13] See Appendix IV; George B. Peck, "Homoeopathy in the United States," *Hahnemannian Monthly* 35 (1900): 560–61.

[14] "Complete Report of the Board of Censors," *Transactions of the American Institute of Homoeopathy*, 25th session (1872): 121–22; "Complete Report of the Board of Censors," *Transactions of the American Institute of Homoeopathy*, 26th session (1873): 152–53.

new members were generally older than the homeopathically educated new members, suggesting that they turned to homeopathy after practicing as regular physicians, perhaps because they had been unsuccessful in their first efforts.

HOMEOPATHIC MEDICAL INSTITUTIONS

The wealth and influence of their clientele enabled homeopaths to amass an impressive number of institutions during the last decades of the century. In 1898, homeopaths had 9 national societies, 33 state societies, 85 local societies and 39 other local organizations, 66 general homeopathic hospitals, 74 specialty homeopathic hospitals, 57 homeopathic dispensaries, 20 homeopathic medical colleges, and 31 homeopathic medical journals.[15] Considering that there were fewer than ten thousand homeopaths at the time, these numbers are remarkably large.

Medical Societies. Homeopathic medical societies were structured in the same way as regular medical societies, with national, state, and local societies. Of course the AIH had its own code of ethics. A committee which revised the AIH code in 1884 reported that its code duplicated the form and language of the AMA code, "modifying it where changes seemed to be demanded by a proper regard for liberality and for justice, both to patient and to physician, or by a due concern for the freedom of medical education, opinion and action."[16]

Specialties. Specialization developed among homeopaths at about the same rate and in the same directions as among regular physicians. Some homeopathic surgeons were quite famous, and a visiting British physician reported in 1891 that a homeopathic surgeon had the largest practice in Chicago. Homeopaths also managed a variety of specialty hospitals, and one homeopathic ophthalmic hospital in New York City was particularly well known. The relatively small number of homeopaths made independent specialty societies impractical, so specialty sections were established in the AIH to bring specialists together. These developed in the AIH considerably more rapidly than their counterparts in the AMA. By 1882, AIH specialty sections included obstetrics, gynecology, pediatrics, surgery, psychological medicine, ophthalmology,

---

[15] Bradford, *Homoeopathic Medical College*, p. 895. Peck also enumerated the institutions described in Bradford. The two sets of data correspond closely, with minor discrepancies. Peck's data also show that most hospitals controlled by homeopaths were public ones, and that homeopaths staffed a proportion of the beds in about 100 other hospitals: Peck, "Homoeopathy in the United States," pp. 561–62.

[16] Carroll Dunham, *et al*, "Report on a Complete Code of Medical Ethics," *Transactions of the American Institute of Homoeopathy*, 37th session (1884): 681.

otology, and laryngology, as well as public health and all the basic medical sciences.[17]

Hospitals. Homeopaths were the only non-regular sect to establish private hospitals and to be placed in charge of state and local hospitals. This development occurred to its greatest extent in New York State, where in 1905 homeopaths managed 22 hospitals, including a state mental hospital. Many of the private homeopathic hospitals throughout the country were amply supported by wealthy homeopathic patrons.[18]

Medical Schools. Although the numerous homeopathic medical schools varied in quality in the same way as the medical schools of the other sects, several of them were among the best and the wealthiest medical schools in the country. In 1900, for example, three of the four largest medical school libraries were in homeopathic medical schools, and two of the five medical schools with the greatest assessed value of buildings and grounds were homeopathic. The exclusion of homeopaths from regular hospitals encouraged the wealthiest homeopathic medical schools to establish their own hospitals. The 1907 announcement of the Homeopathic Medical College of New York declared that "ours is the only medical college in the City of New York which owns its own hospital—except the [New York Medical College for Women], also homeopathic; our students have clinical instruction at as many hospital beds—about fifteen hundred—as have the students from all the other colleges in the city combined."[19]

Homeopaths also operated several university affiliated medical schools. One was established in 1873 in Boston University, a privately endowed university. The others were affiliated with state universities in Michigan, Iowa, Minnesota, Nebraska, California, and Ohio. In all instances the state-supported homeopathic medical schools were located in the same universities as the regular medical schools, and regular and homeopathic medical students often took their basic science and

[17] William Tod Helmuth was the best known of the homeopathic surgeons, and he was head of surgery at the New York Homeopathic Medical College for many years: Wershub, *New York Medical College*, pp. 75, 158; for a history of the New York Ophthalmic Hospital, see "New York Ophthalmic Hospital and its Schools," in King, *History of Homoeopathy* II: 215–18; "Constitution and By-Laws," *Transactions of the American Institute of Homoeopathy*, 35th session (1882): 763.

[18] For a description of these institutions, see Thomas Lindsley Bradford, "Homoeopathy in New York," in King, *History of Homoeopathy* I: 51–59; and James J. Walsh, *History of Medicine in New York* (New York: National Americana Society, 1919), vol. III.

[19] Henry L. Taylor, *Professional Education in the United States* (Albany: 1900), I: 18, 21; Walsh, *History of Medicine in New York* II: 550.

specialty courses together, much to the consternation of regular physicians.[20]

The content of homeopathic medical education differed little from that of regular (or eclectic) medical education in the scientific subjects, a situation recognized by informed physicians of all sects. William Osler, for example, described the curriculums of the three sects in this way in 1891:

> The homeopathists and the eclectics, will, I think, concur in the necessity of a full and proper curriculum of study in the great branches of medicine. Anatomy, physiology, chemistry, histology, embryology, medicine, surgery, obstetrics, gynecology, and medical jurisprudence know no "isms." The differences only become glaring when we touch the subject of Therapeutics, a subject in which amongst members of each of the so-called schools the greatest individual differences of opinion exist. So strong, however, is the feeling (largely an ethical one), that the divergence of opinion on this one branch separates absolutely the different classes of practitioners from each other. . . .[21]

Homeopathic medical schools pioneered in improving medical education after the Civil War. The major determinants of the quality of a medical school program at that time were generally acknowledged to be the length of the total course of instruction and the use of the graded curriculum instead of the repetitive one. Several homeopathic

[20] The homeopathic medical school at the University of Michigan was founded in 1875; that at the University of Iowa in 1877; that at the University of Minnesota in 1888, when all the private medical schools in the state were merged into a state medical school; that at the University of Nebraska in 1884, but it ceased operation before 1890. The homeopathic medical schools at the University of California at Berkeley and at Ohio State University were originally private medical schools which were incorporated into the state university medical schools in or after 1909 and in 1914 respectively. It is difficult to provide data on the termination of instruction in homeopathic medicine at these schools, because the courses in homeopathic therapeutics were gradually phased out, as, indeed, were those in regular materia medica. For the Boston University medical school, see John Preston Sutherland, "Boston University School of Medicine," in King, *History of Homoeopathy* III: 185; for Michigan see Wilbert B. Hinsdale, "Homoeopathic Medical College of the University of Michigan," in King, *History of Homoeopathy* III: 89–97, and Burr, *Medical History of Michigan* I: 535–36; for Iowa, see George Royal, "College of Homoeopathic Medicine of the State University of Iowa," in King, *History of Homoeopathy* II: 189–90; for Minnesota, see "The College of Homoeopathic Medicine and Surgery of the University of Minnesota," in King, *History of Homoepathy* III: 244–47; for Nebraska, see *Transactions of the American Institute of Homoeopathy*, 40th session (1887): 804–5, 43d session, (1890): 729; for California, see Henry Harris, *California's Medical Story* (San Francisco: Stacey, 1932), pp. 245–46; for Ohio see Waite, *Western Reserve School of Medicine*, p. 333.

[21] William Osler, "The License to Practice," *Transactions of the Medical and Chirurgical Faculty of Maryland*, 91st Annual Meeting (1889): 72. For statements on the widespread use of regular textbooks in homeopathic medical schools, see John B. Roberts, *Modern Medicine and Homoeopathy* (Philadelphia: Edwards and Docker, 1895), pp. 10–11; William E. Quine, "The Medical Profession," *Journal of the American Medical Association* 32 (1899): 905.

medical schools were among the first to adopt a three year graded curriculum and one of them (Boston University School of Medicine) was the first medical school in the country to offer a four year graded curriculum (which it did on a voluntary basis). The AIH was a decade in advance of its regular counterpart when it recommended in 1870 that homeopathic medical schools adopt a three-year graded course with six-month terms. Homeopathic medical schools were also more prompt than their regular counterparts in achieving these goals. An 1888 survey by the president of the American Medical Association disclosed that 39 percent of the 13 homeopathic schools, with 30 percent of the students, used three-year graded courses, compared to only 24 percent of the 89 regular schools, with 19 percent of the students (eclectic schools ranked considerably below the regular schools).[22]

THE CONFLICT OVER HAHNEMANN'S LAWS

Throughout homeopathy's history in America, one conflict pervaded every homeopathic institution, setting homeopath against homeopath, medical society against medical society, medical school against medical school. On one side were the small number of high-dilutionists, who accepted and even exceeded Hahnemann's most extreme teachings, using the thirtieth, the one-thousandth, and even the one-millionth dilution. They approached medical science and specialization cautiously and reluctantly. The low-dilutionists, on the other side, not only used the low dilutions, but also often disregarded Hahnemann's laws and used non-homeopathic doses and drugs. They accepted medical science and specialization in the same manner as the regular physicians did.

MEDICAL SOCIETIES

Rancorous debates between low- and high-dilutionists recurred almost annually at the meetings of homeopathic societies. For example, one high-dilutionist said at the 1872 AIH meeting:

There seems to be an "irrepressible conflict" here. There seems to be a party determined that nothing shall pass unless it has the mark of allopathy upon it. I hold that any physician who has passed five, ten, or twenty years, and has used nothing but cold water, if it be the forty-thousandth [dilution] of

---

[22] Bradford, *Homoeopathic Medical College*, pp. 162–63; Wershub, *New York Medical College*, pp. 68–69; "Boston University School of Medicine Forty-Seventh Annual Announcement and Catalogue, 1919," *Boston University Bulletin* VIII (1919): 9; Alvin E. Small, "Annual Address," *Transactions of the American Institute of Homoeopathy*, 26th session (1873): 25; A. Y. P. Garnett, "The Mission of the American Medical Association," *Journal of the American Medical Association* 10 (1888): 576. Only one eclectic school with 4 percent of eclectic students had a graded curriculum.

cold water, and he has succeeded, is a better doctor than he who has used opiates and palliatives, and has not succeeded. . . . The gift in Hahnemann's discovery was, to cure without killing. . . .[23]

Later in the debate, a low-dilutionist who was a former president of the institute replied:

Now, is there such a thing as a self-limiting disease? With our habit of dosing everything—it is so easy to dose—and because we know we do no harm in doing it, we hardly know whether there is such a thing as a self-limiting disease. . . .

Of what force is it for a person to say he has cured hooping-cough after he has dosed it for twelve weeks? . . . Nobody wishes to derogate aught from the honors of any physician, but we should, if we would be good physicians, be reasonably critical in these matters, and not claim too much for our medicines. It seems to me that the ground that most of the speakers have taken in this matter demands of us altogether too much. Suppose I have one of these cases of puerperal convulsions to treat, and I give . . . the two-hundredth [dilution] of cold water, or the forty-thousandth of nothing, are you obliged to believe me, or are you obliged because I give it to attribute the results to my having done so? I trow not.[24]

Speaking to this point, a high-dilutionist responded, "If this principle is going to prevail, all we have to do as strict Hahnemannians is, to organize another society, if our reports are not respected."[25]

Hahnemann, the master, was always brought in as the authority in these debates, and in short order the low-dilutionists began to attack the high-dilutionists as exceeding his rules. In 1866, one important homeopath said that some of Hahnemann's "disciples have gone far beyond the limits of the master. . . . Imagination remains abashed at the contemplation of these inconceivable infinitessimals." The same writer said that, "in the beginning of his homeopathic career, Hahnemann regarded the dose as a subject of minor importance, and for a long time he continued to use tolerably large doses of the appropriate remedy."[26] Gradually, some of the low-dilutionists began to attack Hahnemann himself. One well-known homeopath, H. M. Paine, read a paper before the Homeopathic Medical Society of the State of New York in 1879 in which he questioned some of Hahnemann's major principles:

Hahnemann promulgated a great *central principle* in medicine, viz.: that of effecting cures by the application of medicines, whose toxical effects

23 "Proceedings," *Transactions of the American Institute of Homoeopathy*, 25th session (1872): 79.

24 *Ibid.*, pp. 82–83.

25 *Ibid.*, p. 84.

26 Professor Hempel, "What Might and Should be the Social and Political Relations of Homoeopathy to the Dominant School of Medicine," *American Homoeopathic Observer* 3 (1866): 416.

closely resemble the symptoms of the diseases for which they are usually the more appropriate and natural remedies. He then attempted to deduce from this principle or natural law two corollaries—the *doctrine of the minimum dose* and the *theory of the dynamization of the medicine.*

Although Hahnemann claimed that these two [corollaries] were essential and necessary, in order to secure the proper application of the central or governing principle, is it not probable that he promulgated thereby *two fundamental errors?* [27]

With regard to the minimum-dose corollary, Paine argued that Hahnemann advocated doses "so inconceivably minute as not to possess, by any known method of examination, the least possible quantity of medicine in a material form." With regard to the theory of dynamization (shaking a drug renders it more potent), Paine called it "a theory which has no relation whatever to the proper application of the homeopathic principle; one which is as pernicious as it is false, and might be properly treated with entire indifference were it not positively harmful." [28]

The attacks on Hahnemann's basic theories soon led the high dilutionists to separate themselves from the main body of homeopaths. In 1880, a number of them organized the International Hahnemannian Association to revive the waning interest in Hahnemann's teachings. However, the organization was too small to have any impact on homeopathy. The association had only about two hundred members, and one of its presidents conceded in 1892 that there were probably not more than three hundred true Hahnemannians in the world. [29]

MEDICAL SCHOOLS

The occasional conflicts between low and high dilutionists in homeopathic medical schools involved somewhat different issues than the conflicts in the homeopathic medical societies. In these cases the high dilutionists questioned not only the teaching of non-homeopathic therapeutics, but also the emphasis on the basic medical sciences and clinical specialties.

The Homeopathic Medical College of Pennsylvania, founded in Philadelphia in 1848, adhered strictly to Hahnemann's teachings, as shown by the dismissal in 1854 of a faculty member who advocated more medical science in the curriculum and who used non-homeo-

27 H. M. Paine, "An Examination of the Doctrine of the Minimum Dose and the Theory of Dynamization Promulgated by Hahnemann," *Transactions of the Homoeopathic Medical Society of the State of New York* 15 (1879): 77.

28 *Ibid.*, pp. 77–78.

29 A. C. Allen and J. B. S. King, "Hering Medical College and Hospital," in King, *History of Homoeopathy* II: 423; Roberts, *Modern Medicine and Homoeopathy,* p. 17. The association's membership was listed annually in the *Transactions of the American Institute of Homoeopathy.*

pathic drugs.[30] By 1867, the low dilutionists in the city had become sufficiently numerous to organize a rival medical school, the Hahnemann Medical College, whose prospectus read:

We believe a thorough medical education to be even more important to a homeopath than to an old-school practitioner, on account of the deeper and more scientific principles of Homeopathy, and therefore shall make the utmost efforts to give instruction in all medical branches, equally efficient with any allopathic or homeopathic school. . . .

The high standard of scientific attainment requisite to constitute a thorough medical education demands most careful attention; for Homeopathy, however pure, if not based upon general medical science, must, in common with all other modes of practice, end only in quackery.[31]

Another reason given for the establishment of the new school was that "a large number" of homeopathic physicians sent their students to regular medical schools "alleging that general medical science, as well as surgery . . . can be successfully acquired only in that way." Within two years, Hahnemann Medical College became so successful that the older institution was forced to merge with it under its name and using its curriculum.[32]

Another major dispute occurred in Chicago, where two low-dilutionist schools were established in 1860 and 1876, and two high-dilutionist schools in 1892 and 1895. The new schools complained that the older institutions had adopted "new fads, new and unknown medicines, hypnotics, anti-pyretics, sedatives, temporary expedients, unwise palliatives and aggressive surgery" which had "crowded far to the background" Hahnemann's principles. The faculty of one of the new schools stated that "no palliative treatment or repressive measures will be advocated or employed in any of the lectures or clinics of this college," and that surgery would be used only for the treatment of "strictly mechanical conditions and emergency cases." Here also, the high-dilutionist schools were considerably less successful than the low-dilutionist ones.[33]

THE DOMINANCE OF THE LOW-DILUTIONISTS

Once the low-dilutionists gained control of the major homeopathic institutions, they undertook measures which sought to discredit the arguments of the high-dilutionists. In 1881, the AIH commissioned an

[30] The physician involved defended himself in Charles J. Hempel, *Homoeopathy, A Principle in Nature* (Philadelphia, 1860), pp. v–xliii.

[31] Bradford, *Homoeopathic Medical College*, pp. 134, 137.

[32] *Ibid.*, pp. 137, 158–60.

[33] Allen and King, "Hering Medical College," pp. 427–29; Guernsey P. Waring, "Dunham Medical College of Chicago," in King, *History of Homoeopathy* III: 118–20.

analysis of the ingredients of commercial preparations of one widely used homeopathic drug. The report given at the next convention disclosed that the dilution specified on the label of the preparation bore little relationship to the amount of the drug actually in the preparation: both the seventh dilution and the sixtieth dilution contained about the same amount of the drug. Furthermore, adulterants, sometimes with medicinal properties, often exceeded the amount of the drug in the preparation. Another study presented in 1883 asserted that preparations ground with a porcelain or wedgewood mortar were also unsatisfactory. Large amounts of the mortar (chemically, silicate of alumina) would wear off and be ground in with the drug. Because both silica and alumina were widely used homeopathic drugs, any homeopath prescribing a powdered drug was actually prescribing far more silica and alumina than the drug intended. The president of the AIH admitted the next year: "This proposition is startling and worth our immediate and profound attention. As an unavoidable induction from exhaustive scientific researches, it must inaugurate at once a revolution in our drug provings." Of course it had no such revolutionary impact. Few homeopaths were using high dilutions anyway, and these findings must have only confirmed their disbelief in the high dilutions.[34]

HOMEOPATHS AND REGULAR THERAPIES

The great problem for most homeopaths was not the size of the dose; it was the siren call of regular therapies which continually tempted them to abandon homeopathic drugs for palliative medications. As early as 1873, the president of the AIH warned his colleagues against taking up the ways of the regulars:

The great activity that everywhere prevails in the advancement of medical science leads to the pertinent inquiry, viz.: "Are the great central principles that lie at the foundation of homeopathic practice scrupulously maintained? . . . The only known law of remedial action must be permitted to shine as constantly and as brilliantly as the noonday sun. . . .

We know that venesection will remove the intense pain of pleuritis and pneumonia very speedily; but it is fearfully expensive to vitality, while it increases the number of chances against the recovery of the patient. We also know that the painful sufferings can be palliated by overpowering anodynes

[34] J. Edwards Smith, "Remarks and Suggestions Concerning Certain Homoeopathic Triturations," Transactions of the American Institute of Homoeopathy, 35th session (1882): 575–603; Conrad Wesselhoeft, "The Effects of Trituration Upon Wedgewood and Porcelain Mortars," Transactions of the American Institute of Homoeopathy, 36th session (1883): 339–42; John C. Sanders, "Address," Transactions of the American Institute of Homoeopathy, 37th session (1884): 28.

and anaesthesia. . . . [But we must recall] the wickedness of tampering too freely with the complicated machinery of human life.[35]

Most homeopaths did prescribe regular medicines and often felt guilty about these aberrations. Meetings of homeopathic medical societies occasionally sounded like public confessionals, where members rose and confessed their allopathic sins before their brethren. At the New York state society meeting in 1883, one member confessed to using "massive doses" of quinine as an antipyretic whenever he found it necessary, but claimed that he did so "when my knowledge of homeopathy does not suffice to cure properly; I do not call this homeopathic practice." Another was more defensive in his attitude; he stated that "it was some years after I began the practice of homeopathy that I could administer Quinine with other than a bowed head. But thought and study have convinced me that there is consistency in our doing so, even when standing upon the narrowest platform of homeopathy."[36]

The president of the society did not share the contrition of his colleagues with regard either to dosage or type of drug. He asserted in his presidential address:

. . . we have never suggested that . . . ours was an *universal law*. We can demonstrate that it is a law, but it is limited by those other laws of our being, physical and chemical, which sometime hold it in abeyance; sometimes nullify and vitiate it entirely. . . .

Homeopathy can be practiced while using, in some cases, the same doses as the regular physician. . . . ninety-nine out of a hundred of our physicians use the same drugs, and frequently in large doses day after day, only being careful to not do the injury to their patients by the use of their medicines that the regular doctors frequently do. . . .

The question of dose should have no part or lot in the discussion of homeopathy. It has nothing to do with our creed. Thousands of consistent homeopathic physicians have never used infinitesimals.[37]

Most of the greatest therapeutic problems encountered by homeopaths concerned those illnesses whose symptoms could be relieved by regular treatment. The use of large doses of quinine as an antipyretic is one major illustration. The use of laxatives is another. One homeopathic physician related this anecdote told to him by an old man:

One time about thirty years ago I thought I would try little pills myself. I had been eating pretty heartily without taking much exercise, and got all stuffed up, and I thought I would go to a young Homeopathic doctor who had located near me. He asked me a lot of questions and gave me a vial of

[35] Small, "Annual Address," p. 21.

[36] "Report of the Bureau of Clinical Medicine," *Transactions of the Homoeopathic Medical Society of the State of New York* 18 (1883): 4, 6.

[37] John J. Mitchell, "Annual Address," *Transactions of the Homoeopathic Medical Society of the State of New York* 18 (1883): 62.

little pills—they were very strange to me—but I followed his directions strictly and took his pills for four or five days without any apparent effect. Then I went over to my old doctor, who gave me ten grains of calomel, and I was all right in a short time; I have never tried Homeopathy since.

The physician continued:

Now that circumstance as well as a great many others that I have seen since, taught me that there is a business end of medicine. If that doctor had not been quite so faithful to his law, if he had emptied this old man's bowels out first, and satisfied his mind, he might perhaps have kept him and his family as patients instead of sending them back to old school doctors for thirty years.[38]

By the end of the nineteenth century, practically all homeopaths were using regular as well as homeopathic drugs. The editor of the *Homoeopathic Physician* and the president of the regular state medical society of Pennsylvania both wrote in the 1890's that the great majority of homeopaths did not believe in infinitesimal doses, rejected the universality of the law of similars, and willingly used drugs according to the principles of regular medicine. The decline in homeopaths' interest in their materia medica was also accompanied by an increased interest in clinical specialties.[39]

Eventually, these changes altered the ideology of American homeopathy. In 1899 the AIH redefined a homeopathic physician as "one who adds to his knowledge of medicine a special knowledge of Homeopathic therapeutics. All that pertains to medicine is his, by inheritance, by tradition, by right." In the same year, the institute also modified its motto from "similia similibus curantur" to "similia similibus curentur," after it was pointed out that Hahnemann had used the latter term, and that the two spellings produced very different meanings. The old spelling had been translated, "like is cured by like," but the new spelling was translated, "let like be cured by like," a change from a "law of nature" to a "method of treating disease."[40]

---

[38] W. B. Morgan, "Discussion," *Transactions of the American Institute of Homoeopathy*, 57th session (1901): 645.

[39] [John M. Scudder], "Decadence of Homoeopathy," *Eclectic Medical Journal* 52 (1892): 554–55; Roberts, *Modern Medicine and Homoeopathy*, pp. 13, 16–17; Quine, "Medical Profession," p. 903. Quine's article is a detailed examination of this question, and demonstrates how far homeopaths deviated from Hahnemann's writings. The complete article is to be found on pp. 903–8, 980–85. George Royal, "President's Address," *Transactions of the American Institute of Homoeopathy*, 61st session (1905): 33.

[40] "Minutes," *Transactions of the American Institute of Homoeopathy*, 55th session (1899): 102; J. H. McClelland, "Curentur or Curantur?" *Transactions of the American Institute of Homoeopathy*, 55th session (1899): 99–102. McClelland said that if Hahnemann had intended to make his motto a law of healing he would have used "sanantur" as the verb.

Thus, homeopathy prospered in America. Its leaders were eminent men, its ranks were filled with well-educated and prosperous physicians, its institutions were numerous and impressive. Two characteristics of homeopathy account for its prominent place in the American medical profession of the period. The first was a wealthy and powerful clientele, who increased the influence and position of homeopathy far beyond what could otherwise have been expected from a relatively small medical sect. The second was the receptiveness of homeopaths to advances in medical science and to the changing preferences of their clientele.

The zenith of homeopathy as a medical sect in the United States occurred around 1880. After that time, increasing numbers of homeopaths disregarded homeopathic dogma, partly because of their interest in specialization, partly because of dramatic new developments in medical science, partly because of improved relations between homeopaths and regular physicians. Indeed, new developments in specialization and medical science altered all of American medical practice in the last decades of the nineteenth century.

PART V THE RISE OF
SCIENTIFIC MEDICINE

PHYSICIAN I: "And what is a disease? The lodgment in the system
of a pathogenic germ, and the multiplication of that germ. . . .
Can you, for instance, shew me a case of diphtheria without the
bacillus?"
PHYSICIAN II: "No, but I'll shew you the same bacillus, without
the disease, in your own throat."
PHYSICIAN I: "No, not the same. . . . It is an entirely different
bacillus; only the two are, unfortunately, so exactly alike that
you cannot see the difference. . . ."
PHYSICIAN II: "And how do you tell one from the other?"
PHYSICIAN I: "Well, obviously, if the bacillus is the genuine
Loeffler, you have diphtheria; and if it's the pseudo-bacillus,
you're quite well. Nothing simpler."

BERNARD SHAW, *The Doctor's Dilemma*

CHAPTER 13 THE BEGINNINGS OF SCIENTIFIC MEDICINE: SURGERY

SURGERY WAS affected more profoundly by medical science than any other area of nineteenth-century medical practice. The discovery of useful anesthetics during the middle of the century and the development of means to prevent wound infection during the last decades revolutionized surgical procedures. From a crude and dangerous art, surgery rapidly became the most influential and prestigious of all medical specialties.

SURGERY BEFORE ANESTHESIA

From earliest antiquity to the nineteenth century, surgery had changed little and improved less. Haggard has written:

> The earliest known pictures of surgical operations are engraved on the stones over a tomb near Memphis, Egypt. These engravings were made 2,500 years before Christ. . . . The pictures show the operation of circumcision and operations on the legs and arms, and these operations, with the addition of castration, included all the surgical procedures performed by the Egyptians. At this early period all surgery was wound surgery, which included the dressing and treatment of wounds, the opening of abscesses, and, as a last resort, the amputation of limbs. All operations were on the surface of the body or the extremities. . . .
>
> Forty-three centuries after these pictures were made surgery was still wound surgery. . . . Operations were still performed only on the surface of the body, and operations still involved as much suffering, and wounds were as universally infected, as in the early Egyptian period.[1]

The high mortality rate made surgery a dreaded procedure. At the Massachusetts General Hospital, 173 major amputations were performed between 1822 and 1850 with a mortality of 19 percent. Com-

[1] Howard W. Haggard, *Devils, Drugs, and Doctors* (New York: Harper, 1929), p. 127.

pound fractures were so dangerous that amputation of the limb was the approved, less hazardous procedure.[2]

Haggard has described four prerequisites to the development of surgery as a useful medical procedure: "(1) a knowledge of anatomy; (2) a method for controlling hemorrhage; (3) anesthetics to deaden pain; and (4) a knowledge of the nature of infection and methods for its prevention." The first two problems were solved in Europe well before the nineteenth century, but the absence of medical schools in America delayed their transmission to colonial physicians. A history of medicine in Louisiana found no references to any operations other than amputations before the nineteenth century. By the turn of the nineteenth century, however, the growing number of formally trained American physicians began to perform more complex operations. One South Carolina physician declared in 1807 that "the inhabitants who from misfortunes need the performance of the most difficult and uncommon operations in surgery, are at present under no necessity of seeking foreign operators; for what can be done for them in London or Paris can also be done in Charlestown."[3]

Despite the problems caused by sepsis and the lack of anesthesia, surgery became the most important medically valid therapy in the first half of the nineteenth century. One physician observed in 1851 that in surgery alone "the well-instructed aspirant treads on certain ground, and has nothing to fear from the rivalry or impertinent interference of quackery." No unskilled practitioner, he continued, would "venture to perform a capital operation in surgery, at the risk of having his head broken by the by-standers."[4]

ANESTHESIA AND SURGERY

The lack of anesthesia was the most terrifying surgical problem before the second half of the nineteenth century. Patients refused or delayed surgery if at all possible; tumors, for example, were allowed to grow to fifty or one hundred pounds before removal. Surgical operations themselves reflected the horror of the event:

[2] Table XIII.1; John Brooks Wheeler, *Memoirs of a Small-Town Surgeon* (New York: Garden City, 1935), p. 10.

[3] Haggard, *Devils, Drugs, and Doctors*, p. 128; John Duffy, ed., *The Rudolph Matas History of Medicine in Louisiana* (n.p.: Louisiana State University Press, 1958), I: 148, 290; David Ramsay, *History of South Carolina* (Charleston: 1809), quoted in Joseph Ioor Waring, *A History of Medicine in South Carolina 1670–1825* (n.p.: South Carolina Medical Association, 1964), p. 151.

[4] "Senex," "The Past and Present State of the Medical Profession—Homoeopathy," *Boston Medical and Surgical Journal* 44 (1851): 339.

In case of amputation, it was the custom to bring the patient into the operating room and place him upon the table. [The surgeon] would stand with his hands behind his back and would say to the patient, "Will you have your leg off, or will you not have it off?" If the patient lost courage and said, "No," he had decided not to have the leg amputated, he was at once carried back to his bed in the ward. If, however, he said "Yes," he was immediately taken firmly in hand by a number of strong assistants and the operation went on regardless of whatever he might say thereafter. If his courage failed him *after* this crucial moment, it was too late and no attention was paid to his cries of protest. It was found to be the only practicable method by which an operation could be performed under the gruesome conditions which prevailed before the advent of anesthesia.[5]

Various means of reducing pain were employed. Soporifics like opium, hemp, hashish, and whiskey were widely used. In amputations, the limb was tightly bound above the part to be amputated to dull all sensations below the binding. What was lacking, however, was an anesthetic which (1) would affect everyone similarly; (2) would consistently lead to complete insensibility to pain for a predetermined period of time; and (3) was safe.[6]

In the years between 1842 and 1847, the anesthetic properties of nitrous oxide (laughing gas) and ether were discovered by American physicians, and those of chloroform by a British physician. Ether in particular became world-famous within weeks after its first public clinical demonstration at the Massachusetts General Hospital in Boston in 1846. Henry J. Bigelow claimed that "no single announcement ever created so great and general excitement in so short a time. Surgeons, sufferers, scientific men, everybody, united in simultaneous demonstration of heartfelt mutual congratulation."[7]

Although both ether and chloroform were rapidly and widely adopted, their use did not produce major advances in either the scope or the safety of operations. An 1864 review of developments in surgery over the preceding three decades listed almost none which required an incision into the abdomen, thorax, or cranium.[8] With regard to the safety of operations, data from the Massachusetts General Hospital showed that the mortality from operations actually increased after the introduction of anesthesia (Table XIII.1).

[5] J. Collins Warren, *To Work in the Vineyard of Surgery*, ed. Edward D. Churchill (Cambridge, Mass.: Harvard University Press, 1958), p. 37.

[6] Henry J. Bigelow, "A History of the Discovery of Modern Anaesthesia," in Edward H. Clarke, *et al., A Century of Modern Medicine* (Philadelphia: Lea, 1876), pp. 79–80.

[7] Haggard, *Devils, Drugs, and Doctors*, pp. 98–105; Bigelow, "Discovery of Modern Anaesthesia," p. 80.

[8] J. Mason Warren, "Recent Progress in Surgery," *Medical Communications of the Massachusetts Medical Society* 10 (1864): 267–340.

TABLE XIII.1
MORTALITY FROM MAJOR AMPUTATIONS AT THE MASSACHUSETTS GENERAL HOSPITAL,
1822–60

Limb Amputated	Number of Amputations		Percent Fatal	
	1822–50	1850–60	1822–50	1850–60
Thigh	88	86	22	22
Leg	60	84	17	29
Arm	12	19	8	16
Forearm	13	18	15	6
TOTAL	173	207	19	23

SOURCE: J. Mason Warren, "Recent Progress in Surgery," *Medical Communications of the Massachusetts Medical Society* 10 (1864): 299.

Nevertheless, surgical operations became much more frequent after 1850. The average of 6.2 amputations performed annually in the hospital from 1822 to 1850 increased to 20.7 annually from 1850 to 1860. This increase in the number of operations (which probably also reflects an increased use of hospitals for surgery), together with the extensive experience obtained by surgeons during the Civil War, raised the caliber of American surgery to the level of its European counterpart by the end of the Civil War. Furthermore, surgeons were able to refine their skills by proceeding deliberately and carefully during operations. One British surgeon reminisced: "when I was a boy, . . . surgeons operating upon the quick were pitted one against the other like runners on time. He was the best surgeon both for the patient and onlooker, who broke the three-minute record in an amputation or a lithotomy. The obvious boon of immunity from pain, precious as it was, when we look beyond the individual, was less than the boon of time. With anesthetics ended slap-dash surgery. . . ."[9]

Nonetheless, surgery as a full-time specialty was still rare in the United States. Samuel Gross, an eminent American surgeon, said in 1876 that it was "safe to affirm that there is not a medical man on this continent who devotes himself exclusively to the practice of surgery." Surgery's development was retarded because of two problems. First, anesthetics were not yet well understood. As late as 1895, it was not uncommon for inexperienced students or nurses to administer anesthetics, sometimes so deeply that death occurred. These fatalities dis-

[9] Courtney R. Hall, "The Rise of Professional Surgery in the United States: 1800–1865," *Bulletin of the History of Medicine* 26 (1952): 261; Max Kahn, "History of Modern Medicine," in Frederick Tice, ed., *Practice of Medicine*, vol. 1 (New York: Prior, 1920), p. 92.

suaded many patients from using anesthesia, and in Kansas, for example, it was used only in hospital surgery, while most physicians continued to rely on whiskey.[10] The second reason for the slow growth of full-time surgical practice was the persistent and increasing problem of post-operative infection brought about by unsterile procedures.

BACTERIOLOGY AND ANTISEPTIC SURGERY

The last great problem of surgery—infection—historically had been most formidable in the treatment of wounds, whether inflicted by accident, combat, or operative surgery. Until the eighteenth and nineteenth centuries, the healing of wounds which were not excessively deep, bruised, or lacerated was never a major problem. Surgeons joined the two lips of the wound by adhesion and usually produced union "by first intention," as it was called, even though they used no antiseptic procedures. Some suppuration occurred, to be sure, but this did not normally lead to putrefaction or seriously retard the healing process. Deep wounds, however, posed more difficult problems for the surgeon. Joining the superficial parts of the wound by adhesion would often leave a cavity in the interior of the wound which would collect blood, putrefy, and break down the healing process, especially in the absence of antiseptic procedures. Physicians learned that healing in these wounds could occur only from the interior outward, and consequently undertook measures to prevent the superficial parts of the wound from adhering until the interior had begun to heal. This was done by inserting objects like setons, pieces of cloth, or irritating salves into the wound. The open wound would suppurate, which was called "laudable pus," and often putrefy. The healing process could be long and painful and lead to serious or fatal complications.[11]

The incidence of wounds which would not heal by first intention became a major problem among civilians only after the urbanization of the population in the nineteenth century in America and the increased surgery and crowding in hospitals. The presence of large num-

[10] S. D. Gross, "Surgery," in Clarke, ed., *A Century of American Medicine*, p. 117; John F. Fulton, *Harvey Cushing: A Biography* (Springfield, Ill.: Thomas, 1946), p. 93; Thomas Neville Bonner, *The Kansas Doctor* (Lawrence: University of Kansas Press, 1959), p. 24.

[11] Astley Paston Cooper Ashhurst, "The Centenary of Lister (1827–1927): a Tale of Sepsis and Antisepsis," *Annals of Medical History* 9 (1927): 205–11; Edward D. Churchill, "Healing by First Intention and with Suppuration: Studies in the History of Wound Healing," *Journal of the History of Medicine and Allied Sciences* 19 (1964): 193–214; Edward D. Churchill, "The Pandemic of Wound Infection in Hospitals: Studies in the History of Wound Healing," *Journal of the History of Medicine and Allied Sciences* 20 (1965): 390–404.

bers of patients with open wounds in the same ward led to many cases of "hospitalism," or cross-infection from one patient to another. Hospitalism could take the form of hospital gangrene, erysipelas, pyemia, etc., all of which were frequently fatal. Contemporary physicians recognized the cause of the problem and complained that it was much more difficult to achieve union by first intention in urban hospitals than in rural private homes. Hospitalism sometimes became so severe that hospitals were forced to shut down their operating rooms and surgical wards until the epidemics abated. By the end of the century, many physicians were advocating separate small cottages or open air pavilions or barracks for the hospital treatment of wound patients, in order to minimize hospitalism.[12]

Thus by the middle of the nineteenth century, surgeons were acutely aware of cross-infection, and a number of physicians undertook experiments to prevent it, some with considerable success.[13] The problem, however, was that no one knew what caused cross-infection.

About the same time, developments in bacteriology were providing insight into the nature and cause of this problem. The early nineteenth-century bacteriologists had discovered that micro-organisms, or germs, were present in organic matter. They also found that if an organic substance like meat or milk was left standing, the number of micro-organisms contained in it would multiply and soon become visible as a mold. Heating the substance would kill all the micro-organisms, but they would mysteriously reappear if the substance was left standing again. The conclusion drawn from these findings was that the reappearance of the micro-organisms was the product of spontaneous generation of life in the substance itself.

Louis Pasteur (1822–95) demonstrated that the reappearance of micro-organisms was due not to spontaneous generation, but rather to the presence of germs in the dust that settled on the substance. He described his classic experiment in the following manner:

Here . . . is an infusion of organic matter, as limpid as distilled water. . . . It has been prepared to-day. To-morrow it will contain little animalculae, little infusories, or flakes of moldiness.

I place a portion of that infusion in a flask with a long neck, like this one. Suppose I boil the liquid and leave it to cool. After a few days, moldiness or animalculae will develop in the liquid. By boiling I destroy any germs contained in the liquid or against the glass . . . . Now suppose I repeat

12 Churchill, "Pandemic of Wound Infection," pp. 390–98; John Eric Erichsen, "Impressions of American Surgery," *Lancet* 2 (1874): 718–19; Warren, *Vineyard of Surgery*, p. 42.

13 Owen H. Wangensteen, "Preludes to Lister and the interdependence of the sciences," *Surgery* 58 (1965): 931–34.

this experiment, but that before boiling the liquid I draw . . . the neck of the flask into a [curved] point, leaving, however, its extremity open. This being done, I boil the liquid in the flask, and leave it to cool. Now the liquid in this second flask will remain pure, not only two days, a month, a year, but three or four years—for the experiment I am telling you about is already four years old, and the liquid remains as limpid as distilled water. What difference is there, then, between those two vases? They contain the same liquid; they both contain air, both are open! Why does one decay and the other remain pure? The only difference between them is this: in the first case, the dust suspended in the air and their germs can fall into the neck of the flask and arrive into contact with the liquid, where they find appropriate food and develop; thence microscopic beings. In the second flask, on the contrary, it is impossible, or at least, extremely difficult, unless air is violently shaken, that dusts suspended in air should enter the vase; they fall on its curved neck. When air goes in and out of the vase through diffusion or variations of temperature the latter never being sudden, the air comes in slowly enough to drop the dusts and germs that it carries at the opening of the neck or in the first curves.

This experiment is full of instruction; for this must be noted, that everything in air save its dusts can easily enter the vase and come into contact with the liquid. Imagine what you choose in the air—electricity, magnetism, ozone, unknown forces even, all can reach the infusion. Only one thing cannot enter easily, and that is dust, suspended in air. And the proof of this is that if I shake the vase violently two or three times, in a few days it contains animalculae or moldiness. Why? Because air has come in violently enough to carry dust with it.

And therefore, gentlemen, I could point to that liquid and say to you, I have taken my drop of water from the immensity of creation, and I have taken it full of the elements appropriated to the development of inferior beings. And I wait, I watch, I question it, begging it to recommence for me the beautiful spectacle of the first creation. But it is dumb, dumb since these experiments were begun several years ago; it is dumb, because I have kept it from the only thing man cannot produce, from the germs which float in the air, from Life, for Life is a germ and germ is Life. Never will the doctrine of spontaneous generation recover from the mortal blow of this simple experiment.[14]

This eloquent statement is illustrative of the revolution occurring in the life sciences during this period. The analogistic reasoning of the eighteenth and early nineteenth centuries, with its rationalism and flights of logical fancy, had given way to empirical relationships— demonstrable, consistent, and indisputable.

Joseph Lister (1827–1912) was a British surgeon who read Pasteur's work in 1865 and realized that air-borne germs caused putrefaction in wounds in the same way that they produced molds in organic matter.

[14] Kahn, "History of Modern Medicine," pp. 86–87.

His conclusion from this brilliant insight was obvious: simply destroy the germs on the wound during the operation and prevent their entrance into the wound during the healing process, and no putrefaction will occur. Lister chose carbolic acid as his antiseptic or germ destroyer and devised a method for antiseptic operations. He soaked the sponges, instruments, ligatures, and sutures in a carbolic acid solution. He washed his hands, particularly the finger tips, in a carbolic acid solution. He used an atomizer to spray a carbolic acid vapor over the wound during the operation and irrigated the wound with carbolic acid solution during the operation. He endeavored to prevent the wound from becoming infected after the operation with an elaborate system of dressings dipped in carbolic acid solution or otherwise treated with antiseptics.[15]

Although Lister believed that these procedures would prevent sepsis, neither he nor many of his supporters realized how inadequate they were and how thoroughly prevailing operating procedures had to be altered to insure sterility. These surgeons failed to realize that dipping the hands in carbolic acid solution was inadequate to sterilize them, and that a thorough cleaning, including careful brushing under the nails, was essential. The surgeons operated using their bare hands and wearing street clothes or, more often, blood-stained coats which were kept in a closet in the operating room and rarely cleaned. Surgical instruments with wooden handles which could not be sterilized were often placed on unsterile towels after being baked or dipped in the carbolic acid solution. The bowls containing the carbolic acid solution were not sterilized and sponges were simply rinsed out and dipped in the carbolic acid solution between uses. Surgeons would drop instruments, pick them up from the floor, and use them again without sterilizing them; they would not hesitate to wipe their faces or touch unsterile objects with their hands during operations, confident that simply dipping the hands in the solution again would suffice to disinfect them, if they bothered to do that. Consequently, these limited antiseptic procedures were not particularly successful in preventing wound infections, even when surgeons followed them conscientiously. Surgeons using antiseptic measures were rarely able to produce sta-

15 Ashhurst, "Centenary of Lister," pp. 214–15; for contemporary accounts of this stage of antiseptic surgery, see Robert F. Weir, "On the Antiseptic Treatment of Wounds, and its Results," *New York Medical Journal* 26 (1877): 561–77; W. W. Keen, "Recent Progress in Surgery," *Harper's New Monthly Magazine* 79 (1889): 703–13; Herbert L. Burrell and Greenleaf R. Tucker, "Aseptic Surgery," *Medical Communications of the Massachusetts Medical Society* 14 (1889): 551–94.

tistics more favorable than those of capable and careful surgeons not using antiseptic measures.[16]

Other problems aggravated these difficulties and made many surgeons unwilling to adopt Lister's system. The myriad small details seemed like meaningless rituals whose legitimacy was rendered suspect by Lister's frequent modifications of them. Carbolic acid was a deadly poison, often drunk by suicides. Spraying it around the room unceasingly during an operation adversely affected the wound, the patient, the operators, and the assistants alike (Lister abandoned it in 1887). Other antiseptics, like bichloride of mercury, were found to affect adversely the delicate membranes of the wound and could not be used in place of carbolic acid. More basically, many physicians strongly opposed the germ theory on which Lister's procedures were based. Last, many American physicians believed that hospitalism was a greater problem in Europe than in America and that antiseptic procedures were therefore less necessary here.[17]

Given the inevitable lack of any clear-cut success by Lister's supporters and the numerous valid objections to elements of Lister's method, it is hardly surprising that many surgeons refused to accept antiseptic surgery. Gross stated in 1876 that "little, if any faith, is placed by any enlightened or experienced surgeon on this side of the Atlantic in the so-called carbolic acid treatment of Professor Lister, apart from the care which is taken in applying the dressing, or, what is the same thing, in clearing away clots and excluding air from the wound." This state of affairs continued for some time, for speakers at the American Surgical Association conventions in the early 1880's claimed that neither they nor most other surgeons in their communities used antiseptic surgery.[18]

Gradually, however, increased knowledge of the modes of infection and better means of preventing them made antiseptic surgery of

16 J. M. T. Finney, A Surgeon's Life (New York: Putnam, 1940), pp. 74–76; Gert H. Brieger, "American Surgery and the Germ Theory of Disease," Bulletin of the History of Medicine 40 (1966): 139–40; John J. Morton, "The Struggle against Sepsis," Yale Journal of Biology and Medicine 31 (1959): 401–3; Ashhurst, "Centenary of Lister," pp. 217–20.

17 Weir, "Antiseptic Treatment of Wounds," pp. 561–62; New International Encyclopedia (New York: Dodd, Mead, 1914), 2nd ed., s.v., "Carbolic Acid"; Rudolph Matas, "Surgical Operations Fifty Years Ago," American Journal of Surgery, n.s. 51 (1941): 50–51; Erichsen, "Impressions of American Surgery," p. 719.

18 Gross, "Surgery," p. 213; Henry E. Sigerst, "Surgery at the Time of the Introduction of Antisepsis," Journal of the Missouri State Medical Association 32 (1935): 173–76; Fritz Linder and Hugh Forrest, "The Propagation of Lister's Ideas," British Journal of Surgery 54 (1967): 420 (supplement).

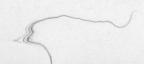

consistent and demonstrable medical value. It was learned that germs coming into contact with the wound from the air were less of a problem than germs on the body of the patient, the hands of the surgeon, and the instruments and devices used in surgery. Methods of steam and dry-heat sterilization were developed and found to be superior to carbolic acid. Surgeons devised methods for sterilizing their hands, yet without subjecting them to the harshness of carbolic acid. Caps, gowns, masks, and rubber gloves were designed, made sterile, and popularized. Metal instruments replaced the wooden-handled ones. Last, it was learned that the wound could be kept dry and yet free from infection, and thus asepsis replaced antisepsis. In addition, the X-ray was discovered in 1895 and brought an entirely new dimension to the surgeon's ability to operate accurately and effectively.[19]

Thus, through the cumulative efforts of many different individuals, surgery was transformed from an act of desperation to a scientific method of dealing with illness. In the 1880's, surgeons began to operate on the head, chest, and abdomen for the first time. An American physician, Reginald Fitz, described the nature of and surgical treatment for appendicitis in 1886. By the end of the decade, surgeons were even performing exploratory surgery in the abdomen and undertaking cranial surgery. Specialization soon made general surgery almost completely abdominal surgery, and surgery involving other organs was delegated to other specialists.[20]

The growing demand for surgery induced many physicians to become full-time surgeons. The number of operations performed annually at the Massachusetts General Hospital increased from an average of 37 in the years between 1841 and 1845 (immediately before the use of anesthesia), 98 per year between 1847 and 1851, and 3700 in 1898. Enough surgeons were practicing full-time by 1880 to warrant the establishment of the American Surgical Association in that year and other specialty surgical societies in subsequent years. Full-time surgeons also developed new relations with general practitioners, on whom they depended increasingly for referrals of their patients. This produced a novel ethical problem—surreptitious fee-splitting between the surgeon and the referring physician. Fee-splitting became such a problem

[19] Matas, "Surgical Operations," p. 53; Morton, "Struggle against Sepsis," pp. 404–5; Linder and Forrest, "Propagation of Lister's Ideas," pp. 420–21.

[20] Matas, "Surgical Operations," p. 52; Keen, "Recent Progress in Surgery," pp. 707–10; Hyman Morrison, "The Chapter on Appendicitis in a Biography of Reginald Heber Fitz," *Bulletin of the History of Medicine* 20 (1946): 259–69; James J. Walsh, *History of Medicine in New York* (New York: National Americana Society, 1919), I: 277.

by 1912 that the AMA code of ethics was amended to condemn com-
missions to physicians for referring patients and to prohibit the secret
division of fees. One surgeon observed that "it was not difficult, however, for the determined physician to devise a method to obviate the
limited proscriptions which were set down."[21]

ANTISEPTIC SURGERY AND THE NON-REGULAR SECTS

Homeopathic surgeons adopted antiseptic and aseptic surgical procedures at the same time as their regular counterparts. The president
of the American Institute of Homeopathy said of surgery in 1882: "the
common interest taken in this field by the physicians of all schools of
medicine has resulted in a degree of advancement, or perfection, that
argues strongly for the cause of unity in the profession." In 1876, a
homeopathic surgeon, William Tod Helmuth, performed one of the
earliest antiseptic operations in the United States (an ovariotomy).
Because he was head of surgery at the Homeopathic Medical College
of New York, it is quite probable that he instructed his students in
antiseptic techniques. In 1883, the AIH's Bureau of Surgery presented
a long and generally favorable report on antiseptic surgery. In 1890,
it reported: "in brief, the year's experience has seemed only to
strengthen the general faith in antiseptic surgery. Indeed, its practice
may be said to have had almost no opposition, at least so far as open
demonstration against it is concerned."[22]

With respect to the eclectic sect, A. J. Howe, whom a medical
historian has called the "foremost surgeon" of eclectic medicine, stated
in 1882 that, although he disagreed with many details of Lister's
method, he believed that "sepsis is the bane of our art," and had believed that for many years. There were few eclectic surgeons, however,
and no eclectic hospitals of consequence. Therefore, the question was
not a major one in the sect and there are few references to it in the
Eclectic Medical Journal.[23]

21 Ibid., p. 274, Loyal Davis, *Fellowship of Surgeons* (Springfield, Ill.: Thomas,
1960), p. 138. For a discussion of AMA policies toward fee-splitting, see Donald E.
Konold, *A History of American Medical Ethics 1847–1912* (Madison, Wis.: State
Historical Society of Wisconsin, 1962), pp. 65–66, 71.

22 W. L. Breyfogle, "Annual Address," *Transactions of the American Institute
of Homoeopathy*, 35th session (1882): 31; William Tod Helmuth, "Antiseptic
Ovariotomy," *Medical Record* 11 (1876): 837–38; "Antiseptic Surgery," *Transactions
of the American Institute of Homoeopathy*, 36th Session (1883): 701–839; Charles M.
Thomas, "Address of the Bureau of Surgery," *Transactions of the American Institute of Homeopathy*, 43rd Session (1890): 630.

23 A. J. Howe, " 'Listerism'," *Eclectic Medical Journal* 42 (1882); 9–13; Otto
Juettner, *Daniel Drake and His Followers* (Cincinnati: Harvey, 1909), p. 378.

Thus, during the nineteenth century surgery rose to the pinnacle of professional esteem and influence, as shown by the succession of surgeons to the AMA presidency in the last two decades of the century. This transformation was due solely to surgery's success in curing the sick. Other aspects of bacteriology were not so readily applicable to therapeutics, and their impact on the profession was correspondingly diminished.

CHAPTER 14 BACTERIOLOGY AND THE MEDICAL PROFESSION

THE DISCOVERIES that produced antiseptic surgery were the forerunners of other major scientific developments, which culminated in the 1880's with the findings that specific bacteria constituted a necessary although not a sufficient cause of many diseases. While these bacteriological discoveries revolutionized medical science, they had a much more limited impact on medical practice. Physicians at the end of the nineteenth century, like those at the beginning, were particularly interested in therapeutics, and these findings contributed primarily to etiology and diagnosis. The indifference and even resistance of physicians to developments in bacteriology widened the gap between medical science and medical practice at the end of the nineteenth century.

SCIENTIFIC PRECURSORS OF BACTERIOLOGY

The first great scientific advances in the etiology of disease were made in the middle of the nineteenth century, primarily through the development of cellular pathology, the study of body tissues altered by disease. Cellular pathology had little practical utility for many years, and most pathologists were medical scientists rather than physicians. The limited interest of physicians in pathological tissue specimens was evident in their neglect of the microscope, which was necessary to examine them. A homeopathic physician was far ahead of his time when he wrote in 1867:

Medicine has reached a point at which we may fearlessly assert that the microscope is its only true touchstone. [For] . . . almost all that we have learned that is truly reliable in medical science, we are indebted to the microscope. Yet how many professed medical men are there who never examined into the structures of a compound microscope—how many of them never used one in pursuing their studies—how very few of them possess such an instrument, or rely upon its use in their daily investigations of the phenomena of health and disease. It may truly be affirmed that there is no physiology

261

but cellular physiology and we may just as safely declare that there is no pathology but cellular pathology.[1]

Only a small number of medical schools, like the Harvard Medical School and the Homeopathic Medical College of New York, used the microscope intensively in their courses in the 1880's. The great majority of schools taught neither microscopy nor the sciences which depended on microscopic analysis until the 1890's. Consequently, their graduates were often ignorant of the latest discoveries in medical science. One pathologist claimed about 1875 that "if what is really known of the laws of disease were told to the members of the profession, more than half of them would indignantly discredit it."[2]

New developments in diagnostics were also disregarded by most physicians, partly because they were impractical, but largely because they too contributed little to therapeutics until they had been in use for some time. Rosenberg found in his study of medical practice in New York in the 1860's that auscultation and percussion were neither taught in medical schools nor used in routine house-calls. Thermometers were not commonly used in urban areas until the 1880's, primarily because they were impractical and unwieldy. The best thermometer available in 1870 was nine or ten inches long, not self-registering, and had no magnification of the mercury column. It was cumbersome to use and difficult to read in a darkened sick room. The ophthalmoscope and laryngoscope were used routinely for many years after their invention in the 1850's only by specialists of the eye, ear, nose, and throat. These instruments had little practical utility for the average physician. One physician observed shortly after the discovery of the ophthalmoscope, "what the ophthalmoscope discloses are morbid conditions which are not for the most part more curable by being seen." It required many years of collective professional experience before physicians could relate what they saw through these instruments to treatments which they could use on patients.[3]

1 Leonard Paul Wershub, *One Hundred Years of Medical Progress: A History of the New York Medical College Flower and Fifth Avenue Hospital* (Springfield, Ill.: Thomas, 1967), p. 9.

2 Russell L. Haden, "The Early Use of the Microscope in Ohio," *Ohio State Archaeological and Historical Quarterly* 51 (1942): 277–78; Wershub, *New York Medical College*, pp. 74–75; Charles Rosenberg, "The Practice of Medicine in New York a Century Ago," *Bulletin of the History of Medicine* 41 (1967): 228.

3 *Ibid.*, pp. 241–42; Samuel B. Ward, "History of Medicine in the State of New York in the Last Hundred Years," *Albany Medical Annals* 27 (1906): 193–94; Arthur J. Bedell, "The First Ten Years of Ophthalmoscopy, 1851–1861," *Transactions of the American Ophthalmological Society*, 86th meeting (1951): 39.

THE DEVELOPMENT OF BACTERIOLOGY

In the second half of the nineteenth century, many European biological scientists turned their attention to the numerous micro-organisms which had been discovered in living matter. During this period Pasteur discovered the role of air-borne germs in fermentation, and he and other scientists, most notably Robert Koch (1843–1910), examined the relationship between bacteria and disease. In 1876, Koch showed for the first time that a bacillus bore a specific etiological relationship to a disease, in this case anthrax. Koch had first duplicated the work of others by inoculating into healthy animals blood containing anthrax bacilli from animals who had died of anthrax. Like the others, he found that the inoculated animals died of anthrax and that their blood also contained the anthrax bacilli. But, as Koch realized, this did not necessarily mean that the bacilli were the cause of the disease; other components of the blood might have been the causal factors. Koch therefore developed a novel method of growing the bacilli on a solid culture medium (in contrast to the liquid culture media used previously). He found that the bacilli reproduced on the solid medium, but that the other constituents of the blood did not. Furthermore, the bacilli could be transferred from one solid culture medium to a new one and grown there. This could be done numerous times in order to remove any trace of other constituents of the blood. Koch then injected these pure anthrax bacilli into healthy animals and they too died from the disease. Thus he proved that anthrax bacilli were directly responsible for the disease.[4]

In 1879, Louis Pasteur discovered that old cultures of fowl cholera bacilli which were injected into healthy chickens failed to produce the lethal disease. He then injected fresh cultures of the bacilli into the previously inoculated and some uninoculated chickens; the uninoculated chickens contracted fowl cholera, but the inoculated ones did not. Later, while working with anthrax bacilli, he discovered that old anthrax bacilli could prevent anthrax in animals in the same way that old fowl cholera bacilli prevented fowl cholera in chickens. Pasteur realized the parallel of these discoveries with Jenner's use of cowpox vaccine to prevent smallpox (as well as, undoubtedly, the immunizing value of inoculations of smallpox), and adopted "vaccination" as a

[4] H. J. Parish, *A History of Immunization* (Edinburgh: Livingstone, 1965), p. 42; Hubert A. Lechevalier and Morris Solotorovsky, *Three Centuries of Microbiology* (New York: McGraw-Hill, 1965), pp. 85–86.

generic term for this form of inoculation, in recognition of Jenner's achievement.[5]

During the rest of the century, bacteriologists discovered microorganisms to be the causes of many diseases, including tuberculosis, diphtheria, cholera, typhoid, and tetanus.[6] Although these discoveries are often attributed to individual men, actually dozens of scientists throughout the world replicated and improved the original experiments to produce scientifically valid, demonstrable, and consistent results. Within a year after Koch presented his findings on the tubercle bacillus, for example, other scientists attempted to replicate his work with varying degrees of success.[7] This concentration of effort by many men on the same problem was often considered to be the most significant feature of the period. Alfred Loomis observed in 1888:

> In looking over the field of bacteriological research for the past ten years, one is struck by the continuous, painstaking investigation of a vast number of observers. Never before has there been so little theorizing with so much work, and the facts which have finally been accepted are such as have come to light only after a long series of carefully made and oft-repeated experiments. One investigator makes a statement; immediately, in a dozen different countries, and by hundreds of observers, his experiments are repeated, his statement of facts proved or disproved, and his conclusions accepted or discarded. . . .[8]

These discoveries were made possible by technological developments which occurred after the middle of the nineteenth century. Two technological refinements were of paramount importance. One was the development of a microscope which would produce an undistorted high-level magnification of the bacteria. The achromatic lens became practical in the 1830's, water immersion lenses were devised in the late 1860's and in the 1870's, and oil immersion lenses were developed in 1878 and 1879. The importance of the immersion lens system is indicated by Koch's use of it for all his major discoveries in the 1880's. The second technological improvement was the manufacture of chemicals to stain the bacteria to make them visible. Aniline dyes revolutionized microscopic technique and contributed to virtually all of the major bacteriological discoveries of the period. They were first produced by the German dye industry in 1856, but were used in micro-

[5] Parish, *History of Immunization*, pp. 43–45.

[6] For a chronology of the major developments, see Frederick P. Gorham, "The History of Bacteriology and its Contribution to Public Health Work," in Mazyck P. Ravenel, ed., *A Half Century of Public Health* (New York: American Public Health Association, 1921), pp. 71–72.

[7] Harold C. Ernst, "A Contribution to the Study of the Tubercle-Bacillus," *Medical Communications of the Massachusetts Medical Society* 13 (1883): 126.

[8] Alfred L. Loomis, "Anniversary Address," *Transactions of the Medical Society of the State of New York* (1888): 56.

biology only in the 1860's and 1870's. These technological prerequisites in turn depended on countless discoveries and inventions in such fields as chemistry, physics, optics, glass-making, machine tools, metallurgy, engineering, etc., which also occurred during the nineteenth century. Indeed, technological barriers were a far greater impediment to progress in microbiology than were the intellectual problems of research or the vagaries of professional research interests. This is clearly shown by the astonishing rapidity with which bacteriology developed once the technological impediments were overcome.[9]

THE REACTIONS OF PHYSICIANS TO BACTERIOLOGY

Because the bacteriological diseases were among the most common and terrifying causes of death in the period, physicians might have been expected to accept the discoveries readily and gratefully. Now, for the first time in history, the causes of these diseases were known. However, the immediate reaction of physicians to developments in bacteriology was often hostile. James J. Walsh recalled that it was not unusual in New York "for well known physicians to get up and leave the hall when medical papers were being read which emphasized the germ theory of disease. They wanted to express their contemptuous scorn for such theories and refused to listen to them." Medical histories of New Jersey, Kansas, and Louisiana also found widespread opposition to the germ theory.[10]

There were several reasons for this hostility to bacteriology. One was the average physician's distrust of most scientific medicine. As late as 1902 Cathell warned physicians not to get involved in medical science:

Do not allow yourself to be biased too quickly or too strongly in favor of new theories based on physiological, microscopical, chemical, or other

---

[9] Thomas D. Brock ed., *Milestones in Microbiology* (Englewood Cliffs, N.J.: Prentice-Hall, 1961), pp. 1, 5–6, 211; S. Bradbury, *The Evolution of the Microscope* (Oxford: Pergamon Press, 1967), pp. 200, 248–49, 257; G. L'E. Turner, "The Microscope as a Technical Frontier in Science," in S. Bradbury and G. L'E. Turner, eds., *Historical Aspects of Microscopy* (Cambridge, Eng.: Heffer, 1967), pp. 191–92; Harold Joel Conn, *Biological Stains* (Geneva, N.Y.: 1925), pp. 7–10. See also N. S. Davis, Jr., "Internal Medicine in the Nineteenth Century," *Medical Record* 59 (1901): 888–89. For a general statement of the interdependence of inventions, see S. C. Gilfillan, *The Sociology of Invention* (1935; reprint ed., Cambridge, Mass.: M.I.T. Press, 1970).

[10] James J. Walsh, *History of Medicine in New York* (New York: National Americana Society, 1919), I: 258–59; David L. Cowen, *Medicine and Health in New Jersey* (Princeton; N.J.; Van Nostrand, 1964), p. 39; Thomas Neville Bonner, *The Kansas Doctor* (Lawrence: University of Kansas Press, 1959), p. 57; John Duffy, ed., *The Rudolph Matas History of Medicine in Louisiana* (n.p.: Louisiana State University Press, 1962), 2: 347.

experiments, especially when offered by the unbalanced to establish their abstract conclusions or preconceived notions, or by those who have blindly identified themselves with the latest medical novelty.

Also do not allow yourself to be led too far from the practical branches of your profession into histology, pathology, microscopical anatomy, refined diagnostics, bacteriomania . . . comparative anatomy, biology, psychology, the arrangements of electrical currents in muscular fiber and analogous wide and digressive subjects that merely interest or create a fondness for the marvelous; else it may impair your practical tendency, give your mind a wrong bias and almost surely make your usefulness as a practicing physician diminish. The first question for you, as a practitioner, seeking additional and better tools, to ask yourself in everything of this kind is "What is its use to me?"

We would not apply these remarks to scholars and scientists . . . who . . . are not looking to their practice for . . . bread and butter. . . .[11]

Physicians sometimes refused to believe that the horrifying effects of many diseases could be traced to an almost invisible micro-organism. One elderly Illinois physician recalled the cholera epidemic of 1849–50, and denied that bacteria could be responsible for such terrors:

I can not imagine and think that the so-called "comma bacillus" is the cause and substance of this dread disease. It is repugnant to my common sense to account for such symptoms as are prevailing in cholera, that this "comma bacillus" could produce such symptoms, as, for instance, the changed voice, the vox cholerica, consisting in nothing but a mere whisper without all tone and strength, the hollow, sunken eye with a black halo, the sharp-pointed ice-cold nose, the continual audible rolling of the gas in the bowels, the cramps in the legs, the asphyate condition, the paralytic condition of the skin, which will keep standing if elevated, above all, the unquenchable thirst, with a cold-pointed tongue, a continual effort to vomit or purge, of what? of a rice-water stool, colorless, odorless. No, such grave symptoms are not the result of the "comma bacillus," at least I do not believe it. I cannot adhere to such a doctrine, which, if true, has done so far no good at all in promoting a more successful treatment.[12]

All these physicians were agreed on one point. As Cathell stated: "The great test of medical skill is curing the sick, and your usefulness will depend more on the successful treatment of your cases than upon familiarity with the ultra-scientific." Bacteriology, as one physician observed, "rendered great service to the art by adding to the power of preventive medicine. It has not done much for the drug treatment of disease." So long as bacteriology remained divorced from medical

11 D. W. Cathell and William T. Cathell, Book on the Physician Himself (Philadelphia: Davis, 1902), 11th ed., p. 109.

12 Dr. Trude, quoted in Lucius H. Zeuch, History of Medical Practice in Illinois, vol. I (Chicago: 1927), pp. 431–32.

therapeutics, the crucial feature of medical practice, physicians would look upon it without enthusiasm.[13]

Another reason for physicians' skepticism was that nineteenth-century bacteriology raised more methodological and substantive questions than it answered, so that its findings were often based on less than conclusive evidence. Skepticism was neither irrational nor reactionary; it was a reasonable position, taken by many leaders of the profession.[14] This point is best illustrated by analyses of the two major bacteriological contributions of the nineteenth century—tuberculosis and diphtheria.

TUBERCULOSIS

Tuberculosis was the major cause of adult deaths during the nineteenth century in the United States, particularly in the urban areas. Hermann Biggs, the eminent public health authority, estimated in 1894 that one-seventh of the total population and one-quarter of the adult population died from it. Even more striking, he found that more than sixty percent of the autopsies in charity hospitals in New York City showed evidence of tuberculosis, although only about half of the tubercular group actually died of tuberculosis. In the other half of the group, the tubercular process had stopped and was not the direct cause of death. It would not be unreasonable to assume from these data that close to half of the adult population of large cities contracted tuberculosis to some degree in the course of their lives. For reasons which are still not fully understood, the mortality rate from tuberculosis in large cities declined after the middle of the century, and especially after 1880. Nonetheless, tuberculosis remained, in the words of William Osler, "the Captain of the Men of Death."[15]

[13] Cathell and Cathell, *Physician Himself*, pp. 110–11; John T. G. Nichols, "The Misuse of Drugs in Modern Practice," *Boston Medical and Surgical Journal* 129 (1893): 263; see also William H. Draper, "The Principles and the Progress of Modern Therapeutics," *Medical Record* 30 (1886): 591.

[14] For a discussion of some widely accepted alternatives to the germ theory, see Phyllis Allen Richmond, "Some Variant Theories in Opposition to the Germ Theory of Disease," *Journal of the History of Medicine and Allied Sciences* 9 (1954): 290–303.

[15] Hermann M. Biggs, "To Rob Consumption of its Terrors," *Forum* 16 (1894): 763; Wilson G. Smillie, *Public Health* (New York: Macmillan, 1955), pp. 150–55, 379; H. R. M. Landis, "The Reception of Koch's Discovery in the United States," *Annals of Medical History*, n.s. 4 (1932): 532. The difficulty of attributing the decline in tuberculosis morbidity and mortality to any specific causal factors is illustrated by the observation of the distinguished public health authority, Charles V. Chapin. Chapin observed in 1906 that the decline in the incidence of tuberculosis in New York City, which had an active program of prevention and public

Numerous experiments in the late 1860's and 1870's showed that a specific germ was apparently responsible for tuberculosis and that the germ was present in the sputum of tubercular patients. Edwin Klebs and others claimed to have isolated the tubercle bacillus, but none of their claims was substantiated. This was not at all surprising because the tubercle bacillus was only a tenth the size of the anthrax bacillus, very difficult to stain, and very slow-growing on solid media.[16]

In 1882, Koch claimed to have successfully isolated the bacillus. Because of the difficulties involved, the immediate reaction was quite cautious. George M. Sternberg, the eminent American bacteriologist, wrote a series of articles in which he argued for a "spirit of scientific conservatism," and cautioned physicians not to accept Koch's findings without replication. Sternberg himself tried to repeat Koch's work but was not consistently successful. Gradually, as Koch's techniques were more closely followed, and after a new method of staining the bacillus was discovered by Ehrlich, other scientists were able to replicate Koch's work with sufficient success to support the validity of his finding.[17]

Most physicians reacted quite critically to this discovery. Many had believed that tuberculosis was hereditary rather than communicable, partly because of the frequency with which cases occurred in the same families, and partly because physicians and nurses in frequent contact with consumptives were not believed to have higher rates of infection than those not so exposed. Many other physicians were indifferent to the discovery because they saw no therapeutic benefits to be derived from it. Consequently, as late as 1902, Hermann Biggs stated that "a comprehension of the full meaning of the discovery of Koch on the prevention of tuberculosis has very slowly found its way into the minds of the medical profession, and even now, after

---

health measures, was only slightly greater than the decline in Chapin's community of Providence, Rhode Island, where very little had been done. He concluded that "race, age and numberless other factors so complicate the problem that almost nothing is known of the cause of the world-wide decrease in this disease." James H. Cassedy, *Charles V. Chapin and the Public Health Movement* (Cambridge, Mass.: Harvard University Press, 1962), p. 128.

16 Lawrason Brown, *The Story of Clinical Pulmonary Tuberculosis* (Baltimore: Williams and Wilkins, 1941), p. 24; William T. Councilman, "Tuberculosis as an Infectious Disease," *Maryland Medical Journal* 9 (1882): 289–94; Brock, *Milestones in Microbiology*, p. 115.

17 George M. Sternberg, "Is Tuberculosis a Parasitic Disease?" *Medical News* 41 (1882): 6–7, 87–89, 311–314, 564–66, 730–31; Ernst, "Study of the Tubercle-Bacillus," p. 126; for a discussion of Koch's method, see the description of his laboratory by J. T. W., "The Bacillus Tuberculosis . . . ," *Medical News* 41 (1882): 189–93.

twenty years, a large proportion of the profession have failed to grasp its vast significance."[18]

The negative attitudes of many physicians were intensified by the aftermath of Koch's announcement in 1890 that he had discovered tuberculin, which he claimed was a cure for tuberculosis. This statement immediately attracted world-wide attention. One physician said: "no discovery in medicine or surgery ever found such ready introduction and universal acceptance. The discoverer, the distinguished Koch, the father of bacteriology, had scored so many victories on this modern field of research that every word he uttered brought conviction." Within a few months, however, it was found that while tuberculin had some value in a few cases, in others it was of no benefit, and in many it even aggravated the disease. Early in 1891, Rudolph Virchow, the great German pathologist, disclosed that he had found fresh tubercles in autopsies of patients who had been treated with tuberculin, and faith in the therapy rapidly dissipated after this announcement. This disastrous episode was only grist to the mill of physicians hostile to the germ theory. One physician blamed the "wild enthusiasm" on the "credulity which too often accepts conclusions without adequate investigation or proof," and concluded that "this failure and revulsion, because of disappointment, will have a salutary influence." As late as 1899, another physician said that the profession had not yet "recovered from the shock of the failure of tuberculin to do what its most ardent and hopeful supporters claimed for it."[19]

[18] C.-E. A. Winslow, *The Life of Hermann M. Biggs* (Philadelphia: Lea and Febiger, 1929), pp. 55–56; Councilman, "Tuberculosis," p. 294; Hermann M. Biggs, "Sanitary Measures for the Prevention of Tuberculosis in New York City and their Results," *Journal of the American Medical Association* 39 (1902): 1635.

[19] N. Senn, "Away with Koch's Lymph," *Medical News* 58 (1891): 625. One American medical journal put out a special edition with Koch's report: Robert Koch, "A Further Communication on a Cure for Tuberculosis," *Medical News* 57 (1890): 521–26; "Virchow on the Injurious Effects of Koch's Methods," *Medical News* 58 (1891): 85–86; Harold C. Ernst, "Preliminary Report on the Clinical Use of Tuberculin," *Boston Medical and Surgical Journal* 125 (1891): 5–7, 25–28, 55–58, 76–79, 131–35; William Hunt, "A View of Koch's Remedy for Tuberculosis," *Medical and Surgical Reporter* 64 (1891): 295–97; A. S. Coe, "Therapeutics," *New York Medical Journal* 54 (1891): 240; T. J. Happel, "Quo Vadis?" *Journal of the American Medical Association* 32 (1899): 271.

To the writer's knowledge, there is no detailed account of this significant episode in medical history. Hermann Biggs justified Koch's work by saying that the "sensational and extravagant claims made by the daily press or by interested charlatans" and the "frequent use in unsuitable cases, its administration in too large doses, and the neglect of certain precautions, which had been specifically described" were the causes of the demise of tuberculin. Both he and Trudeau felt that the treatment was useful under certain limited situations. Trudeau, however, observed that Koch's announcement departed "from the rigid methods of presenting scientific evidence which in his previous work he had always adhered to

The discovery of the tubercle bacillus also did not contribute much to the diagnosis of the disease. Tuberculosis was relatively easy to diagnose through physical signs in its advanced stages, but was often extremely difficult to diagnose in its incipient stage, when the patient's chances for a complete recovery were best. Many patients confused the early symptoms of tuberculosis—cough, fluctuation of the daily temperature, and slight hemoptysis—with other illnesses, and did not consult a physician until the incipient stage was passed. Physicians also often failed to diagnose the disease when confronted with it in its incipient stage. Edward Trudeau, a major innovator in sanitarium treatment of tuberculosis, blamed this partly on "the apathy of the profession"; others felt it was due somewhat to the physician's "want of skill, but largely to erroneous teachings of the past and to carelessness and want of thorough investigation." While these factors were often important, the nature of the disease itself made accurate diagnosis by even a conscientious physician a problematic one. The physical signs mentioned above were often absent in the earliest stage of the disease, or, if present, were easily confused with those of other diseases. Bacteriological examination of a patient's sputum, which could provide a definite diagnosis, was often ineffective. The patient frequently did not expectorate in the incipient stage of the disease so that no sputum was available for examination. If he did expectorate, tubercle bacilli were often absent from the sputum so that negative findings were inconclusive, even after repeated examinations of sputum samples. Trudeau and others advocated the subcutaneous inoculation of tuberculin, which produced fever and other positive reactions in tubercular patients. However, small doses of tuberculin did not always produce positive reactions and large doses sometimes produced reactions in non-tubercular patients. Even worse, large doses of tuberculin sometimes aggravated the tubercular process in a patient. Trudeau suggested that tuberculin be administered in graded doses, beginning with very small ones, until a positive reaction was obtained. Many physicians felt that any use of tuberculin was excessively risky, and one said that using it was "like hunting for a gas leak with a lighted candle." Thus, bacteriological analysis was not consistently

so strictly" and that Koch did not disclose the nature of tuberculin until many months after his original announcement. Trudeau stated that he had experimented with "practically the same substance" as tuberculin before 1890 and had found it ineffective. Thus there seems little doubt that Koch had to share some of the blame for the failure of tuberculin. Hermann M. Biggs, "Robert Koch and His Work," *American Monthly Review of Reviews* 24 (1901): 326; Edward Livingston Trudeau, *An Autobiography* (Garden City, N.Y.: Doubleday, 1916), pp. 212–15.

useful in the diagnosis of incipient cases of tuberculosis, and therefore many physicians were reluctant to accept it.[20]

The bacteriological discoveries in tuberculosis did have important consequences in two major respects: the recognition that tuberculosis was a communicable disease which could be minimized by proper prophylaxis, and an increased interest in the treatment of tubercular patients by isolating them in hospitals and sanitaria. During the last years of the nineteenth century, but more commonly during the first years of the twentieth century, private and public action was taken to increase public awareness of the tuberculosis problem and to establish sanitaria and hospitals for the treatment of tubercular patients. Interested laymen and physicians organized the National Tuberculosis Association in 1904 and regional voluntary associations in many states about the same time. Municipal and state governments established tuberculosis hospitals and sanitaria, and began to make the control and treatment of tuberculosis a government responsibility. In 1907, the Pennsylvania state legislature appropriated one million dollars for sanitaria and other measures, following a political campaign which stressed the government's role in the treatment of tuberculosis. Before the turn of the century, the New York City board of health examined sputum samples without cost, disinfected residences where tubercular patients had lived, and otherwise undertook to prevent the spread of tuberculosis, particularly in tenement districts where the incidence of the disease was highest.[21]

The medical profession often adopted a passive or even opposing role in many of these activities, which they found were unrelated to their professional concerns. The AMA, for example, showed little interest in the National Tuberculosis Association, and even the physicians who participated in it were more concerned with the study of tuberculosis than with public health measures or sanitarium treatment. The organized medical profession often strongly resisted at-

[20] E. L. Trudeau, "The Adirondack Cottage Sanitarium for the Treatment of Incipient Pulmonary Tuberculosis," *Practitioner* 62 (1899): 138; Llewellyn P. Barbour, "The Diagnosis of Early Phthisis," *Medical Record* 49 (1896): 829–33; Charles G. Wilson, "Circular of Information from the New York City Health Department," *Medical News* 69 (1896): 222–23; E. L. Trudeau, "The Tuberculin Test in Incipient and Suspected Pulmonary Tuberculosis," *Medical News* 70 (1897): 687–90. C. P. Ambler, "A Few Remarks Upon the Early Diagnosis of Pulmonary Tuberculosis," *New York Medical Journal* 67 (1898): 205–7.

[21] James Alexander Miller, "The Beginnings of the American Antituberculosis Movement," *American Review of Tuberculosis* 48 (1943): 361–67; S. Adolphus Knopf, *A History of the National Tuberculosis Association* (New York: 1922); Lawrence F. Flick, *The Crusade Against Tuberculosis in* Pennsylvania (n.p.: 1908), pp. 4–12; Biggs, "Sanitary Measures," pp. 1635–36.

tempts by boards of health to require physicians to report cases of tuberculosis. Every important medical society in New York City opposed compulsory reporting when it was instituted by the local board of health in 1897. In the next year, some of the New York City medical societies tried to have the state enact legislation denying the city board of health the power to treat tuberculosis as an infectious disease. The Philadelphia board of health passed a compulsory reporting ordinance in 1893, but rescinded its action in 1894 because of opposition from influential elements of the profession. As late as 1902, the physicians of Chicago were so strongly opposed to reporting the disease that the health commissioner refused to require it. Practicing physicians felt that the compulsory reporting provisions were unnecessary for their middle-class clients who resided in private dwellings. The boards of health wanted to quarantine all tuberculosis patients in order to reduce the incidence of tuberculosis in the tenement districts where professional medical care was almost nonexistent. Biggs observed that "the medical profession sometimes forgets that ... many measures which are not demanded or necessary in the best portions of the city are required for the well-being of the inhabitants of the tenement-house districts."[22]

DIPHTHERIA

The significance of therapeutics in influencing physicians' attitudes about bacteriology is most clearly manifested in the bacteriological developments in diphtheria, a virulent children's disease which was especially prevalent during the latter half of the nineteenth century. Diphtheria was an epidemic disease which produced high fever, affected the heart, frequently caused paralysis, and often produced a distinctive membrane across the throat that asphyxiated its victim. The mortality rate was terrifyingly high, and not infrequently two or more children in the same family succumbed during a single epidemic, often within the same week. Diphtheria had always been a notoriously difficult disease to diagnose because many of its symptoms were easily confused with those of other diseases, especially croup. There was no effective therapy of any kind for it; physicians even tried to tear off the membrane, but this and other therapies were useless. A. J. Howe declared: "In the less severe types of the disease, the recuperative

22 Robert G. Paterson, "The Tuberculosis Movement in the United States of America, 1882–1904," *Past and Present Trends in the Tuberculosis Movement* (n.p.: 1942), pp. 24–26; Biggs, "Sanitary Measures," pp. 1636, 1638; Flick, *Crusade against Tuberculosis*, p. 3; Hermann M. Biggs, "Sanitary Science, the Medical Profession, and the Public," *Medical News* 72 (1898): 48.

forces of the body are alone able to tide the patient over safely.... But all bad cases of diphtheria die; and no doctor is to be blamed for losing them."[23]

The discovery of the etiology of diphtheria was far more complex than that of tuberculosis. Friedrich Loeffler, one of Koch's assistants, isolated the diphtheria bacillus in 1884, after Edwin Klebs had done preliminary work in the previous year. This, however, was only a beginning, because Loeffler was unable to produce paralysis in laboratory animals inoculated with diphtheria bacilli. It remained for Pierre Roux and Alexandre Yersin, who worked with Pasteur, to produce all the symptoms of diphtheria in inoculated animals in their work, published in 1888. They discovered that the bacilli themselves remained localized, but produced a toxin which spread through the body and caused the disease. Two years later, analyses of the tissues of animals who died of diphtheria were shown to be similar to their counterparts in humans. Thus, while the initial discovery of a diphtheria bacillus was made in 1883, a real understanding of the nature of the disease was not achieved until 1890, and this date rather than the earlier one should be considered the time when the diphtheria bacillus began to have significance for the medical profession.[24]

These developments created a considerable amount of confusion in the profession. Initially, it was found that major discrepancies existed between clinical and bacteriological diagnoses of diphtheria. Park and Beebe[25] investigated 5,611 suspected cases in New York City in 1893–94 and reached these conclusions: (1) Clinical diagnoses of diphtheria often failed to identify many cases lacking the most common clinical symptoms, such as the membrane in the throat. (2) Eighty percent of the cases diagnosed as membranous croup were actually diphtheria. (3) A large number of cases with a pseudo-membrane in the throat diagnosed as diphtheria were in fact caused by streptococcus, and the two diseases were so similar clinically that they could not be differentiated except by bacteriological examination. Park and Beebe called the streptococcus disease "pseudo-diphtheria." Overall,

23 Cowen, *Medicine in New Jersey*, pp. 43–45; Harry H. Moore, *Public Health in the United States* (New York: Harper, 1923), p. 104; D. S. Fairchild, *History of Medicine in Iowa* (n.p., 1927), p. 139; [A. J. Howe], "Croup, Diphtheria, and Malignant Tonsilitis," *Eclectic Medical Journal* 38 (1878): 148. For a detailed description of therapy during the period, see H. W. Berg, "The Treatment of Diphtheria, Including Serum Therapy," *Medical Record* 47 (1895): 33–43.

24 William Hallock Park and Alfred L. Beebe, "Diphtheria and Pseudo-Diphtheria," *Medical Record* 46 (1894): 386–87; Lechevalier and Solotorovsky, *Three Centuries of Microbiology*, pp. 122–35, 138–41; Parish, *History of Immunization*, p. 119.

25 Park and Beebe, "Diphtheria and Pseudo-Diphtheria," pp. 385–401.

only about 60 percent of the suspected cases were true diphtheria cases. The obvious conclusion from these major findings was that the clinical definition of diphtheria was so inadequate as to require wholesale revision.

Park and Beebe also found, however, that bacteriological diagnosis suffered from some extremely significant problems. Bacteriological analyses of a large number of throat swabs identified three major types of bacilli: (1) The diphtheria bacillus in its virulent state was found not only in cases of diphtheria but also in one percent of the throats of healthy persons examined in New York City during the study. The great majority of these healthy persons never contracted the disease, but were able to transmit it to others. (2) The diphtheria bacillus in a non-virulent state was found in the throats of many diphtheria patients, most often during the patient's recovery. The two states of the bacillus could not be differentiated except by animal inoculation, a long and laborious procedure which was usually impractical because of the rapid progress of the disease. (3) A different, non-virulent bacillus, physically similar to the diphtheria bacillus, was also found in one percent of the throats of healthy persons examined in the study. This bacillus, which was discovered in 1888, was shaped like the diphtheria bacillus, but had somewhat different chemical properties. It was called the "pseudo-bacillus" (not to be confused with pseudo-diphtheria).

These findings, which were made and confirmed by many researchers after 1888, raised a number of extremely serious questions. If the diphtheria bacillus was found in the throats of healthy individuals, how could it be the cause of diphtheria? If the diphtheria bacillus existed in both virulent and non-virulent states, what was the diagnostic value of bacteriological analyses without animal inoculation? Even Park and Beebe were forced to admit that the diagnostic problems were significant. They concluded that bacteriological diagnosis "can be thoroughly relied on in cases where there is visible membrane in the throat, if the culture is made during the period in which the membrane is forming, and no antiseptic, especially no mercurial solution, has lately been applied." In the large number of other cases, Park and Beebe concluded that bacteriological diagnosis was "surprisingly accurate" but conceded that "absolute reliance" could not be placed on it. Under these circumstances, many physicians refused to abandon their clinical experience for this new and confusing bacteriological approach, a decision which could hardly be called obdurate conservatism.

During this same period, work was being carried on by Emil von

Behring and S. Kitasato, two of Koch's assistants. They found that animals inoculated with the diphtheria toxin gradually built up a resistance to it by generating some substance in the blood (which they failed to isolate) called an "antitoxin." Inoculation of the serum of these animals into other animals or into human beings would protect the recipients from the toxin. Even more important, this serum could actually cure cases in which the disease already existed. After numerous experiments, Roux, Yersin, and Louis Martin concluded in 1894 that horse serum was especially useful for large scale production, and anti-toxin was soon being produced in reasonably large quantities. These great discoveries—the results of the cumulative effort of dozens of scientists—made diphtheria, according to Parish, "the first infectious disease to be studied fully—its clinical and bacteriological identification, its cure by a specific serum (antitoxin), and [later] its prevention by a specific vaccine (toxoid)."[26]

The announcement of the diphtheria antitoxin early in 1894 aroused considerable professional interest, but little enthusiasm. Having been disappointed by tuberculin, many physicians adopted a skeptical attitude toward the antitoxin. Leading proponents of the antitoxin, like Biggs and Park, took considerable pains to point out the different principles behind the two therapies, but with little apparent success. Attempts were also made to demonstrate the value of antitoxin by means of clinical statistics, and many articles in all the leading medical journals documented its effectiveness in hospitals throughout the world.[27]

These efforts to prove the validity of diphtheria antitoxin through clinical statistics led the skeptical physicians to produce contrary evidence of their own. Because the statistics of the proponents of the antitoxin were based on bacteriologically diagnosed cases, the critics attacked the validity of the diagnoses. They observed that the presence of diphtheria bacilli in a patient's throat was not proof of the presence of the disease, and that pseudo-diphtheria bacilli were easily confused with real diphtheria bacilli. They also questioned the legitimacy of the rapid increase in the number of reported diphtheria cases which

26 Hermann M. Biggs, "The New Treatment of Diphtheria," *McClure's Magazine* 4 (1895): 361–62; Parish, *History of Immunization*, pp. 118, 120–22.

27 W. H. Thomson, "How the Facts about the Antitoxin Treatment of Diphtheria Should be Estimated," *Medical Record* 49 (1896): 896; Biggs, "New Treatment of Diphtheria," p. 360; William Hallock Park, "Comments on Some of the Objections Offered to the Use of Antitoxin in the Treatment of Diphtheria," *Medical News* 68 (1896): 213–15; John H. McCollom, "Antitoxine in the Treatment of Diphtheria" *Medical Communications of the Massachusetts Medical Society* 17 (1896): 193–208.

occurred after the introduction of bacteriological diagnosis (which proponents attributed to the superiority of the new diagnostic procedures). They felt this was an attempt to make the antitoxin appear more effective by reporting its success in many cases which were not really diphtheria. One physician called the increase a "singular coincidence" and claimed: "My personal experience showed me that many persons never presented clinical evidence of disease." The critics were even able to produce clinical statistics from well-known hospitals, showing that the use of the antitoxin had little or no perceptible effect on diphtheria mortality. This was possible because diphtheria was an epidemic disease which fluctuated markedly in its severity from year to year, so that lower or higher mortality rates in selected previous years were easily obtained. Furthermore, the diphtheria antitoxin was not administered correctly during the first year of its production. The doses were too small for maximum effect. In addition, it was not realized for some months that the effectiveness of inoculations of antitoxin decreased markedly after the second day of the patient's illness. Because most cases of diphtheria inoculated with antitoxin in hospitals did not enter the hospitals until they had been ill for several days, hospital statistics were often unfavorable. These unfavorable statistics from well-known hospitals raised serious doubts about the antitoxin's effectiveness.[28]

Proponents of the antitoxin did not successfully rebut these attacks. Although they recognized the importance of both the size of the dose and the stage of the patient's illness when the antitoxin was administered, they failed to present statistics which took both these factors into account simultaneously. Neither did they resolve the diagnostic problems. Rather, they deemphasized clinical statistics altogether. Park conceded in 1895 that some of the clinical statistics had a "very confusing effect upon the profession." Biggs admitted in the same year that clinical evidence did not offer conclusive proof of the antitoxin's effectiveness and advised physicians to examine antitoxin experiments on laboratory animals for proof of its effectiveness. Supporters of the antitoxin urged physicians to use the drug in the proper dose and at the proper stage of the disease to see its value for themselves. One homeopath told his colleagues in 1901: "Statistics are not

[28] "Diphtheria Germs in the Normal Throat . . . ," *Medical News* 70 (1897): 316; William L. Stowell, "Diphtheria with and without Antitoxin," *Medical Record* 49 (1896): 903; for other critical views of diphtheria antitoxin, see Joseph E. Winters, "Clinical Observations Upon the Use of Antitoxin in Diphtheria . . . ," *Medical Record* 49 (1896): 877–93; Dowling Benjamin, "The Treatment of Diphtheria," *Journal of the American Medical Association* 27 (1896): 850–57; William Galloway, "Conservative Views of Antitoxin," *Medical Record* 47 (1895): 379–80.

necessary to convince any one of the value of antitoxin in diphtheria. It is simply necessary to employ it a few times properly. It may be stated, however, without fear of successful contradiction, that nothing in therapeutics is as well supported by figures as this antitoxin treatment of diphtheria. . . . It is the most brilliant, towering fact of modern applied therapeutics, standing out boldly above every other fact."[29]

Diphtheria antitoxin did work, and it often worked miraculously. However incongruous the findings of clinical studies, the decline in the crude death rate from diphtheria after the widespread use of the antitoxin in a region showed beyond any doubt that its use was strongly correlated with reduction in the diphtheria mortality. In Illinois, the diphtheria death rate dropped from 113 per 100,000 of the total population in 1886 to 22 per 100,000 in 1902; in Massachusetts the trends were very similar.[30]

Popular demand for adoption of the antitoxin put pressure on government public health authorities, who in turn were able to induce physicians to use the therapy. Parents with children dying from diphtheria were eager to accept a therapy which had been recommended by so many illustrious physicians and public health authorities. As early as 1895, the commissioner of health of New York City and State spoke of the "great interest taken by the laity . . . and their appreciation of the valuable discovery." He asserted that public interest enabled the *New York Herald* to raise large sums through a popular subscription and helped the New York City board of health to obtain an appropriation of $30,000 in 1895 for diagnosis and manufacture of serum. Other cities throughout the country also provided funds and facilities for bacteriological diagnosis of diphtheria and for manufacture of the antitoxin. By 1895, when the profession was still sharply divided, bacteriological diagnosis was being employed in New York City, Brooklyn, Washington, Boston, Philadelphia, Buffalo, Cincinnati, Detroit, St. Louis, New Orleans and other cities; antitoxin was also being manufactured in many of them In 1895. Antitoxin was supplied free to the indigent in New York and Philadelphia in 1895 and

[29] Park, "Objections to the Use of Antitoxin," p. 214; "Society of Alumni of Bellevue Hospital Meeting of December 4, 1895," *New York Medical Journal* 63 (1896): 221 (this article presents an excellent discussion by a number of important physicians who bring out most of the major issues: pp. 217–227); William C. Goodno, "The Antitoxin Treatment of Diphtheria," *Hahnemannian Monthly* 36 (1901): 371, 376.

[30] Hermann M. Biggs, "Antitoxine in Diphtheria," *Maryland Medical Journal* 36 (1897): 297–98; Isaac D. Rawlings, *The Rise and Fall of Disease in Illinois*, vol. I (Illinois State Department of Public Health, 1927), pp. 354–55; Moore, *Public Health*, p. 104; Cassedy, *Chapin and the Public Health Movement*, p. 71.

in California in 1896. Physicians found it difficult to resist the combined influence of the public and public health authorities. In Illinois, for example, physicians were unwilling to adopt the antitoxin when a diphtheria epidemic struck in the fall of 1895. The state health department used its medical staff to administer the antitoxin and to teach physicians how and when to use it. As a result, it was generally adopted by the end of the year.[31]

The success of the diphtheria antitoxin brought about the triumph of bacteriology in medicine. Widespread interest in the application of bacteriology to the treatment of tuberculosis occurred only in the last years of the century, and was undoubtedly due to the impetus given to the field by the antitoxin. In short order, public health authorities turned their attention to other bacteriological diseases. Typhoid fever, which became a major epidemic disease as cities grew without providing for pure water, sewage disposal, inspection of dairies, etc., also benefited from the application of bacteriological principles. By the beginning of the twentieth century, public health had become a dynamic new field based on the principles of bacteriology.[32]

HOMEOPATHIC AND ECLECTIC PHYSICIANS AND BACTERIOLOGY

Homeopathic physicians reacted to the bacteriological discoveries in much the same manner as did regular physicians. At the 1882 session of the AIH, for instance, two homeopaths read papers that were highly critical of Koch's discovery of the tubercle bacillus. In 1883, however, papers presented to the AIH accepted Koch's ideas; one of these concluded: "Should therapeutics remain unbenefited, prophylaxis and hygiene *must* derive great profit from it." By 1886, bacteriology appeared to have been largely accepted in the AIH; in that year numerous papers praising bacteriological discoveries were read, and Hahnemann was even referred to as a forebear of bacteriology. In the early twentieth century, homeopathic tuberculosis sanitaria were established. Although some homeopaths, like some regular physicians,

---

[31] Cyrus Edson, "Antitoxin in Diphtheria," *Medical Record* 47 (1895): 424; Winslow, *Life of Biggs*, pp. 110–15; Henry W. Bettmann, "Diphtheria: Its Bacteriological Diagnosis and Treatment with the Antitoxin," *Medical News* 67 (1895): 5; Henry Harris, *California's Medical Story* (San Francisco: Stacey, 1932), pp. 289–90; Frederick P. Henry ed., *Standard History of the Medical Profession of Philadelphia* (Chicago: Goodspeed Bros., 1897), p. 301.

[32] Erwin H. Ackerknecht, "Diseases in the Middle West," *Essays in the History of Medicine* (Chicago: University of Illinois Press, 1965), pp. 172–73; George M. Kober, "The Progress and Tendency of Hygiene and Sanitary Science in the Nineteenth Century," *Medical Record* 59 (1901) 898–906; L. Emmett Holt, "Infant Mortality and its Reduction, Especially in New York City," *Journal of the American Medical Association* 54 (1910): 682–90.

remained unconvinced of the value of the germ theory and questioned its validity as late as 1901, the better educated homeopaths undoubtedly accepted bacteriology at about the same time as their regular counterparts.[33]

A similar process occurred among eclectic physicians. The leaders of the older generation, including men like John Scudder and Alexander Wilder, never accepted bacteriology. Scudder stated in 1891, three years before his death: "I had examined [bacteriology thirty years ago] and my mind was made up—there was but little in it." Wilder called it a "dogma" in 1901 and said that it would "pass out of sight" in a generation. These men were products of an earlier generation and it was not surprising that they should have been reluctant to accept such an innovation. Other eclectics, however, were more positive in their appraisals. A prominent eclectic physician in Kansas stated in 1883 that the "preponderance of testimony" favored the germ theory. After Scudder died in 1894, the Eclectic Medical Institute taught medicine and surgery "in a thoroughly modern manner." Therefore, it seems likely that the better educated eclectic physicians adopted bacteriology at about the same rate as did the better educated regular and homeopathic physicians.[34]

OTHER EFFECTS OF BACTERIOLOGY ON PHYSICIANS

The developments in bacteriology made physicians aware of the importance of cleanliness and sterility in all their relations with patients. This was tempered by an ignorance of exactly what was necessary for cleanliness or sterility. An examination of several editions of Cathell's book showed that his interest in this question increased after the editions of the early 1880's. However, Cathell's advice betrayed an ignorance of what was necessary to achieve sterility. In

[33] J. S. Mitchell, "Clinical Aspects of Koch's Discovery," *Transactions of the American Institute of Homeopathy*, 35th session (1882): 235–43; Rollin R. Gregg, "Professor Koch's Bacteria in Tubercles a Great Fallacy," *Ibid.*, pp. 649–57; W. Albert Haupt, "The Bacteria Question," *Transactions of the American Institute of Homeopathy*, 36th session (1883); 956; A. R. Wright, "Resume of the Foreign Literature of 1885 on Bacteriology," *Transactions of the American Institute of Homeopathy*, 39th session (1886): 696–713; John C. Morgan, "The New Bacillus of Diphtheria," *ibid.*, pp. 714–26; W. Albert Haupt, "The Cholera Bacillus, *ibid.*, pp. 727–48; Rawlings, *Disease in Illinois*, p. 368; Goodno, "Antitoxin Treatment of Diphtheria," p. 374.

[34] [John M. Scudder], "Why Have We Not Taken as Much Interest in Bacteriology as other Medical Journals?" *Eclectic Medical Journal* 51 (1891): 190; Alexander Wilder, *History of Medicine* (New Sharon, Me.: 1901), p. 385; Bonner, *Kansas Doctor*, pp. 57–58; Ralph Taylor, "The Formation of the Eclectic School at Cincinnati," *Ohio State Archaeological and Historical Quarterly* 51 (1942): 288.

1902, for example, he suggested to his colleagues that they cater to the public concern for cleanliness in this manner:

Never omit to call for a glass of water and napkin with which to cleanse your thermometer, both before and after you make use of it. . . .
A knife, probe, needle, or other pocket-case instrument can be readily cleaned and disinfected, both before and after using, by thrusting it several times through a wet, well-soaped towel or rag, or into a cake of wet soap.[35]

At the same time, he cautioned physicians not to carry these measures to excess, especially where the patient might be embarrassed:

Should you ever notice [bedbugs, fine-tooth-comb insects, roaches, and other vermin] about a respectable patient's body, clothing, or bedroom, show inattention and affect not to see them, for nothing is more deeply mortifying than to have anything of the kind noticed and pointed out by the physician.[36]

Obviously, Cathell and many other physicians of his generation failed to realize how deeply bacteriology affected all facets of medical practice. These physicians probably never adopted all that was discovered by bacteriologists, and a whole new generation of physicians was needed to understand fully the manifold implications of bacteriology for every aspect of medicine.

At the same time, other physicians reacted to bacteriology by carrying it to the same excesses as some early homeopaths had carried homeopathy, and discarded much previously discovered knowledge. One physician cautioned his colleagues not to abandon all of the older diagnostic aids in favor of laboratory analyses. He observed that many diagnoses continued to require "the trained eye, the skilled touch, and the well-attuned ear, and, above all, the careful training of the reasoning faculties, which comes only with patient observation and investigation." Many physicians also believed that all diseases were bacteriological in origin, and that it would be only a matter of time before vaccines and antitoxins were discovered for all of them. Once again, as in the past, some physicians tended to accept a discovery as a panacea which would render obsolete all previous diagnostic and therapeutic knowledge.[37]

Perhaps the most surprising aspect of physicians' reaction to bacteriology was not their opposition, but—on the contrary—their rapid acceptance of a dramatic new concept of disease that few of them

[35] Cathell and Cathell, *Physician Himself*, p. 27.
[36] *Ibid.*, pp. 233–34.
[37] N. P. Dandridge, "An Address," *Cincinnati Lancet-Clinic*, n.s. 48 (1902): 427; L. Emmett Holt, "Medical Tendencies and Medical Ideals," *Journal of the American Medical Association* 48 (1907): 845.

had anticipated and no one understood completely.[38] The flaws in nineteenth-century bacteriology were evident to everyone. Why did diphtheria bacilli cause disease in one person and not in another whose throat cultures showed the presence of virulent bacilli? How did bacilli actually cause disease? All physicians were ignorant of the answers to these and many other fundamental questions. One of Koch's students once asked him why anthrax bacilli caused death in an animal. Koch said, "Why its vessels are plugged with bacilli!" The student asked, "A mechanical death?" to which Koch replied, "Certainly." The student, who later became an eminent medical scientist, commented when recalling the incident, "There was I fancy at that date very little chemistry in his pathology."[39] These questions, which should have raised serious doubts about all bacteriology, do not appear to have disturbed physicians very deeply. Physicians were less concerned with how and why a therapy worked than with the demonstrable fact that a therapy was medically valid, demonstrable, and consistent. Thus they accepted antitoxin in much the same way that they had accepted quinine and smallpox inoculation and vaccination. Medical science was never a major interest of physicians; medical therapeutics and all that contributed to medical therapeutics was their overriding and singular concern.

The influence of bacteriology, like that of specialization, extended beyond therapeutics to medical schools, licensing, medical societies, and medical sectarianism. All of these institutions were altered by the developments in medical science.

[38] Duffy, *History of Medicine in Louisiana*, p. 336. The eminent physician, Austin Flint, said in 1876: "The great event in the seventeenth century was the discovery of the circulation of the blood, in the eighteenth century the discovery of vaccination, and in the present century the discovery of anesthesia. Events like these are not to be expected to recur at much shorter intervals." Austin Flint, "The First Century of the Republic; Medical and Sanitary Progress," *Harper's New Monthly Magazine* 53 (1876): 83. Phyllis Allen Richmond has shown the paucity of references to bacteriology in American medical literature prior to 1880: Phyllis Allen Richmond, "American Attitudes Toward the Germ Theory of Disease (1860–1880)," *Journal of the History of Medicine and Allied Sciences* 9 (1954): 442–46.

[39] Charles Scott Sherrington, "Marginalia," in E. Ashworth Underwood, ed., *Science, Medicine and History*, (London: Oxford University Press, 1953), II: 549.

CHAPTER 15 DEVELOPMENTS IN MEDICAL EDUCATION AFTER THE CIVIL WAR

MEDICAL SCHOOLS proliferated after the Civil War and became increasingly stratified in their quality and cost. Some of them appealed to wealthy students who could afford a lengthy and expensive education, others to poorer students seeking a short and inexpensive education. The development of scientific medicine so increased the cost of medical education that the low-quality schools were unable to continue operating on a self-supporting basis. They either merged with other medical schools or suspended their activities. The same pressures also eliminated most non-regular medical schools. Consequently, the number of medical schools decreased after the turn of the twentieth century.

The educational programs of most medical schools improved considerably during the period from the middle of the century to the end of the Civil War. In 1845, most colleges had terms of 13 to 16 weeks; in 1865, most had terms of 18 weeks, with some having terms of five or six months. In 1845, most schools had either no clinical instruction at all or clinical instruction but no hospital instruction. By 1865, two-thirds of the schools had both clinical and hospital instruction. One major reason for this progress was the internal differentiation among schools, which occurred as the 30 regular medical schools in 1840 increased to 47 in 1860 and to 60 in 1870.[1] The leading schools appealed to wealthy students with considerable preliminary education; the others appealed to the poorer students with less preliminary education. The best schools were able to raise their standards because they were not competing directly with the less prestigious ones. Many of their above average competitors were thereupon forced to raise their standards in order to maintain their reputations as superior institutions. Another

[1] Nathan S. Davis, "Address," *Transactions of the American Medical Association* 16 (1865): 76; see Table V.1 in Chapter 5 for the number of regular medical schools.

282

reason was the great expansion of public secondary education during this same period and the increased wealth of the country, which provided a favorable environment for a general improvement in the quality of medical education.

The AMA and the Medical Schools

The AMA's contribution to these innovations in medical education was insignificant. J. Marion Sims stated in 1876 that "the standard of medical education has been raised in the last twenty-five years. But the most ardent friend of the cause must admit that this has not been achieved by the efforts of our Association.... we have ... signally failed in this." The failure of the AMA can be illustrated by the aftermath of one of the most important resolutions enacted at its first meeting in 1847—that the medical school term should be extended from four to six months. Only one of the almost three dozen existing medical schools adopted something approximating this standard: the University of Pennsylvania medical school increased its term to five and one-half months. In fact, however, the school merely formalized an existing program. The faculty had gradually lengthened the term since 1836, first by extending it by a month, later by adding a month of preliminary lectures before the term. The Pennsylvania school continued its solitary course until no later than 1853, when it retrenched to a five month term, because the other leading schools would not extend their terms.[2]

Even though the AMA's early efforts to reduce the number of medical schools had no real impact, relations between the AMA and the medical schools remained discordant, primarily because the AMA continued to enact resolutions which the medical schools felt were ill-advised and unfeasible. Austin Flint, a medical-school faculty member, said in his AMA presidential address in 1884: "Hitherto the Association has been content with reports, addresses, and communications pointing out existing defects in medical education, and recommending changes and improvements, the immediate adoption of some of which [by the colleges] was impracticable. Too often a predominant spirit of animadversion has been apparent."[3]

[2] J. Marion Sims, "Address," *Transactions of the American Medical Association* 27 (1876): 92; A. H. Stevens, *et al.*, "Report of the Committee on Education," *Transactions of the American Medical Association* 1 (1848): 237; Joseph Carson, *A History of the Medical Department of the University of Pennsylvania* (Philadelphia: Lindsay and Blakiston, 1869), pp. 171–72.

[3] Austin Flint, "Annual Address," *Journal of the American Medical Association* 2 (1884): 508.

In the early 1870's, the role of the medical schools as members of the AMA came under scrutiny as part of another problem. The original AMA constitution provided for representation not only from medical societies and medical schools, but also from large asylums, hospitals, dispensaries, boards of health, and some other organizations whose members were physicians. The proliferation of delegates from these organizations gradually aroused resentment among the delegates of the medical societies. Furthermore, prolonged debates occurred around 1870 over the seating of women and Negro delegates from some medical organizations. Consequently, a constitutional amendment was enacted in 1874 that effectively limited AMA membership to delegates of state medical societies and other societies recognized by them.[4]

The most important consequence of this new membership system was that the medical schools were no longer permitted representation in the AMA. After stating at its first meeting that the AMA was established in large measure to improve medical education, and after enacting numerous resolutions regarding medical education over the years, the AMA summarily expelled the medical schools from the association without any real concern being expressed by its leaders or members in the published records of the association. Years later, in 1888, a president of the association justified the expulsion by claiming that the representatives from the medical schools had manifested "a determined and successful opposition" to all efforts to improve medical education. He conceded, however, that in the years following the expulsion of the medical schools, the association had "unquestionably failed" to enact any important measures concerning medical education. Therefore, other factors must have been involved in the purge of the medical schools from the AMA.[5]

In fact, the schools were expelled because of the intensification of the problems which had affected their relations with the AMA from the start. The AMA continued to have no effective sanctions to impose on schools which violated its standards. Whatever the merits of its resolutions, an AMA president conceded in 1878, "there were no powers in the Association to carry them out, and they remained upon

4 James G. Burrow, *AMA: Voice of American Medicine* (Baltimore: Johns Hopkins Press, 1963), pp. 15–16; Donald E. Konold, *A History of American Medical Ethics 1847–1912* (Madison: State Historical Society of Wisconsin, 1962), pp. 23–24; "American Medical Association," *Medical Record* 9 (1874): 311. Sims stated that the debate over women and Negro delegates was resolved in their favor: Sims, "Address," p. 93.

5 A. Y. P. Garnett, "The Mission of the American Medical Association," *Journal of the American Medical Association* 10 (1888): 574.

the record as mere mementos of the praiseworthy zeal of their authors."[6] Furthermore, the schools were growing larger, more prosperous, and more independent of the association. The demise of the
apprenticeship system eliminated the major link between the schools
and the medical societies. Hospitals and clinics gave the medical
schools increased influence and independence in their communities.
Thus the schools and the societies moved further apart in their interests, and the formal relationship between them weakened and was
severed.

CHANGES IN MEDICAL EDUCATION

In the second half of the century, American medical schools adopted
their first significant innovation—replacing the two-year repetitive
curriculum with a three-year graded curriculum. Antecedents of the
graded curriculum can be traced back to the 1830's and 1840's, when
many medical students attended one session of shorter and less difficult courses at rural schools, and a second session of the same subject
matter offered at a more advanced level at urban schools. A few medical schools adopted a two-year graded curriculum in the 1850's, but
these were isolated events. In the late 1860's and the 1870's, a number
of medical schools offered optional graded curricula, but few students
selected this option. The first compulsory three-year graded curriculum was instituted at Harvard Medical School in 1871, when a nine-
month term was also adopted. These changes reduced the school's
enrollment, which induced the university to place the medical school
faculty on a salaried basis, a radical departure from traditional medical school practice. (The University of Michigan had paid salaries to
its faculty since the 1850's, making Harvard the second medical school
to adopt this mode of payment.) Altogether, ten medical schools—eight
regular and two homeopathic—adopted compulsory three-year graded
curricula during the 1870's, and 33 medical schools—one-quarter of
the total number—adopted a three-year graded curriculum by 1889.[7]

Also during this period, regular medical schools tried to establish
standards of medical education through a voluntary association. Representatives from 22 medical schools formed the American Medical

[6] T. G. Richardson, "Address," *Transactions of the American Medical Association* 29 (1878): 94.

[7] M. Paine, "Medical Education in the United States," *Boston Medical and
Surgical Journal* 29 (1843): 332–33; Frederick C. Waite, "Advent of the Graded
Curriculum in American Medical Colleges," *Journal of the Association of American
Medical Colleges* 25 (1950): 316–20; C. Sidney Burwell, "The Evolution of Medical
Education in Nineteenth Century America," *Journal of Medical Education* 37 (1962):
1163.

College Association in 1876. The Association made its first major effort to improve medical education in 1880, by requiring all members to adopt a three-year graded course, divided into six-month terms. By 1880, however, only 17 American medical schools, some of them non-regular, had adopted this curriculum, and only a few others were willing to follow their lead. Consequently, the number of schools represented in the association dropped to 18 in 1881 and to 11 in 1882, and the organization thereupon suspended its activities until 1889.[8]

The majority of medical schools were reluctant to raise their graduation requirements because of increasing competition in medical education. Medical schools proliferated at a dramatic rate after the nation recovered from the Civil War (Table XV.1).[9] The total number of schools increased by 16 percent from 1860 to 1870, by 23 percent from 1870 to 1880, and by 34 percent from 1880 to 1890. Many of these schools appealed to lower-middle and working class students and consequently were opposed to higher standards.

Eventually, some kind of graded curriculum was adopted by all medical schools after the enactment of many new licensing laws. These laws required applicants for licenses to possess diplomas from colleges which met certain minimum entrance, term length, and length of course requirements. Some degree of uniformity among states in these requirements was established with the creation of the National Conference of State Medical Examining and Licensing Boards in 1891. In that year, the conference established a three-year graded course as a standard. This forced virtually all medical schools to increase the length of their courses to comply with the regulations (Table XV.2). These increases were often only nominal, because many schools permitted students to study one year with a preceptor in lieu of formal clinical training at the college. William Osler estimated in 1891 that the preceptorship year was a *"bona-fide* period of medical instruction" for less than five percent of the students in these schools.[10]

[8] Dean F. Smiley, "History of the Association of American Medical Colleges, 1876–1956," *Journal of Medical Education* 32 (1957): 512–14; Waite, "Graded Curriculum," p. 319.

[9] A comparison of this table with Table V.1 in Chapter 5 reveals a larger number of medical schools in the table in this chapter for 1850 and 1860. Furthermore, tabulations by contemporary sources after the Civil War do not agree with this table either. One tabulation in 1880 listed 72 regular, 7 homeopathic, and 5 eclectic schools, with 9,876, 950, and 518 students respectively. Charles McIntire, *The Percentage of College-Bred Men in the Medical Profession* (Philadelphia: 1883), pp. 8–9. The data seem close enough to warrant generalizations about trends, which is the major concern in this study.

[10] Smiley, "Association of American Medical Colleges," pp. 515–16; William Osler, "The License to Practice," *Transactions of the Medical and Chirurgical Faculty of Maryland*, 91st Annual Meeting (1889): 75.

Table XV.1

Medical Schools, Students, and Graduates; by Sect, 1850–1920

Year	Regular			Homeopathic			Eclectic			Other			Total		
	Schools	Students	Graduates	Schools	Students	Graduates	Schools	Students	Graduates	Schools	Students	Graduates	Schools	Students	Graduates
1850	44	—	—	3	—	—	4	—	—	1	—	—	52	—	—
1860	53	—	—	6	—	—	4	—	—	2	—	—	65	—	—
1870	60	—	—	8	—	—	5	—	—	2	—	—	75	—	—
1880	76	9776	2673	14	1220	380	8	830	188	2	—	—	100	11826	3241
1890	106	13521	3853	16	1164	380	9	719	221	2	—	—	133	15404	4454
1900	126	22710	4715	22	1909	413	9	522	86	3	—	—	160	25171	5214
1903	126	24930	5088	20	1498	420	9	848	149	5	239	41	160	27615	5698
1906	130	23116	4841	19	1085	286	8	644	186	5	359	51	162	25204	5364
1910	109	20136	4113	12	867	183	8	455	114	2	68	30	131	21526	4440
1913	92	15919	3679	10	850	209	5	256	93	0	0	0	107	17015	3981
1916	82	13121	3274	10	638	166	3	263	78	0	0	0	95	14012	3518
1920	76	13220	2826	5	386	97	1	93	30	3	389	94	85	14088	3047

Source: "Medical Education in the United States," Journal of the American Medical Association 79 (1922): 629–33.

287

TABLE XV.2
LENGTH OF COURSE OF MEDICAL SCHOOLS, 1875–99

| | Schools with Course Requiring | | | | | |
Year	4 years %	3 years %	2 years %	1 year %	Total %	Number of Schools
1885	0	5	95	0	100	108
1897	66	33	0	1	100	150
1898	71	29	0	0	98	145*
1899	91	7	1	1	100	155**

* Six schools not reporting.
** One school not reporting.
SOURCE: Henry L. Taylor, *Professional Education in the United States* (Albany, N.Y.: University of the State of New York, 1900), I: 13.

The Association of American Medical Colleges was revived under this new name in 1889, with membership restricted to schools with a three-year graded course of six-month terms, entrance requirements, and other educational standards. By 1894, 71 of the approximately 115 regular colleges in the country were members. In that year, the association adopted a four-year course as a membership requirement (at about the same time that the licensing boards were setting the same requirement), and expanded their other requirements for membership by specifying the minimum entrance requirements. Apparently, not all the member societies adhered to the latter requirement because the association's president stated in 1894 that "a suspicion prevailed that the rules as to entrance requirements were more honored in the breach than in the observance." Nonetheless, the better schools made marked improvements in their standards of medical education during this period.[11]

DIFFERENCES AMONG MEDICAL SCHOOLS

The continuing improvements in the better medical schools increased the disparity between the quality of their educational program and that of the poorer schools. The discoveries in bacteriology and the developments in the specialties made the difference between the well-educated and the poorly educated physician a meaningful one: in John Billings's words, it now paid a physician to become well educated. This permitted the better medical schools to disregard completely the competition of their competitors offering cheaper and shorter courses.

[11] Smiley, "Association of American Medical Colleges," pp. 515–18.

Traditionally, all American medical schools had emphasized a practical, clinically oriented education. The faculty were practitioners who taught on a part-time basis, and the students wanted a short, vocational education. Norman Walker, a British physician who toured American medical schools in 1891, wrote:

The Americans . . . endeavour to make all their lectures practical. . . . The American teachers are practitioners first and professors afterwards; and every subject, from anatomy to micro-organisms, is illustrated by reference to "cases I have seen." No subject is kept to itself. . . . A lecturer on Pathology will branch off to a clinical picture of a case of pneumonia, while a lecturer on Anatomy will discuss the treatment of Pott's disease. . . . The number of practical lectures is enormous. When you consider that the course only lasts three years, and that in this are included courses on the nervous system, ophthalmology, otology, laryngology, diseases of the urinary organs, diseases of the chest, and maybe one or two other special subjects, it is plain that the time must come off the more elementary subjects, which are the only true foundation of a good education.[12]

This clinically oriented education suffered from a major defect: the absence of what Walker called a "thorough grounding in Anatomy, Physiology, Pathology, and Therapeutics," the basic medical sciences. Anatomy, physiology, and pathology in particular were stagnant backwaters of the curriculum of most medical schools; Walker found that the basic scientific courses were "almost always badly put together" and provided insufficient laboratory instruction. He observed that "very many schools have no class of Practical Histology, and a man may actually take his degree without ever having looked through a microscope."[13] Anatomy courses also suffered from a lack of adequate organization and thorough instruction. Abraham Flexner, the author of a classic study on medical education in 1910, wrote:

The professor is a busy physician or surgeon. He lectures to ill prepared students for one hour a few times weekly, in a huge amphitheater, showing a bone between his finger-tips or eloquently describing an organ which no one but the prosecutor distinctly sees; at the close of which oratorical performance he snatches his hat and, amid mingled applause and cat-calls, makes for his automobile to begin his round of daily visits. In the afternoon "demonstrators" supervise the dissecting, where eight or ten inexpert boys hack away at a cadaver until it is reduced to shreds. The actual emphasis falls on the didactic teaching and the quiz-drills. . . . The really effective work is not infrequently done by [private] quiz-masters, who drill hundreds of students in memorizing minute details which they would be unable to

[12] Norman Walker, "The Medical Profession in the United States," *Edinburgh Medical Journal* 37 (1891): 240–41.
[13] *Ibid.*, pp. 241–42.

recognize if the objects were before them. This is a flourishing industry in "great medical centers" like Chicago and Philadelphia.[14]

This poor preparation led instructors in the clinical subjects to complain, according to an American physician, that students coming to them were "utterly unprepared as regards the structure and functions of the normal body and almost totally ignorant of the changes which take place in disease."[15]

Another defect of virtually all medical schools was the inadequacy of bedside clinical training. The clinical teaching was usually done in public or private hospitals unaffiliated with the medical school and sometimes located miles away. The hospital physicians and surgeons often were placed on the medical school faculty to insure harmonious relations, even though they were otherwise unqualified. Furthermore, the hospitals considered teaching to be a secondary activity, and the clinical training invariably suffered.[16]

The first effort to eliminate all these defects in American medical education was the formation in the late 1880's of The Johns Hopkins Medical School, which Flexner considered the first American medical school with substantial endowment, well equipped laboratories, a full-time faculty for the basic scientific courses, and its own teaching hospital. Hopkins was the first American medical school to require a baccalaureate degree as an admission requirement, and its course was geared to a high level of individual attainment. Every student possessed his own microscope and reagents and, according to Flexner, "was responsible for a patient's history and for a trial diagnosis, suggested, confirmed, or modified by his own microscopical and chemical examination of blood, urine, sputum, and other tissues." During the same period, other leading medical schools took similar steps to incorporate scientific medicine into their curriculum through both increased scientific laboratory training and the direct application of scientific tools into clinical education. This necessitated hiring faculty in the basic medical sciences who were neither practitioners nor part-time teachers, but instead trained scientists who devoted their entire activities to teaching and scholarship. The increasing number of these medical scientists is shown by the formation of professional societies

[14] Abraham Flexner, *Medical Education in the United States and Canada*, Bulletin No. 4 (New York: Carnegie Foundation for the Advancement of Teaching, 1910), pp. 83–84.

[15] Lewellys F. Barker, "Medicine and the Universities," *American Medicine* 4 (1902): 144.

[16] *Ibid.*, p. 143; Walker, "Medical Profession," p. 240.

and scholarly journals in anatomy, physiology, and pathology in the last fifteen years of the century.[17]

While these developments were occurring in the best schools, the low-grade schools proliferated and prospered in the years immediately before the turn of the century. Medicine had become an attractive and popular vocation as a result of the developments in the specialties and bacteriology, and students flocked to the schools as never before. The one hundred schools with 11,826 students in 1880 increased to 160 schools with 27,615 students in 1903. Even though the number of schools increased by 60 percent, the average number of students per school increased from 118 to 173. Furthermore, as the better schools improved their education to include more clinical and laboratory work, the difference between their fees and entrance requirements and those of the poorer schools also increased. In 1910 in Chicago, which had more medical schools than any other city in the country, one of the two most expensive schools cost $185 per year, while the least expensive one cost $100 per year. The former school required two years of college as an entrance requirement; the latter had no stated entrance requirement.[18]

The licensing requirements served only as a minimal restraint to the worst excesses of the low-grade schools. Some of the requirements, like the four-year course, were profitable to the schools. Others were disregarded without any action being taken by the licensing agencies. Furthermore, the licensing examinations, if they were required, were not at all difficult. The school whose students obtained the best record of all Chicago schools on the licensing examinations in 1906 had, according to Flexner, "no entrance requirement, no laboratory teaching, no hospital connections." A few years later it was declared "not in good standing" by the state board of health.[19]

The major distinguishing feature of the worst schools was their unrestrained commercialism. Probably the most extraordinary example was the Harvey Medical College in Chicago, which maintained in the same building a day college, an evening college, a hospital, a free dispensary, a training school for nurses, a dime drug store, and an

[17] Flexner, *Medical Education*, pp. 12, 22; Barker, "Medicine and the Universities," p. 144. The American Physiological Society was founded in 1887; the American Association of Anatomists in 1888; and the American Association of Pathologists and Bacteriologists in 1900: Margaret Fisk, ed., *Encyclopedia of Associations*, 6th ed., vol. 1 (Detroit: Gale Research Co., 1970).

[18] "Medical Colleges of the United States," *Journal of the American Medical Association* 55 (1910): 668–69; Thomas Neville Bonner, *Medicine in Chicago 1850–1950* (Madison, Wis.: American History Research Center, 1957), p. 112.

[19] Flexner, *Medical Education*, p. 170.

"out practice." The drug store furnished drugs for ten cents to the dispensary and out-practice patients. The medical school students were taught pharmacy by the drug store pharmacist, who provided instruction in "the practical as well as the theoretical compounding of drugs." These schools resorted to blatant and often flagrantly false advertising to attract students, and Flexner observed that their deans occasionally knew "more about modern advertising than about modern medical teaching." Commercialism was possible because medicine attracted many working and lower-middle class young men who exemplified what Walker described as the "American characteristic of trying many trades." Walker observed that many young men in their twenties, dissatisfied with their vocations, would try their luck at medicine, and, if they failed, would return to their previous vocations.[20]

The major problem caused by these schools was not their poor educational programs, because most of them produced very few graduates (the great majority of students never completed the course), but rather that they tended to drag the medium-grade schools down to their level. For example, there were six medical schools in San Francisco in 1900. Harris claimed that "all of these schools showed the stain of commercialism, faculties practiced in exclusive gangs, college dispensaries were likely to be the stalking fields for financial prey, and students in the poorer schools became cappers and steerers for their teachers." The quality of the graduates of the average schools can be ascertained by the failure rates of the physicians taking the examinations for admission to the medical corps of the armed services. Between 1900 and 1909, the Naval medical corps failed 46 percent of the M.D.s taking the examination; between 1904 and 1909, the Marine hospital service failed 81 percent; and between 1888 and 1909, the Army medical corps failed 72 percent. Furthermore, Flexner wrote that "very few of the applicants examined came from the unmitigatedly bad schools."[21]

THE DEATH OF COMMERCIAL MEDICAL EDUCATION

Virtually all medical schools were self-supporting during the nineteenth century, with the exception of a very few elite institutions. This

[20] Frances Dickinson, "History of Harvey Medical College," in H. G. Cutler, ed., *Medical and Dental Colleges of the West: Chicago* (Chicago: Oxford Publishing Co., 1896), pp. 495–96; Flexner, *Medical Education*, pp. 18–19; Walker, "Medical Profession," p. 243.

[21] Henry Harris, *California's Medical Story* (San Francisco: Stacey, 1932), p. 235; Flexner, *Medical Education*, p. 170. The paucity of graduates of the lowest grade of schools is shown by any of the tabulations of those taking and passing the licensing examinations, such as those listed yearly around 1900 in the *Bulletin of the American Academy of Medicine*, e.g., vol. 4 (1900): 808–12.

was often true of the state schools. When the California legislature established a state medical school in 1897, they provided no funds for furnishings and permitted the students' fees to be distributed to the faculty in lieu of salaries. They assumed that the medical school would be largely self-supporting. Throughout most of the nineteenth century these expectations had been valid. The schools had no laboratories and little clinical instruction, the faculty was small, costs were minimal, and profits were common. Even if the faculty earnings were small, the prestige and additional patronage obtained by faculty members compensated for their efforts. These indirect benefits were sometimes so great that professorships were sold for as much as two thousand dollars per chair. In many instances, the number of applicants for vacant faculty positions far exceeded the number of vacancies.[22]

By the turn of the century, the situation was changing radically. In order to comply with the state licensing requirements and to attract students, medical schools were forced to make heavy investments in expensive laboratory equipment and to hire faculty on a full-time basis to teach the basic science courses. These additional expenses soon proved an enormous drain on the finances of the schools. Frank Billings said in his AMA presidential address in 1903:

> The laboratory method . . . involves an expense which is appalling when compared with the methods of teaching formerly practiced in all schools, and still adhered to in many medical schools. The method is expensive, inasmuch as it involves more extensive buildings, much expensive apparatus and an increase of the teaching force. The instruction must be individual or to small groups of laboratory workers, and this involves also an extension of the time of instruction. . . . The teachers of these fundamentals must . . . give their whole time to the instruction of students and to original investigation. . . . The salaries of such professors and of the corps of assistants which the laboratory method implies makes the cost of the university or college far beyond the income which could be derived from the tuition of students.[23]

Abraham Flexner concluded from this in his 1910 study:

> It has, in fact, become virtually impossible for a medical school to comply even in a perfunctory manner with statutory, not to say scientific, requirements and show a profit. The medical school that distributes a dividend to its professors or pays for buildings out of fees must cut far below the standards which its own catalogue probably alleges. Nothing has perhaps done more to complete the discredit of commercialism than the fact that it has ceased to pay. It is but a short step from an annual deficit to the conclusion that the whole thing is wrong anyway.[24]

[22] Harris, *California's Medical Story*, pp. 241–42; Barker, "Medicine and the Universities," p. 143.

[23] Frank Billings, "Medical Education in the United States," *Journal of the American Medical Association* 40 (1903): 1273.

[24] Flexner, *Medical Education*, p. 11.

Three courses of action were open to medical schools in financial difficulty. One was to seek a university sponsor to underwrite the costs of the institution. Many schools were able to do this in the short run because universities had not yet realized the financial burden of a medical school. However, these medical schools often failed to survive. A second course of action was to merge with other medical schools, which was very common early in the twentieth century (Table XV.3). The third course of action was to suspend operations, which occurred with increased frequency after 1906. The two latter trends were masked before 1907 by the large number of new schools being founded, but once this ceased, the number of medical schools showed a dramatic decline.[25]

CHANGES IN THE HOMEOPATHIC AND ECLECTIC SCHOOLS

The pressures which struck down the commercial regular schools bore down the homeopathic and eclectic schools much more forcefully. Only a small proportion of the homeopathic and none of the eclectic

TABLE XV.3
CHANGES IN NUMBER OF MEDICAL SCHOOLS, 1900–1910

Year	Medical Schools Involved in Mergers or Absorbed into Other Schools	New Schools Created by Merger	Schools Suspending Operations	Newly Organized Schools	Net Change
1900	0	0	1	6	+5
1901	3	1	2	2	−2
1902	5	2	0	5	+2
1903	3	0	2	5	0
1904	2	0	1	2	−1
1905	8	3	1	5	−1
1906	0	0	0	5	+5
1907	6	2	4	5	−3
1908	5	0	4	2	−7
1909	5	2	8	0	−11
1910	6	2	4	0	−8

SOURCE: "Changes in Colleges in Ten Years," *Journal of the American Medical Association* 55 (1910): 691–92.

25 *Ibid.*, p. 196. It is frequently argued that the extensive publicity resulting from the highly critical Flexner report was the major cause of the decline in the number of medical schools after 1910. Table XV.3 and Flexner's own statement above show that many schools merged or suspended operations in the decade before the report was published, and that many others were on the verge of suspension. The impetus generated by Flexner's report merely added to a clearly established trend.

schools were affiliated with universities, compared to a large proportion of regular schools. Furthermore, the relationship between the
homeopathic and eclectic schools and the practitioners in these sects
changed greatly. This can be illustrated more readily for the homeopaths.

Because homeopathy was a relatively small and geographically
localized sect, it lacked the broad base of public support available to
the regular sect. Homeopathic medical schools depended on the support of homeopathic physicians, and when that support declined, they
were unable to survive. The major source of students for homeopathic
medical schools was referrals by homeopathic physicians. A 1907 survey of 100 homeopathic students in one school found that 96 of them
attended a homeopathic school because they had been directly or
indirectly influenced by homeopathic physicians. As scientific medicine
developed, many homeopaths became uninterested in homeopathy
and stopped recommending homeopathic schools to students. A
speaker at the 1907 AIH convention complained of an "astonishing
apathy in Homeopathy," which he traced to the discoveries in scientific medicine and the growth of specialization. The president of the
AIH stated in 1906 that many homeopaths were sending their students
to regular medical schools, not because they felt the teaching was superior in regular schools, "but largely through a spirit of indifference."
Other homeopaths observed that a regular medical education was
more useful in obtaining appointments to boards of health and the
army and navy, in being admitted to regular medical societies, and in
all the other institutional arrangements of the profession.[26]

At the same time, the homeopathic medical schools were becoming increasingly similar to regular medical schools, which antagonized
the more dedicated homeopaths. One homeopath complained that
"hundreds of young men have been graduated who are therapeutic
skeptics. They may have much knowledge of microscopy, bacteriology,
serum-therapy, chemistry, suggestion, manual and electro-therapeutics,
but in the essential principles of healing the sick [homeopathy] they
are remarkably weak and ignorant." Another homeopath confessed to
having noticed that "more and more each succeeding year ... [our
graduates] know less about homeopathic materia medica than they do

26 William Harvey King, "By What Means Can We Place Ourselves in Touch
with Prospective Students of Medicine," Transactions of the American Institute
of Homoeopathy, 63rd Session (1907): 163–68; H. E. Beebe, "The Attitude of the
Profession—How to Correct the Indifference of Homeopathic Physicians and its
Effects," Transactions of the American Institute of Homoeopathy, 63rd Session
(1907): 195–201; William E. Green, "American Institute of Homoeopathy," Transactions of the American Institute of Homoeopathy, 62nd session (1906) 1: 710.

about anything else pertaining to the general practice of medicine." The combined influence of these changes drastically reduced the number of homeopathic medical schools. From 1900 to 1910, the number of homeopathic medical schools declined from 22 to 12, while the number of regular schools declined from 126 to 109.[27]

The decline in the number of eclectic schools was more gradual, but ultimately much more severe than in the homeopathic schools. These schools did not have the wealthy patronage of the homeopathic schools and therefore were almost totally unable to survive. In 1910, Flexner spoke of the "utter hopelessness of the future of these schools."[28] Although eight of the nine eclectic schools in 1900 survived to 1910, seven of the eight were defunct before 1920. Only the Eclectic Medical Institute remained, until it too closed its doors in 1939.

CONVERSION OF HOMEOPATHIC SCHOOLS TO REGULAR SCHOOLS

The three high-grade homeopathic medical schools in Boston, New York, and Philadelphia were able to survive the great wave of closures, but the decline of sectarianism in medicine made their future unpredictable, and they began to consider discarding the homeopathic label entirely. The first homeopathic school to do so was the Boston University School of Medicine. In 1917, at the instigation of the university's president, the medical school faculty undertook a study and concluded:

Times have changed. The arts of medicine have changed. Surgery, electro-therapeutics, serology, the specialties of eye, ear, nose and throat have forced themselves to the front, while drug therapy has been pushed further and further into the background until it occupies a relatively minor position, especially in the dominant school. In the homeopathic school, the study of homeopathy occupies but a small proportion of the curriculum. Nevertheless, we designate our school as homeopathic because within its walls homeopathy is taught. We are singling out one specialty to dominate and characterize the whole. Inasmuch as drug therapy does not occupy the conspicuous position which it formerly held and the general belief in the efficacy of drugs is diminishing rather than increasing, are we not attributing too much importance to our particular method of prescribing when we brand our broad and comprehensive medical training as distinctly homeopathic?[29]

27 Guernsey P. Waring, "Dunham Medical College of Chicago," in William Harvey King, ed., *History of Homoeopathy* (New York: Lewis, 1905), III: 120; W. J. Martin, "Is Our Materia Medica Becoming One of the Lost Arts?" *Hahnemannian Monthly* 35 (1900): 680.

28 Flexner, *Medical Education*, p. 163.

29 *History of the Reorganization of the Boston University School of Medicine* (n.p., 1918), p. 11.

Inquiries made to the AMA Council on Medical Education in 1918 ascertained that the association would certify the school as a regular medical school, even though it taught homeopathy, provided that the homeopathic courses were "not overemphasized." In 1919, the university offered to subsidize the medical school, which then abandoned its homeopathic designation.[30]

The New York Homeopathic Medical College and Hahnemann Medical College of Philadelphia retained their homeopathic designation for some time thereafter. Morris Fishbein wrote in 1932 that they taught "modern medicine with some reflection of the history of homeopathy." The New York Homeopathic Medical College obtained legislative approval to drop the word "homeopathic" from its title in 1936 and in that year greatly reduced the number of homeopathic courses in the curriculum. All remaining courses in homeopathy were eliminated in the 1940's. The Hahnemann Medical College in Philadelphia also reduced the number of courses in homeopathy in 1936, but it continued to award the degree of Doctor of Homeopathic Medicine to its graduates along with the M.D. degree until the late 1940's. Required courses in homeopathy were eliminated in the early 1950's, and the last elective course in homeopathy was taught in the early 1960's. The demise of homeopathy in these institutions was due to two factors. First, students were no longer interested in homeopathy, and courses in the subject were consequently discontinued. Second, the decreasing number of faculty members competent to teach homeopathy made it difficult to replace those who retired or left the faculty, and the courses were dropped from the curriculum.[31]

Thus, under the overpowering influence of scientific medicine, medical education lost both its proprietary and its sectarian nature. Somewhat more slowly, but equally arduously, the medical societies also abandoned their sectarian designations and opened their portals to all physicians.

[30] *Ibid.*, pp. 23–24; "Boston University School of Medicine . . . Forty-Seventh Annual Announcement and Catalogue," *Boston University Bulletin* 8 (1919): 10.

[31] Morris Fishbein, *Fads and Quackery in Healing* (New York: Covici, Friede, 1932), p. 27. The information on the New York Homeopathic Medical College was obtained from the *Annual Announcements* of the College and personal correspondence from Linn J. Boyd, Professor Emeritus of Medicine. The information on the Hahnemann Medical College was obtained from the *Announcements* of that college and from a conversation with Acting Dean Joseph R. DiPalma. The writer would like to thank both Professor Boyd and Dean DiPalma for their kindness in sharing their knowledge with him.

CHAPTER 16 THE DEATH OF SECTARIAN
MEDICINE

CONFLICT BETWEEN regular physicians and homeopaths and eclectics continued to be a dominant feature of the organized profession in the later years of the century. Many regular physicians viewed members of the other sects as renegades and heretics, moral reprobates who were not signatories to the sanctified code of ethics. Many specialists and some other regular physicians, however, realized that non-regular physicians could be a profitable source of referrals and could add to the economic and political strength of the profession in such areas as licensing and public health. The efforts of these physicians brought about increased cooperation among the sects and eventually destroyed sectarian boundaries. These changes in turn weakened the traditional code of ethics of the regular sect and led to the complete reorganization of the AMA and its constituent societies from exclusive to inclusive organizations.

CONFLICT BETWEEN REGULAR AND HOMEOPATHIC PHYSICIANS

During the last half of the century, relations between regular and non-regular physicians continued to deteriorate. The regulars viewed the homeopaths—the strongest and most influential competing sect—in especially vituperative terms. "How long, O Lord!" exclaimed one regular physician, after two of his colleagues had been replaced by homeopaths on the local board of health, "how long must poor suffering humanity continue to pay tribute to those vile pretenders, those truculent speculators upon credulity, those sycophantic parasites of fraud and villainy that infest our state and nation."[1] D. W. Cathell reserved his most severe censure for non-regular physicians, particularly homeopaths. "Where stand quacks and irregulars of every kind

[1] Henry Harris, *California's Medical Story* (San Francisco: Stacey 1932), pp. 195–96.

298

in the upward track of scientific medical progress?" he demanded. "What have they done for science? 0 0 0 0—nothing!"[2] The inconsistency in these arguments was nowhere better illustrated than in Cathell's own book, where, scarcely a dozen pages later, he conceded that homeopathy still was a useful counterbalance to the tendencies of regular physicians to use excessive medication:

So strong has been the reaction against old-timed medication, that Hahnemann's silly system has secured a large and earnest following, and enjoys the sunshine of popular favor among the susceptible to such an astonishing degree that it may be regarded as the grand delusion of the nineteenth century,—"How long, O Lord, how long!"—and there is to-day no (lawful) human occupation that yields so large a return for the amount of capital and brains required as the practice of homeopathy, and that so few have deserted the crowded paths of rational medicine to seek its shekels is a monument to man's preference of the true and noble path. There can be no doubt that its prosperity would have already terminated had the profession not been so slow to accommodate itself to the demands of fashion, particularly with reference to medication in slight and imaginary cases. But rational physicians are arousing to the importance of this feature, and are rapidly conforming to it. They are also administering more concentrated and palatable forms of medicines in serious cases . . . . Determine that you will bear your share in the good work by devoting time and study to rendering therapeutics useful and at the same time cheap, pleasant, and acceptable to patients. If you will carry a small pocket vial-case of your favorite pills, tablets, granules, etc. both strong and weak, for use on suitable occasions, you can meet homeopaths in the matter of free-dispensing, and also have as much benefit as they of the mystery that envelops the name and nature of the drugs thus employed. Besides, you will escape the drugstore "repeats," and if there be any repeating you will do it yourself.[3]

The greatest sin conceivable to many regular physicians was to consult with a homeopath. Cathell advised his regular colleagues:

Do not refuse to consult with foreign physicians, doctresses, colored physicians, or any other regular practitioners; for you, as a physician . . . should know nothing of national enmities, race prejudices, political strife, or [religious] differences. RESCUE! is our battle-cry, and you, as a physician . . . have no moral right to turn your back on sick and suffering mankind, by refusing to add your knowledge and skill on a plane of real and brotherly equality, to that of any honorable, liberal-minded person who practices medicine, if his professional acquirements and ethical tenets give him a claim to work in the professional field. . . .
But while you bid "All Hail!" and give the right hand of fellowship to every honorable, unrestricted physician, and become the friend and brother of all the friends of rational medicine, no matter what their misfortunes or

2 D. W. Cathell, *Book on the Physician Himself* (Philadelphia: Davis, 1895), 10th ed., p. 229.
3 *Ibid.*, pp. 243–44.

how great their deficiencies; you must, on the other hand, remember that medicine is a liberal profession and not a mere trade, and refuse to extend the hand of brotherhood to any one belonging to a party or association whose *exclusive system*, narrow creed, or avowed or notorious hostility to our profession, prevents him from accepting every known fact and employing all useful remedies . . . [and] who cannot honestly say his mind is wide open for the reception of all medical truths . . . ; as that constitutes a voluntary disconnection from the profession. When called in a case in which the medical attendant cannot do this, you cannot agree with him, and must let his retirement be one of the conditions on which you will assume charge.

You may, however, be called to a case of pressing emergency, such as an alarming hemorrhage, poisoning, drowning, choking, convulsions, or difficult labor, and find on your arrival that an irregular practitioner or quack is in attendance, with whom you are thus brought face to face. In such urgent cases the path of duty is plain, for, owing to the great danger to life, the higher law of humanity will require you temporarily to set aside ethics and etiquette, and to unite your efforts—head, heart and hand—with those of your chance associate. Treat him with courtesy, but studiously avoid formal consultations, or private professional dealings, or whispering conversation with him, or any other act that might imply association in consultation.

Thus, you see, there is not only no antagonism between medical ethics and humanity, but that they overlook all questions of etiquette, and allow and cover any and every act honestly performed for the benefit of humanity. . . . it is a duty which you owe both to yourself and to your profession that you terminate the accidental and unnatural connection—in a gentlemanly way, of course—as soon as the pressing urgency will admit.[4]

These illustrations are sufficient to suggest the highly emotional and moral manner in which many regulars viewed their homeopathic and eclectic competitors. Cathell even opposed social contacts with non-regular physicians: "Shun this and every other contaminating alliance that would confound them with us before the public." Many medical societies treated any regular physician who had any contact with non-regular physicians as contaminated and fallen from grace. One unfortunate regular physician actually married a homeopath. This anonymous martyr to love was expelled from the Fairfield County (Conn.) Medical Society for professionally consulting with his wife. At least the society thought he consulted with his wife. The state society set aside the decision for lack of evidence and remanded the case to the county society for further hearings. No more is known of the matter.[5]

[4] *Ibid.*, pp. 214–16. Cathell oversimplified the problem in this description. In 1885, the AMA resolved that no "emergency" could make it "necessary or proper to enter into formal professional consultations" with non-regular physicians. The situation described by Cathell was permissible only if the consultations were informal. "Society Proceedings," *Journal of the American Medical Association* 4 (1885): 551–52.

[5] Cathell, *Physician Himself*, pp. 10–11; "Connecticut Medical Society," *Medical Record* 13 (1878): 510. Homeopathy, like the other non-regular sects, had many more female practitioners than regular medicine did. In 1900, women constituted 5

These controversies frequently involved interpretations of the AMA code and, in several instances, the AMA enacted specific resolutions defining relations between regular and non-regular physicians. The most important of these concerned the homeopathic medical course at the University of Michigan. When the legislature incorporated the course into the university medical school in 1875, it did not appropriate sufficient funds to establish a completely separate homeopathic medical school. Consequently, the homeopathic students took all their courses, except those concerning the materia medica and the practice of medicine, in classes with the regular students. Thus regular medical-school faculty members were teaching future homeopathic physicians. The AMA judicial council examined the question and found no violation of the code of ethics. The AMA convention, however, enacted a resolution in 1881, stating that no regular physician should sign any diploma or certificate of any persons "whom they have good reason to believe intend to support and practice any exclusive and irregular system of medicine." This resolution was to have an important impact on the association in the next two decades.[6]

These actions, which intensified the ostracism of non-regular physicians, antagonized some regular physicians. The *Medical Record* called the resolution referred to above unenforceable and undesirable. "Unless we are willing to admit that the teaching of truth is harmful, that education is dangerous, that true science can be misconstrued, and that the right will not always prove itself such," the editor observed, "we are forced to acknowledge that the association has taken a step backward." The editor added that it was in the interest of the public to insure that all physicians receive a proper education.[7]

THE MEDICAL SOCIETY OF THE STATE OF NEW YORK AND THE CODE OF ETHICS

Differences within the regular profession over relations with non-regular physicians soon became so significant that they disrupted the nation's largest medical society, the Medical Society of the State of New York. Some of the most eminent members of the society under-

---

percent of the students in regular medical schools, 9 percent of the students in eclectic schools, and 17 percent of the students in homeopathic schools. George M. Kober, "The Progress and Tendency of Hygiene and Sanitary Science in the Nineteenth Century," *Medical Record* 59 (1901): 906. In the same year, 12 percent of all homeopathic physicians were women. George B. Peck, "Homoeopathy in the United States," *Hahnemannian Monthly* 35 (1900): 560.

6 "American Medical Association," *Medical Record* 13 (1878): 464; "American Medical Association," *Medical Record* 19 (1881): 537.

7 "The Meeting of the American Medical Association," *Medical Record* 19 (1881): 551.

took an attack on the code of ethics, and particularly on the restrictive consultations clause, that culminated in 1882 with the society's revision of the code and its expulsion from the AMA.

These physicians advanced a number of arguments in opposition to the restrictive consultations clause. They observed that the clause had been adopted to ostracize the homeopaths and to reduce public confidence in them, and thereby to suppress the sect. However, the ostracism had precisely the opposite effect. In a detailed history of the whole question, Henry Piffard, a well-known physician of the time, pointed to the prosperity and popularity of the homeopaths and stated that "the general effect of the 'code' was, in many ways, to build up and strengthen the sectarian societies, not only by forcing men into them, but by exciting public sympathy in their favor, and thus aiding them politically." He concluded, "if the object of this code were the suppression of quackery, its success can hardly be described as brilliant." A second argument was that the regular societies' ostracism of users of homeopathic medicines made the regular physicians more sectarian than the homeopaths. Piffard stated that while regular societies expelled any of their members who used homeopathic medicines, no homeopathic society had ever expelled one of its members for using regular medicines. Sectarianism was more characteristic of the regular physicians than the homeopaths. Third, consultations between homeopaths and regulars had not only become frequent, but were overlooked and covertly accepted by regular medical societies. Thus the clause was disregarded in practice. Another argument was that the doctrinal differences between regular and homeopathic physicians had virtually disappeared, and no longer were grounds for ostracism. Abraham Jacobi stated in his presidential address to the New York state society in 1882 that if regular physicians believed that medical science was "one and indivisible," they should meet homeopaths "with a spirit of reconciliation." The last and undoubtedly the major argument was that the homeopaths were extremely influential in the urban areas of New York state, and no effective licensing laws or laws regulating medical schools could be enacted without their support. Seventeen percent of the physicians in Brooklyn (then a separate city) and ten percent of the physicians in New York City were homeopaths. Jacobi said that cooperation between the homeopaths and regular physicians was "absolutely necessary" if higher standards of medical education were to be realized.[8]

[8] Henry G. Piffard, "The Status of the Medical Profession in the State of New York," *New York Medical Journal* 37 (1883): 401–2, 569; Abraham Jacobi, "Inaugural Address," *Transactions of the Medical Society of the State of New York* (1882): 11. A thorough discussion of these and other arguments can be found in Alfred C. Post, *et al.*, *An Ethical Symposium* (New York: Putnam, 1883).

Those opposed to changing the code replied to these charges with two arguments. In a detailed discussion of the code of ethics, Austin Flint wrote that the reason for the ostracism of homeopaths was that "under no circumstances can there consistently be fellowship with any class of practitioners who adopt a distinctive title as a trade-mark, and who are banded together in order to impair the confidence of the public in the medical profession."[9] If the homeopaths would abandon the designation "homeopath" in their medical societies and medical schools, they would be welcome in the regular profession. Proponents of repeal replied to this by saying that homeopaths could not be admitted to regular societies without demeaning themselves:

> If they were allowed to come into the regular societies without going down on their knees and confessing that they had been sinners, and being forced to renounce their previous faith, they would soon after admission stop preaching homeopathy, as they became accustomed to their new positions, with the gradual change of mind that good fellowship produces. The majority of them now do not practice homeopathy, but they are forced to preach it in self defense.[10]

A second point made by the opponents of the change was that the reformers only wanted to "break down the barriers that ... prevented them from coming into possession of certain consultation fees that the homeopathists might throw into their hands," according to an editorial in the New York Medical Journal. There was considerable validity to this argument. A New York correspondent of a Chicago medical journal wrote that in New York City "the proportion of specialists among the anti-code men is relatively considerable." One specialist justified the proposed change by claiming that thousands of dollars and many lives were being lost by the prohibition against consultations with homeopaths.[11]

The issue soon came to a head. In 1881, the Medical Society of New York County admitted to membership two homeopathic medical school graduates who had subsequently abandoned homeopathy. Some members of the state society challenged this breach of the code. The Committee on Medical Ethics of the state society examined the question and concluded:

> It seems to us eminently desirable and proper, that all homeopaths and other irregular practitioners should be advised and encouraged to renounce

9 Austin Flint, "Medical Ethics and Etiquette," New York Medical Journal 37 (1883): 372.

10 Quoted in John B. Roberts, Modern Medicine and Homoeopathy (Philadelphia: Edwards and Docker, 1895), p. 67.

11 "The New York Specialist," New York Medical Journal 35 (1882): 484; "A Commentary on the Code Controversy," New York Medical Journal 37 (1883): 502: William S. Ely, "The Questionable Features of our Medical Codes," in Post, Ethical Symposium, p. 19.

their errors and qualify themselves for admission to what we esteem to be the regular profession. It would be a singular position for the profession to take, that a person, who had once entered on an erroneous system of medicine, should be considered as having committed a sin against the profession, for which no subsequent repentance could atone.[12]

The state society accepted the report of the committee, which encouraged the advocates of repeal of the code to press their advantage. Under their leadership, the state society revised the code of ethics in 1882 to permit consultations with homeopaths. Support for the change, according to an examination of the balloting on that motion and on an 1883 motion to repeal the revisions, was greatest in the large cities. Physicians in New York City, Brooklyn, Albany, and Rochester all provided majorities for the changes, while physicians in the small towns and villages constituted the greatest opposition to the changes. The four cities named above were the strongholds of homeopathy in the state, suggesting that specialists and those most affected by competition from the homeopaths (who operated hospitals in New York City, Rochester, and Albany) were the major supporters of the revision.[13]

The reaction of the physicians opposed to cooperation with the homeopaths was immediate and vociferous. Most of the county societies in the state, according to the 1883 state society president, "expressed their surprise at and disapproval of the new code adopted by a majority of their respresentatives, as unbecoming the dignity of the profession, and as revolutionary in its nature, and 'disorganizing in its tendency'." The medical press and the profession generally throughout the country also disapproved of the state society's action. A survey taken in November, 1883, of 5,219 members of the society found 46 percent for the old code, 18 percent for the new code, 4 percent for no code at all, and 31 percent uncommitted. Despite the amount of the opposition to the new code, its proponents were sufficiently influential to defeat a motion to repeal it presented at the 1883 convention of the state society.[14]

The 1882 convention of the AMA refused to seat the New York state society delegation because of the latter's repeal of the AMA code, which in effect expelled the society until it conformed to the AMA

12 Thomas Hun and C. R. Agnew, "Report of the Committee on Medical Ethics," *Transactions of the Medical Society of the State of New York* (1881): 54.

13 "Proceedings," *Transactions of the Medical Society of the State of New York* (1882): 18–19, 49; (1883): 73–78.

14 Harvey Jewett, "Inaugural Address," *Transactions of the Medical Society of the State of New York* (1883): 11–12; F. G. Baker in "Proceedings," *Transactions of the Medical Society of the State of New York* (1884): 60.

code. This provided the New York opponents of the new code with an opportunity, and they organized a new state organization, the New York State Medical Association. This organization adhered to the AMA code and was seated at its meetings, and thus attracted all the physicians who wanted to retain their membership in the AMA. For the next two decades New York had two state medical societies and two sets of county and local medical societies, one adhering to the AMA code, the other to the new code. Many physicians joined both societies, but the older one was larger and had the more eminent leaders during the period of their schism.[15]

PATTERNS OF COOPERATION AMONG MEDICAL SECTS

THE REVIVAL OF MEDICAL LICENSING

The medical profession did not continue to grow at an unabating pace after the establishment of many new medical schools in the second quarter of the century. The economic dislocations caused by the Civil War and the depressions which preceded and followed it curtailed the rate of growth of medical practitioners in the 1860–70 decade to less than one-half the rate of growth of the prior decade. By the 1870's, however, medical schools were being founded at an unprecedented rate and the numbers of new graduates were increasing even more rapidly.[16]

Thus, once again as in the 1840's, the medical profession was confronted with the problem of reducing the rate of growth of the profession to what physicians considered a satisfactory level. This time, however, the organized profession realized the futility of direct regulation of medical schools. Medical societies therefore sought to institute compulsory state licensing of all physicians as a means of regulating the number of physicians.

The existence of several medical sects compounded the difficulties of convincing state legislatures to enact licensing measures. The homeopaths and eclectics were convinced that the regular profession would use any state regulation of medical practice to harass them, and they therefore opposed any legislation which did not provide independent licensing boards for each sect. The regular physicians, on their side, usually wanted a single board and were opposed to any form of cooperation with the other sects. Their code of ethics prohibited regular

---

[15] For a brief history of the Association, see Alvin A. Hubbell, "The Reason for the Existence of the New York State Medical Association," *New York State Journal of Medicine* 1 (1901): 94–97.

[16] See Appendix IV and Table XV.1.

physicians from consulting with members of other sects and (after 1881) from signing the diplomas or licensing certificates of members of other sects. This prevented regular and non-regular physicians from serving on the same licensing boards under any circumstances.

In several states the regular physicians endeavored to obtain a legal monopoly over the licensing of all physicians through a single licensing board composed only of regular physicians. Wherever there were even moderate numbers of non-regular physicians, these efforts failed. Charles A. L. Reed, one of the AMA's greatest presidents, stated in 1903 that "it required only a few preliminary skirmishes to discover that the sectarian physicians, stimulated into numbers and influence by the long sustained policy of ostracism, were in a position to thwart every effort at medical legislation."[17]

In some of the states with large numbers of non-regular physicians, the regular physicians were able to obtain legislation which required all physicians beginning practice to have degrees from approved medical colleges. This legislation was acceptable to the homeopaths and eclectics because they had their own medical colleges. However, the statutes were generally so faulty or otherwise amenable to evasion that they were useless in practice. For example, the law passed in Ohio in 1868, according to a historian, created no enforcement officers and "only made extra and often unpopular work for the prosecuting attorney." Whenever a licensed physician preferred charges against an unlicensed one, "the affair smacked of jealousy and envy and not only prevented conviction, but actually enhanced the position of the irregular in the community."[18] Furthermore, when the laws required all physicians (or those with less than ten or so years of practice) to have degrees, the practicing physicians without diplomas usually tried to obtain diplomas by taking a small number of courses at a chartered medical school and paying a large fee. After a law of this type was passed in Michigan, John Scudder wrote in 1883:

The law of Michigan is "driving regulars out of the state"—to buy diplomas. Seven Michiganders have been at my office wanting to graduate in one session (not an eclectic among them), and the seven went [to a regular medical college]. . . . I will wager that from three to five hundred "brannew" diplomas, not one of them honestly earned, will be registered in that state.[19]

17 Charles A. L. Reed, "Medical Organization and the Present Status of the Code of Ethics of the American Medical Association," *New York Medical Journal* 77 (1903): 370.

18 Jonathan Forman, "Organized Medicine in Ohio, 1811 to 1926," *Ohio State Medical Journal* 43 (1947): 279.

19 [John M. Scudder], "What of the Day?" *Eclectic Medical Journal* 43 (1883): 539.

In other states, the regular physicians realized the futility of trying to enact effective licensing legislation without the cooperation of the other sects. Because the regular physicians were unwilling to cooperate with the other sects on a single licensing board, they accepted separate licensing boards for each sect. Each sect thereby remained independent and equal in power, and some form of true licensing— compulsory certification of all physicians by a licensing board—could be enacted. This was sometimes successful, but more often it failed as a form of regulation of medical practice. The laws were frequently loosely drafted and inadequately enforced, problems which could have been overcome if the sects combined their influence, but the opposite usually occurred. For example, a law establishing independent licensing boards was enacted in Kansas in 1879, but it was a weak law. The eclectics contested the law and declared that they would license all candidates regardless of sect. Newspapers accused the regulars, who had sought a single board dominated by them, of trying to monopolize medical practice. The law proved unenforceable and was declared unconstitutional in 1881. This experience did not convince the regulars of the desirability of open cooperation among the sects, because they immediately undertook new efforts to obtain a single licensing board monopolized by them. The result was two more decades without any effective medical practice law.[20]

Eventually, a number of regular physicians realized that the only way to obtain effective, viable licensing legislation was to cooperate with the non-regular physicians on a single board. This sometimes meant having a non-regular majority on the board, even though regular physicians constituted the majority of the physicians in all states. The impetus toward greater cooperation was provided by some of the most eminent men in the profession and a number of leaders of the medical societies. William Osler, probably the most eminent American physician of his day, advised the Maryland state medical society in 1891: "if we wish legislation for the protection of the public, we have got to ask for it together, not singly. I know that this is gall and wormwood to many—at the bitterness of it the gall rises; but it is a question which has to be met fairly and squarely." Reginald Fitz, another eminent physician, advised his colleagues in Massachusetts in 1894 that the Massachusetts Medical Society had made a "decided and decisive error of policy" by ostracizing homeopaths. He argued that the "harmony of action" among educated physicians of all sects had produced the successful medical legislation enacted in other states, and that Mas-

[20] Thomas Neville Bonner, *The Kansas Doctor* (Lawrence: University of Kansas Press, 1959), pp. 75–77.

sachusetts regular physicians also had to cooperate with the other sects to enact similar legislation in their state. A physician who later became president of the state medical society in Pennsylvania went so far as to suggest in 1892 that regular medical societies should admit to membership any physician whose "education and personal character make him a fit associate for intelligent men," regardless of whether he used homeopathic remedies occasionally.[21]

Gradually, these efforts began to bear fruit. Laws were enacted in numerous states providing for "mixed boards" of licensure, in which —in clearcut violation of the AMA code of ethics—regular, homeopathic, and sometimes eclectic physicians sat as members of the same board or, in some states, constituted separate advisory groups to the same board. The extent of the cooperation among the sects can be ascertained by the data in Table XVI.1. Non-regular physicians participated in some way in the licensing process in at least 32 of the 45 states with licensing laws in 1900. Physicians representing at least two sects served on the same licensing board in 20 states. The influence of

TABLE XVI.1

SECTARIAN COMPOSITION OF STATE MEDICAL LICENSING AGENCIES CA. 1900

Licensing Agency*	All States	States with Non-Regular Medical Schools
Single licensing board, composed of regular sect only	3	0
Two or more independent licensing boards, each representing a sect	7	3
Single licensing board, with two or more examining boards, each representing a sect	5	2
Single licensing board, with two or more sects represented	20	9
Other or unknown*	10	2
Total states with licensing boards	45	16

* State boards of health were considered as licensing boards when authorized to license: where composition was known, they were placed in the appropriate category; where composition was unknown, they were placed in the "other" category.

SOURCES: Henry L. Taylor, *Professional Education in the United States* (Albany: University of the State of New York, 1900), I: 516–719; Alexander Wilder, *History of Medicine* (New Sharon, Me.: New England Eclectic Publishing Co., 1901), pp. 776–835.

21 William Osler, "The License to Practice," *Transactions of the Medical and Chirurgical Faculty of Maryland*, 91st annual meeting (1889): 72; Reginald H. Fitz, "The Legislative Control of Medical Practice," *Medical Communications of the Massachusetts Medical Society* 16 (1894): 308, 310; Roberts, *Modern Medicine and Homoeopathy*, p. 7.

the homeopaths, eclectics, and physio-medicalists (the remnants of Alva Curtis's group) was most manifest in the states where they were numerous, which can be estimated by listing separately the states in which schools of those sects were in operation in 1900. In 14 of the 16 states with homeopathic, eclectic, or physio-medical schools, representatives of those sects were included in the licensing systems. It may therefore be concluded that cooperation among the sects was almost always absolutely necessary to obtain licensing legislation in states with many non-regular physicians.[22]

Once these laws were passed, it was usually discovered that the sects were able to work in harmony. For example, the Dean of the school of medicine at Indiana University wrote of the licensing board established in Indiana in 1897:

Of the five members, there was one Homeopath. . . , one Physiomedic, one Eclectic. . . , and two members of the regular medical profession. This organization gave assurance from the start that the minority groups would not be treated unfairly. In fact, the minority groups, if they had united, could have out-voted the regular medical men, three to two. But nothing of this sort happened. The sectarian appointees were very high-grade men who joined the appointees of the regular medical profession in sincerely promoting the best interests of the people of Indiana. The board was a much stronger board than it would have been if composed of five members of the regular profession, for a board so constituted would have had the opposition instead of the co-operation of these sectarian minority medical groups.

This organization, as a mixed board, has been criticized by doctors from states having multiple boards, but the mixed board had some advantages over multiple boards. Under the mixed board students of regular and sectarian schools had to meet the same entrance requirements, and graduates of both regular and sectarian schools had to pass the same examination in preclinical subjects. . . .[23]

The development of effective licensing laws was a slow and laborious procedure, even with the cooperation of the three sects. Frequently, the boards did not carry out their responsibilities fully. Flexner reported in 1910 that appointments to the boards were regarded in many

22 Charles A. L. Reed, "The President's Address," *Journal of the American Medical Association* 36 (1901): 1604. The four states whose licensing boards were composed only of regular physicians were Alabama, North Carolina, South Carolina, and Texas. Very few homeopaths or eclectics practiced in those states. Kansas had no licensing board. Non-regular physicians were often able to influence the licensing laws regardless of their numbers: the fifteen homeopaths in Virginia in 1886 obtained substantial representation on the single licensing board. Wyndham B. Blanton, *Medicine in Virginia in the Nineteenth Century* (Richmond: Garrett and Massie, 1933), p. 201.

23 Burton D. Myers, *The History of Medical Education in Indiana* (Bloomington: Indiana University Press, 1956), pp. 102–3.

states as "political spoils," that faculty members of medical schools were often excluded by law from membership on the boards, and that the boards were sometimes unwilling to carry out their duties. One of the duties of many of the boards was the establishment of standards for medical schools in their states. Flexner stated that the Illinois state board established such standards, but that the medical schools in Chicago "flagrantly violated" them "with the indubitable connivance of the state board." This was often due to the resistance of some schools and physicians to the regulations. Scudder had contended in 1883 that the laxity of the Illinois board was caused by the influence of the regular colleges who "could not stand the pressure, and revolted *en masse.*" Frequently the legislation itself was faulty and provided only minimal penalties for violation, or sometimes had no enforcement provisions at all.[24] Frederick Green stated in 1917:

I venture to assert that there is not a single state in the Union today in which the medical practice act prevents any except the most flagrant quacks and charlatans from carrying on their business unmolested. This is shown by the relatively small number of prosecutions and convictions in each state. There are states in which there has not been a single prosecution under the medical practice act in years, yet does any one believe that this is because there are no violations? In those states in which they are undertaken they are often futile. In different state societies and state journals, the opinion has been repeatedly expressed that prosecutions under the medical practice acts were a waste of time because juries would not convict even when the evidence was overwhelming. . . .[25]

Green observed further that the lists of licensed practitioners compiled and maintained by the state licensing boards were grossly inaccurate, so that the boards were unable to ascertain which physicians were practicing without licenses.[26] Effective licensing legislation was not achieved in many states until well into the twentieth century.

PUBLIC HEALTH

A major area of developing cooperation among the sects analogous to licensing was boards of health, which were established in many cities and states after the Civil War. A survey of one hundred large cities in 1873 found that only five cities had established local boards of health in the years from 1800 to 1830, but that 32 cities did so in the years between 1870 and 1873. Only two states, Louisiana and Massa-

24 Abraham Flexner, *Medical Education in the United States and Canada,* Bulletin No. 4 (New York: Carnegie Foundation for the Advancement of Teaching, 1910), pp. 170–71, 216; Scudder, "What of the Day?" p. 538.

25 Frederick R. Green, *State Regulation of the Practice of Medicine* (Chicago: American Medical Association, 1917), p. 23.

26 *Ibid.,* p. 24.

chusetts, created state boards of health by 1870, but 31 states established them in the next two decades.[27]

Before the 1880's, most physicians showed little interest in public
health. Henry Bowditch said in 1877 that "Public Hygiene seems to
afford less interest to the profession than almost any other topic," and
an AMA president said in the following year that "a very large proportion" of physicians had "never given the subject sufficient systematic
study to enable them to speak with authority upon any of its most
important points."[28]

Once boards of health were established in large numbers, however, physicians realized that they could be used as licensing agencies
to control the supply of physicians. A physician reported to the AMA
convention in 1878 that boards of health were the best means to regulate the practice of medicine. Non-regular physicians immediately
deplored this tactic, and John King, the well-known eclectic physician, said of the effort of Ohio physicians to enact a board of health
with licensing powers: "sanitary regulation, study of epidemics, vital
and mortuary statistics" were only "a thin glossing or sugar coating of
that old scheme to bolster up by legislation a school of medicine thus
confessedly unable to exist by its own merits." These legislative efforts
by regular physicians failed either because legislatures would not enact
them, which occurred in Ohio and Kansas, or because governors appointed members to the boards from all major sects, which happened
in Illinois. Thus regular physicians had to be content with using
boards of health as convenient vehicles for personal advertising and
recognition.[29]

The appointment of homeopaths and eclectics to the boards of
health caused considerable controversy in the ranks of the regular sect.
When a homeopath was appointed to the short-lived National Board
of Health, for example, the subject was a matter for controversy among
regular physicians. The inability of regular physicians to dominate the
boards of health soon forced them to reconsider their opposition to

[27] Charles V. Chapin, "History of State and Municipal Control of Disease," in
Mazyck P. Ravenel, ed., *A Half Century of Public Health* (New York: American
Public Health Association, 1921), p. 137; J. W. Kerr and A. A. Moll, "Organization,
Powers, and Duties of Health Authorities," *Public Health Bulletin*, no. 54 (1912):
12.

[28] Henry I. Bowditch, *Public Hygiene in America* (Boston: Little, Brown,
1877), p. 37; T. G. Richardson, "Address," *Transactions of the American Medical
Association* 29 (1878): 107.

[29] H. O. Johnson, "The Regulation of Medical Practice by State Boards of
Health . . . ," *Transactions of the American Medical Association* 29 (1878): 298, 294;
John King, "Special Medical Legislation," *Eclectic Medical Journal* 44 (1884): 493;
Bonner, *Kansas Doctor*, pp. 77–78.

joint membership of regulars and homeopaths on the same boards. A speaker at the AMA convention said in 1879 that the ban on consultations with non-regular physicians did not apply to joint membership on boards of health, because boards of health did not practice medicine. He also said that it was the duty of regular physicians to serve on boards of health, even if non-regular physicians were also members.[30]

Gradually, the three sects found that they could work amicably and effectively on boards of health, inasmuch as therapeutic conflicts rarely occurred. A president of the AIH said in 1882 that "the united stand taken by the medical profession in sanitary matters has . . . contributed greatly to the advancement of public health." A leading regular physician in New York said in 1901 that regulars, homeopaths, and eclectics "have worked hand in hand, and harmoniously, in securing the enactment of laws for the proper protection of the public health, and doubtless will continue to do so."[31]

Public health programs, however, were of little interest to most nineteenth-century physicians. In the larger cities, relations between boards of health and most physicians were constrained by points of view which were "widely separated," according to Hermann M. Biggs, the outstanding American public health official of his time. Physicians in large cities often opposed the compulsory reporting of contagious diseases desired by boards of health. Biggs attributed this difference of opinion to the boards' concern with the sanitary problems of tenement residents and the physicians' concern with their clients, most of whom were residents of private homes who did not encounter the sanitary problems of tenement residents. Biggs also complained that "only with rare exceptions can physicians be induced to read the circulars of information" issued by the New York City board of health. Furthermore, he stated that public health officials in all but the large cities were "generally physicians without special knowledge, experience, or ability in the performance of the work required." Thus the absence of any direct relationship between the activities of boards of health and the

30 For a history of the National Board of Health (1879–1883), see Wilson G. Smillie, *Public Health* (New York: Macmillan, 1955), pp. 331–39; B., "National Board of Health and Homoeopathy," *Medical Record* 15 (1879): 621; James F. Hibbard, "The Relations of the Code of Ethics to State and Municipal Sanitary Organizations," *Transactions of the American Medical Association* 30 (1879): 383–86.

31 W. L. Breyfogle, "Annual Address," *Transactions of the American Institute of Homoeopathy*, 35th session (1882): 32; Frank Van Fleet, "The History, Aim and Purpose of the Medical Societies of the State and Counties of New York," *Medical News* 78 (1901): 8.

professional interests of physicians led physicians to ignore many aspects of public health.[32]

ADMISSION OF NON-REGULAR PHYSICIANS TO REGULAR MEDICAL SOCIETIES

After the liberal membership policy of the Medical Society of the State of New York and its constituent local societies was shown to be acceptable to large numbers of physicians, other medical societies gradually began to admit both graduates of non-regular medical schools and even practicing non-regular physicians. In 1893, the New York Academy of Medicine, the redoubtable guardian of regular morals for so many years, admitted a graduate of a homeopathic medical college who disavowed his former heresies.[33] Eventually, some regular medical societies, in outright violation of the AMA code, actually admitted numbers of homeopathic and eclectic physicians. This occurred not only in the medical societies on the east coast, but also in some of the traditionally more conservative mid-western societies. John Scudder observed in 1892 that "the Mississippi Valley Medical Association, at its recent meeting, resolved to 'admit all physicians in good standing,' without the qualification *regular*, and I have been told that they would be glad to see Eclectic and Homeopathic applicants for membership."[34] By 1903, Charles Reed was able to report that regular medical societies,

and in many instances very important societies, contrary to the letter and spirit of the code, were receiving men of sectarian antecedents into membership, while many who were already members, contrary to the letter and spirit of the code, were exercising the largest possible liberty in the matter of consultations. The representatives of former sectarianism were, in fact, to be found among both the members and officers of the American Medical Association itself. The Illinois State Medical Society, contrary to the letter and spirit of the code, went so far as to resolve "that the school of gradua-

32 Hermann M. Biggs, "Sanitary Science, the Medical Profession, and the Public," *Medical News* 72 (1898): 48–49.

33 The Academy was more liberal-minded in other areas. A few years later, Roswell P. Flower was named a "Benefactor of the Academy" after he served on a committee which raised $100,000 for the Academy. Some years earlier the same man had contributed a hospital (called the Flower hospital in his honor and still in operation) to the Homeopathic Medical College of New York. Apparently the Academy was willing to overlook his previous indiscretion. Philip Van Ingen, *The New York Academy of Medicine* (New York: Columbia University Press, 1949), pp. 245, 251, 271; Leonard Paul Wershub, *One Hundred Years of Medical Progress: A History of the New York Medical College Flower and Fifth Avenue Hospital* (Springfield, Ill.: Thomas, 1967), pp. 100–101.

34 [John M. Scudder], "The End of the Year," *Eclectic Medical Journal* 52 (1892): 593.

tion shall be no bar to membership in the Illinois State Medical Society, providing that such physician is recognized by the local societies as qualified and not claiming to practice any exclusive system of medicine." Members of the American Medical Association, all over the country, contrary to the letter and spirit of the code, . . . were engaged in the certification and licensure of the avowed practitioners of sectarian medicine. All of this occurred before 1900, from which it will be seen that the code . . . had actually ceased in practice to be the "expression of the ethical sense" of the very organization that had formulated and adopted it.[35]

THE ATTACK ON THE CODE OF ETHICS

The increasing number of code violations encouraged opponents of the code to become more outspoken in their denunciations of it. One of the earliest attacks on the code occurred in 1876 in the AMA presidential address of J. Marion Sims, a world-famous surgeon. Sims had developed an important gynecological device and operation while practicing in a rural southern community. When he moved to New York City, Sims was forbidden by the code to patent his invention or to advertise his presence, and thus was unable to make himself known. He was invited by some leading surgeons to demonstrate his innovations, but, as Sims stated, "As soon as the doctors had learned what they wanted of me, they dropped me. . . . My thunder had been stolen, and I was left without any resources whatever." Sims gradually prospered, but his experiences led him to state that physicians were often forced to violate the code in order to survive. He asked: "Is the Code of Ethics up to the requirements of the times, when it compels honorable men to do dishonorable things to promote an honest action?"[36] He also claimed that the code could be used for personal malice by physicians:

[Do you know that the code] is capable of being used as an engine of torture and oppression?—that men, jealously, maliciously intent upon persecuting a fellow member, may distort the meaning of the Code to suit their malign purposes, thus entering into a regular conspiracy to blacken character, and that under the sanctity of the Code's provisions?[37]

Other critics of the code complained that physicians openly violated many important provisions. The ban on consultations with nonregular physicians was ignored in most large communities. The ban on proprietary medicines (which were then all secret nostrums) was dis-

---

[35] Reed, "Medical Organization," p. 371.
[36] J. Marion Sims, "Address," *Transactions of the American Medical Association* 27 (1876): 96–98; J. Marion Sims, *The Story of My Life* (New York: Appleton, 1884), p. 269.
[37] Sims, "Address," p. 99.

regarded by most physicians, according to Abraham Jacobi: "The vast majority of the physicians accept them, employ them, and recommend them, and their prescriptions are frequently nothing else but the name of an American or a foreign proprietary compound."[38]

Another criticism of the code was that it was enforced inequitably within the profession. The *Medical Record* stated in 1881 that local and state medical societies, and the AMA itself, refused to convict certain violators of the code "simply because such offenders presume upon what they term their high positions in the profession." This led many physicians to believe that "the code, as presently constituted, is nothing more than a convenience for the strong, and little else than a means of discipline for the weak."[39]

Other critics argued that the code weakened medical societies, because many physicians were reluctant to join them and become involved in the squabbles which so often occurred. Cathell stated in 1903 after the code had been revised:

. . . there are numerous [non-members of the regular societies] who are perfectly eligible who doubted their ability to measure up to the code's requirements; others who dissented from this restriction or that feature, and would not affiliate; others knew the code was binding on every member of every society, and would not put themselves under its yoke for fear of unwittingly rendering themselves liable to trial by rivals or enemies; others wished to keep out of code wrangles, and to hold themselves responsible for their own conscience alone . . . ; others had no respect for the effete nonintercourse laws [concerning non-regular physicians] . . . .[40]

Some physicians claimed that the pattern of enforcement of the code had subverted the fundamental purpose of the document. Enforcement had altered the code from an ethical doctrine to a legal one, when its structure and contents rendered it worthless for the latter purpose. Charles Reed stated that the code was originally adopted by the AMA solely as an advisory document. In 1855, the Ohio state medical society enacted a resolution permitting its members to patent medical and surgical instruments, although such patents violated the AMA code. Later in the same year, the AMA convention resolved to require all member societies to adhere to the AMA code as a condition

[38] Abraham Jacobi, "Medicine and Medical Men in the United States," *Journal of the American Medical Association* 35 (1900): 496.

[39] "Shall We Change the Code of Ethics," *Eclectic Medical Journal* 41 (1881): 135. This situation remained a problem in profession for some time. In 1910 a physician observed that the "younger or less influential practitioner" suffered most from the differential enforcement of codes of ethics. Norman Barnesby, *Medical Chaos and Crime* (New York: Mitchell Kennerley, 1910), pp. 39–52.

[40] D. W. Cathell, "Was It Wise for the American Medical Association to Change Its Code of Ethics?" *American Medicine* 6 (1903): 619–20.

of membership. The code was thereupon inserted into the constitution of the association without ever being adopted as a constitutional amendment.[41] Reed continued:

It is important to state in this connection that the Code of Ethics thus enacted into law was a set of rules which, for nearly half a century, assumed to prescribe who were and who were not physicians, and to regulate in detail the conduct of members of the American Medical Association, not only toward each other and to the Association, but toward non-members, while, with equally surprising complacency, it assumed to control the conduct of non-members, of society in general, toward members. . . . Its original status was that of a purely advisory document, the only status that can be given to an ethical declaration and have it remain ethics. With the resolution of 1855, however, or rather with its surreptitious insertion into the constitution, the Code of Ethics ceased to be ethics—by which is meant the science of right conduct—and became law, by which is meant a rule of conduct prescribed by authority and containing a penal clause to be enforced by designated tribunals. The result of this action was that State and local societies all over the country, desiring to avoid the stigma of non-recognition by the national body, imitated its example and made the code a part of their own organic law. Judicial councils were elected, and everywhere men were liable to be subjected, and in many instances were subjected, to inquisitorial proceedings, resulting in the disgrace attending either censure, suspension, or expulsion, for such offenses as offering an opinion out of the prescribed turn at a consultation, or for entering into consultation at all with anyone proscribed by the code. As a further result, many good physicians, with liberal education and with independence of spirit, recognizing the code as an unethical decree that reflected upon their intelligence and interfered with their individual liberty, declined to join the medical societies [subscribing to the code]. . . .

It is well to recall . . . that a code of perfect personal conduct can never be made definite. . . . It thus happened that the Code of Ethics, in its attempted application to diverse conditions, physical, ethical, political, social and professional, became in many instances a most unethical document, with the inevitable result that the idea of ethics in general was brought into corresponding disrepute.[42]

THE REORGANIZATION OF THE AMA

Although the AMA had been founded primarily to alter the system of medical education and to debar practitioners whom its members considered unqualified, the AMA did not contribute to the achievements being made in both areas in the last decades of the century. In its 1904 report, the AMA Committee on Medical Education observed that the association "was founded for the special purpose of obtaining a uniform and elevated standard of requirements for the degree of M.D.

[41] "Minutes," *Transactions of the American Medical Association* 8 (1855): 56.
[42] Reed, "Medical Organization," pp. 370, 372.

The American Medical Association has so far accomplished little toward this end." In fact, those physicians who were working to reform medical education were in breach of the AMA code of ethics. For example, in 1894 the Association of American Medical Colleges, the leading proponent of higher education standards in the profession, violated the AMA code by permitting students transferring to regular medical colleges from homeopathic or eclectic ones to receive credit for their studies at the non-regular institutions.[43] Similarly, the revival of medical licensing laws was due to the cooperation among regular, homeopathic, and eclectic physicians, also in violation of the AMA code of ethics.

Relations between the AMA and its member societies were deteriorating. Although the AMA expelled the New York state society for its actions, three other state societies (Massachusetts, Rhode Island, and Mississippi) retained their memberships despite their nonadoption of the AMA code. Furthermore, dozens of state societies were cooperating openly with homeopathic and eclectic societies in medical licensing, without being sanctioned by the AMA.[44]

The AMA had failed to build a large and respresentative membership. In 1900, only 8,400 of the over 100,000 regular physicians in the nation were members. Around the same time, only about 25,000 physicians belonged to all state and local societies affiliated with the AMA. Furthermore, about 40 percent of the AMA's membership in 1900 resided in seven states situated close to the association's Chicago headquarters. Large areas of the country, including most southern and western states, had few AMA members. The AMA was, in fact, more a regional than a national organization.[45]

The weakness and ineffectiveness of the AMA were nowhere more evident than in national political activities, where the association had been continually unable to secure desired legislation. This was due partly to the association's inability to mobilize the rank and file of the profession to bring their influence to bear on Congressmen, and partly to the absence of professional manpower for gathering data in the national office.[46]

---

[43] Morris Fishbein, *A History of the American Medical Association 1847–1947* (Philadelphia: Saunders, 1947), p. 891; Dean F. Smiley, "History of the Association of American Medical Colleges 1876–1956," *Journal of Medical Education* 32 (1957): 516.

[44] Reed, "President's Address," p. 1604.

[45] James G. Burrow, *AMA: Voice of American Medicine* (Baltimore: Johns Hopkins Press, 1963), pp. 17–19; Reed, "Medical Organization," p. 371.

[46] Reed, "President's Address," pp. 1601–5; Frederick R. Green, *Sixty-Six Years of Medical Legislation* (Chicago: American Medical Association, 1914), p. 8.

STRUCTURAL REORGANIZATION

The association undertook two bold reforms in 1901 and 1903 which completely changed its major features. The 1901 reforms were based on two objectives established in an earlier and unsuccessful attempt to reorganize the AMA in 1887. One objective was to bring back into the AMA the many specialists who had ceased to involve themselves in the affairs of all general medical societies.[47] N. S. Davis, who headed the 1887 reorganization committee, wrote:

[A reorganized AMA should be one] where every legitimate specialist finds an appropriate field for work in some one of the Sections, and at the same time is enabled to mingle in the general sessions with the great body of general practitioners, to the mutual benefit of all. In union there is not only strength and harmony, but the most sure and rapid progress, while exclusive organizations and class distinctions beget prejudice, foster divisions and retard true progress.[48]

A second objective was to reorganize the state and local societies to coordinate their relationship to each other and to the AMA, and to increase the membership of the AMA and its affiliated societies.

To achieve these goals, Charles Reed, who as AMA president was the guiding spirit behind the reorganization, appointed a reorganization committee. The committee reported in 1901 that medical societies were "organized without any common plan and without relationship one to the other." At the local level, multitudes of independent specialty and other societies drew members away from the county societies. A number of "district" societies in metropolitan areas overlapped territories and prevented any one local or county society from being "strong and active." Multi-state regional societies weakened the state societies in a similar manner.[49]

To remedy these problems, the committee proposed that the county society be made the basic organizational unit of the profession: "on the success of the county organization depends all above it; it is the foundation of the whole superstructure."[50] Membership in county societies was to be changed from a privilege to a right; no reputable licensed physician could be refused membership. The committee stated

[47] J. G. Mumford, "The Proposed Boston Academy of Medicine," *Boston Medical and Surgical Journal* 146 (1902): 129–30.

[48] N. S. Davis, *et al.*, "Report of the Special Committee on Changes in the Plan of Organization and By Laws of the Association," *Journal of the American Medical Association* 8 (1887): 715–16. This statement was quoted in the 1901 committee's report.

[49] "Preliminary Report of the Committee on Organization," *Journal of the American Medical Association* 36 (1901): 1445.

[50] *Ibid.*, p. 1450.

that the county society must not have the right to determine its own membership qualifications except under very limited circumstances:

> Membership in a county society must be a right that can be demanded by every reputable physician, and if this right is refused on account of local feeling, the recourse should be had to a higher body, and if on trial it can be shown that the applicant is worthy of membership, it should be accorded him.[51]

The county society was no longer to be an exclusive body, subject to the whims of cliques and the ambition and malice of individual physicians. It was to become an inclusive body in which the applicant had to show only that he was legally qualified to practice and that he was of reputable character (apparently regardless of his sectarian antecedents), and no county society could refuse him membership. The committee even recommended that paid organizers be hired, in a manner similar to those of the "trades unions." These organizers would make registers of all physicians in their areas, organize county medical societies where none existed, and "use every effort, including personal solicitation when necessary, to get all reputable physicians to affiliate themselves with the society."[52]

Having completely altered the basis of membership in the county medical society, the committee proceeded to do the same for the state societies. Every member of a county society would automatically be a member of his corresponding state society by virtue of his membership in the county society. Thus state societies were also denied the right to choose their own members and were made inclusive organizations. The state societies, in turn, would be the only constituent members of the AMA, unlike the previous system in which both state and local societies were represented in the AMA. Furthermore, only a small number of delegates from each state society would be permitted voting rights in the AMA's House of Delegates, which was made the legislative body of the AMA. All members of county societies and only members of county societies would be eligible for membership in the AMA. These alterations would assure a minimum of overlap between levels of the organization and a well-defined role for each level.[53]

The committee's recommendations were both bold and daring— bold because they were so much at variance with the traditional organization of the medical profession, and daring because they constituted a great risk. The reorganization weakened the AMA. Under the old organization, the AMA adjudicated disputes involving local as

---

[51] *Ibid.*, p. 1451.

[52] *Ibid.* A paid organizer was actually hired shortly after the new organization plan was adopted, and he served until 1911; Burrow, *AMA*, pp. 36–41.

[53] "Preliminary Report," pp. 1436–37.

well as state societies and undertook whatever activities it thought desirable. Under the new organization, the AMA was constrained by the prerogatives of the local and state societies and acted only as an appeals body in those areas. The reorganization also excluded all specialty societies from any position in the AMA hierarchy. The specialists therefore were faced with a choice: they could abandon the AMA structure and develop their own independent organizational structure; they could abandon the specialty societies and use the structure of the AMA; or they could maintain a dual loyalty to the AMA organizations and to their specialty societies. The proponents of the reorganization placed their faith not in the role of the AMA in the new system, but in the greater overall strength of the total organization. They estimated that some state societies would increase their membership from three to five times if the full program of the reorganization were implemented. The larger membership and tighter structure together would insure the success of the plan. The committee stated: "It is . . . apparent that such a complete national professional organization would offer the greatest possible facilities for collecting and concentrating the influence of the profession for any great or important object."[54]

The 1901 convention enacted all the recommendations of the committee. The immediate effect was a drop in the membership of the AMA. At the 1902 convention, the president observed that a "considerable number of physicians," including "many of the most loyal and faithful supporters" of the AMA, was dropped from membership because they were not members of the appropriate county societies.[55] Undoubtedly, many of these physicians were specialists. These disruptive effects were short-lived, however, and the specialists soon returned to the fold. They could do little else because they needed the general practitioners more than the latter needed them. Specialists depended on general practitioners for referrals, for consultations, and for effective political action. They therefore had to be content with a dual system of organization, in which they maintained independent specialty organizations, but remained affiliated with the regional organizations in the structure of the AMA.

REVISION OF THE CODE OF ETHICS

The spirit of change affected the AMA code of ethics as well, and a committee was appointed at the 1902 convention to study this question. Its report in 1903 was another landmark in the history of the

54 *Ibid.*, pp. 1446, 1449.
55 John Allen Wyeth, "President's Address," *Medical Record* 61 (1902): 921.

AMA. The revision took the AMA largely out of the code business by changing the code to a set of principles, the effect of which, according to the committee, was to leave the specific details to the state societies,

to form such code, and establish such rules as they may regard to be fitting and proper, for regulating the professional conduct of their members, provided, of course, that in doing so there shall be no infringement on the established ethical principles of this Association. The committee regard as wise and well intended to facilitate the business of the parent organization and promote its harmony this course which leaves to the state association large discretionary powers concerning membership and other admittedly state affairs.[56]

The committee also changed the content of the code in a number of ways. They eliminated the section on obligations of patients to their physicians, and added provisions stating that "every physician should identify himself with the organized body of his profession as represented in the community in which he resides," that county societies should affiliate with their state associations, and the latter with the AMA. The code was judiciously circumspect concerning non-regular physicians. The section on consultations stated only that "the broadest dictates of humanity should be obeyed by physicians whenever and wherever their services are needed to meet the emergencies of disease or accident," and eliminated all references to the other partners to the consultation. The code also stated that sectarianism "is inconsistent with the principles of medical science and it is incompatible with honorable standing in the profession for physicians to designate their practice as based on an exclusive dogma or a sectarian system of medicine." The key word in the new sentence was "designate"; all references to actual mode of practice were eliminated. Physicians who ceased designating themselves as homeopaths or eclectics, regardless of their educational backgrounds or actual basis of practice, would henceforth be considered as regular physicians and entitled to all the rights of regular physicians, including membership in regular medical societies. The 1903 convention adopted these changes, and sectarian medicine suffered its greatest blow.[57]

[56] "Report of the Committee on Medical Ethics," *Journal of the American Medical Association* 40 (1903): 1379. The AMA soon found that this experiment in local self-determination was unsatisfactory. In 1911 it reactivated the judicial council and empowered it to adjudicate disputes, and in 1912 a new AMA code of ethics was enacted which gave the association more direct control over the ethical conduct of its members; Donald E. Konold, *A History of American Medical Ethics 1847–1912* (Madison, Wis.: State Historical Society of Wisconsin, 1962), pp. 70–71.

[57] "Report of the Committee on Medical Ethics," pp. 1379–81.

REACTIONS OF THE STATE AND LOCAL SOCIETIES

Patterns of relationships and sets of beliefs which developed over many years were unlikely to change overnight, and many state and local societies initially refused to accept these modifications in the code of ethics. The Philadelphia County Medical Society, for example, initially refused to make the legal practitioner, regardless of college of graduation, the sole criterion of membership, fearing that non-regular physicians would thereby be admitted. The failure of these holding actions is exemplified by the developments in New York State. Despite the revised AMA code, the New York State Medical Association (the organization affiliated with the AMA) refused to merge with the Medical Society of the State of New York so long as the Society retained its liberal admission and consultation policies with respect to non-regular physicians. The Society, however, was in the stronger position by far. The regular members of the state licensing board were appointed only from its members, according to law. The same was apparently true for appointments to boards of health. Furthermore, after 1903, the Society was eligible for membership in the AMA. The Association's position was thus so weak that it was forced to merge with the Society under the latter's name, constitution, by-laws, and code of ethics. The by-laws of the combined organization stated: "Full and ample opportunity shall be given to every reputable physician to become a member of the society in the county in which he resides," a position completely contrary to that espoused by the Association.[58]

In a remarkably short time, physicians and medical societies throughout the country adjusted themselves to the demands of their new situation. State and local regular medical societies were reorganized, physicians educated in homeopathic and eclectic schools were admitted to membership, and medical sectarianism waned.[59] Once the merits of the new plan were demonstrated, regular physicians often changed their opinions about the value of isolating non-regular physicians. Even D. W. Cathell admitted that the new code was a marked improvement:

That this change inaugurates a better and wiser policy for the profession of our country, I am quite sure. . . .

We, of today, can easily see that if, instead of making [homeopathy] a cause for rejection or expulsion, our predecessors had welcomed into fellow-

[58] William M. Welch, "Medical Advancement," *American Medicine* 6 (1903): 675; "Medical Societies of New York," pp. 9–11; Alvin A. Hubbell, "President's Address," *New York State Journal of Medicine* 2 (1902): 308; "Supreme Court," *New York State Journal of Medicine* 6 (1906): 11.

[59] Reed, "Medical Organization," p. 372.

ship such of these men as were educated and lawfully qualified, when they were but a handful, homeopathy would never have been raised into the dignified position of a rival school, and we would never have had to ask the public to choose between them and us. . . .

[The new code] will free us from the old charge of bigotry; it will kill the old cry of persecution; it will have a great and far-reaching effect on our material interests; it will everywhere promote and foster professional unity; and, far above all else, by putting an end to partisan agitations it will increase the good repute of every worthy medical man in America.[60]

CONCLUSION

Ultimately, the reorganization was successful not because physicians had changed, but because medicine had changed. Dogmas and the consequence of dogmas—sectarianism—were no longer tenable in medical practice. Many aspects of medicine now rested on demonstrable scientific proof, and science, not faith, was to be the arbiter between the valid and the invalid. G. M. B. Maughs stated in 1880:

Now, through the improved means of diagnosis, positive knowledge has taken the place of vague guesses or even probable surmises. So long as physicians depended upon rational signs for their diagnosis, all was uncertainty and doubt where now there is certainty. Then, when all, illuminated by an uncertain light, groped their way to conclusions which could not be demonstrated, a difference of opinion was in many cases inevitable, hence that "doctors disagree" has passed into an adage. Now they agree because the fact is in almost every case capable of demonstration.[61]

Thus while traditional medicine tended to divide physicians, scientific medicine tended to unify them. Scientific medicine made it possible to evaluate the curricula and facilities of medical schools objectively. Scientific medicine also made it possible to evaluate the competence of physicians objectively. These objective standards permitted certification of medical schools and physicians on a uniform basis, which in turn eliminated the justification for sectarianism in medicine.[62]

---

[60] Cathell, "American Medical Association Code of Ethics," pp. 618, 620.

[61] G. M. B. Maughs, "Medical Ultraisms," *Transactions of the Missouri State Medical Association*, 23d session (1880); 22.

[62] Not all forms of medical practice contrary to the organized medical profession disappeared at this time, but sectarianism as defined in this study—acceptance of the valid in medicine and rejection of the invalid as practiced by some other group of physicians—was no longer possible. However, numerous new forms of medical treatment developed in opposition to the major medical sects in the latter part of the nineteenth and early twentieth centuries. These cults, the most important of which were osteopathy, chiropractic, and Christian Science, shared one major feature which distinguished them from the early nineteenth-century sects: their espousal of drugless therapy. Thus they served to complement scientific medicine where it failed to act rather than to challenge the effectiveness of its therapies. Louis S. Reed, *The Healing Cults* (Chicago: University of Chicago Press, 1932), pp. 112–14.

Nowhere are these trends illustrated more clearly than in the incidence of malpractice suits. Malpractice is meaningful only when scientifically determined criteria permit an objective evaluation of the performance of physicians. During the first part of the nineteenth century, the limited nature of scientific medicine made malpractice suits impossible to evaluate, and there is practically no mention of them in contemporary discussions of medical jurisprudence. By the middle of the century, medical knowledge had advanced sufficiently in some aspects of surgery—like amputations, fractures, and dislocations —to permit objective evaluation, and an increasing number of malpractice suits occurred around this time involving precisely those aspects of medicine.[63] As medicine became more scientific, additional areas of a physician's performance could be evaluated objectively. Thus, by the end of the century, malpractice had become a major concern of physicians, as George M. Sternberg, the eminent bacteriologist, observed in his 1898 AMA presidential address:

If [a physician] sees fit to prescribe a bread pill or a hundredth trituration of carbo vegetabilis there is no professional rule of ethics to prevent him from doing so. But if his patient dies from diphtheria because of his failure to administer a proper remedy, or if he recklessly infects a wound with dirty fingers or instruments, or transfers pathogenic streptococci from a case of phlegmonous erysipelas to the interior of the uterus of a puerperal woman, it would appear that the courts should have something to say as to his fitness to practice medicine.[64]

The significance of this change is indicated by the dramatic increase in the number of appellate malpractice suits at the beginning of the twentieth century (Table XVI.2), which the compiler of the table estimated to constitute about one percent of the total number of cases. The number of malpractice suits in the first fifteen years of the twentieth century exceeded the number of suits during the entire nineteenth century.

Malpractice suits induced physicians to band together. Medical societies formed malpractice insurance companies, which would be most economical if the risks were spread over all physicians, rather than a small proportion of the regular physicians. Physicians were confronted with the possibility of testifying against each other in malpractice suits, and those physicians who were ostracized from the organized profession might well be more willing to provide testimony damaging

[63] Chester R. Burns, "Malpractice Suits in American Medicine before the Civil War," *Bulletin of the History of Medicine* 43 (1969): 54, 46.

[64] George M. Sternberg, "The Address of the President," *Journal of the American Medical Association* 30 (1898): 1380.

TABLE XVI.2
APPELLATE COURT DECISIONS IN MALPRACTICE SUITS, 1794–1930

Years	Number of Appellate Court Decisions
1794–1900	224
1900–1905	57
1905–1910	57
1910–1915	117
1915–1920	160
1920–1925	174
1925–1930	226

SOURCE: Andrew A. Sandor, "The History of Professional Liability Suits in the United States," *J.A.M.A.* 163 (1957): 463.

to the practitioner involved. Inclusive organizations would minimize this risk as well. Thus scientific medicine increased interdependence among physicians and fostered inclusive organizations, just as sectarian medicine had increased divisiveness among them and fostered exclusive organizations.

Medical historians have often argued that scientific medicine constituted the triumph of regular medicine over homeopathic and eclectic medicine. Perceptive regular physicians of the period recognized that the situation was far more complex. They saw and knew the opposition which existed to bacteriology within their own as well as the other sects. They saw and knew that specialism developed in all sects. Scientific medicine was not a triumph for any sect; it was the death of all sects. Charles Reed recognized this in his presidential address to the AMA in 1901:

Practice has changed. The depletions, the gross medications [of the regulars], the absurd attenuations [of the homeopaths], the ridiculous antimineralism [of the eclectics] have given way to a refined pharmacy, and to a more rational therapy. Sacrifical surgery has yielded to the spirit of conservatism. Prevention is given precedence over cure. . . . I proclaim, events proclaim, the existence of a new school of medicine. It is as distinct from the schools of fifty years ago as is the Christian dispensation from its Pagan antecedents. It is the product of convergent influences, of diverse antecedents.[65]

William Osler recognized it also and said in the same year:

The nineteenth century has witnessed a revolution in the treatment of disease, and the growth of a new school of medicine. The old schools— regular and homeopathic—put their trust in drugs, to give which was the alpha and the omega of their practice. For every symptom there were a score or more of medicines—vile, nauseous compounds in one case; bland, harm-

[65] Reed, "President's Address," p. 1606.

less dilutions in the other. The characteristic of the New School is firm faith in a few good, well-tried drugs, little or none in the great mass of medicines still in general use. Imperative drugging—the ordering of medicine in any and every malady—is no longer regarded as the chief function of the doctor. . . .

The battle against poly-pharmacy, or the use of a large number of drugs (of the action of which we know little, yet we put them into bodies of the action of which we know less), has not been fought to a finish. There have been two contributing factors on the side of progress—the remarkable growth of the sceptical spirit fostered by Paris, Vienna and Boston physicians, and, above all, the valuable lesson of homeopathy, the infinitesimals of which certainly could not do harm, and quite as certainly could not do good; yet nobody has ever claimed that the mortality among homeopathic practitioners was greater than among those of the regular school. A new school of practitioners has arisen which cares nothing for homeopathy and less for so-called allopathy. It seeks to study, rationally and scientifically, the action of drugs, old and new.[66]

In the short span of one century, American medicine became a vocation for many men, developed institutions, fought and divided over sectarian dogmas, and accepted scientific medicine which cast out the dogmas and transformed medicine from sect to science.

[66] William Osler, *Aequanimitas* (Philadelphia: Blakiston's Son, 1932), pp. 254–55.

APPENDIX I FOUNDING DATES OF IMPORTANT LOCAL AND STATE REGULAR MEDICAL SOCIETIES IN SELECTED STATES BEFORE THE CIVIL WAR

COMMENT: This Appendix tabulates the founding dates of major local and state regular medical societies established before the Civil War in states that were widely settled by 1840. Some of these societies were short-lived, but it is rarely possible to ascertain the date of suspension because of the informal nature of most cessations. For this reason, the tabulations do not mention suspensions in most cases, but state instead which societies are known to have survived into the twentieth century by referring to them as being founded "on a stable basis." The names of currently extant state societies founded during this period are set in italics; their names are given in the form used in 1967, even though several name changes may have occurred between their founding and the present. In some cases, the founding dates of the extant state societies differ from those claimed by the societies; this occurred because some existing state societies trace their formation to an older defunct organization separated from the present organization by a period of long suspension, or to other societies with which the state society merged. The dates given here as founding dates of state societies refer to continuous existence, interrupted only by reasonably short periods of suspension, like those caused by the Civil War.

The names of authors in parentheses refer to the sources listed in Appendix III. Italicized names are general references; other names are listed under the appropriate state. The compilation of medical societies made by J. M. Toner in 1873 was used as a source with some frequency. The societies' founding dates listed by Toner are often in error, but in every instance in which this error has been confirmed, the incorrect founding dates are later than the actual founding dates. In other respects, his data agree with other sources. Therefore, Toner's dates have been used as evidence of the existence of societies at a given time, rather than as evidence of the dates of their foundings.

State	Date	Medical Society
Alabama (Cannon)	1841, 1850	Three local medical societies incorporated.
	1847	State society established, incorporated in 1850, suspended activities in 1855.
Connecticut (Thoms)	1767–71	County society founded and suspended (Stookey).
	1775–93	County societies founded on a stable basis in most counties. Other local and county societies founded in first half of nineteenth century.
	1792	*Connecticut State Medical Society* founded.
Delaware (Bird)	1776	*Medical Society of Delaware* founded, incorporated in 1798.
	1848–63	County societies founded in all three counties.
District of Columbia (Nichols)	1817	*Medical Society of the District of Columbia* founded, suspended 1831–38.
	1833	Medical Association of the District of Columbia founded. Society and Association merged in 1911.
Georgia (Bassett)	1804	Savannah city society founded on stable basis.
	1822–28	Several other local societies founded, some on a stable basis.
	1849	*Medical Association of Georgia* founded.
Illinois (Zeuch)	1817–25	Legislature incorporated medical societies on three different occasions, but societies never survived for any length of time (Camp).
	1840	State society founded, suspended in 1847.
	1846–1850's	Several local societies founded, some on a stable basis (Camp, *Toner*).
	1850	*Illinois State Medical Society* founded (Camp).
Indiana (Kemper)	1818, 1825	Legislature incorporated medical societies, but societies never formed (Clutter).
	1817–35	At least one county and one state society founded.
	1840's and 1850's	Several local societies founded, some on a stable basis (*Toner*).
	1849	*Indiana State Medical Association* founded.
Kentucky (Rawlings)	1802	Local society probably founded in Lexington, definitely established before 1828.
	1819	Local society founded in Louisville.
	1839	Regional society founded.
	1851	*Kentucky Medical Association* founded.
	1850's	Several local societies founded.

State	Date	Medical Society
Louisiana (Marshall)	1817, 1820	Societies of French and English speaking physicians founded in New Orleans; both suspended by the 1830's.
	1845–1850's	Local societies founded throughout the state, a few on a stable basis.
	1849	Louisiana state society founded, defunct in 1855.
Maine (Foster)	ca. 1810	Two local societies established as district societies of the Massachusetts Medical Society (Maine then being part of the state of Massachusetts) (Bartlett).
	1820	State medical society founded, suspended in 1845.
	1853	*Maine Medical Association* founded.
Maryland (Cordell)	1799	*Medical and Chirurgical Faculty of Maryland* founded as state medical society.
	1815–1850's	Several local societies organized.
Massachusetts (Burrage)	1735	Medical society existed in Boston, suspended in 1740's.
	1781	*Massachusetts Medical Society* founded.
	1804–58	Numerous local societies founded.
Michigan (Burr)	1819	Michigan state medical society founded. Incorporating legislation repealed in 1851. Society reorganized in 1853, suspended in 1860.
	1839–56	Numerous county medical societies founded.
Mississippi[1]	1846	*Mississippi State Medical Association* founded.
Missouri (Goodwin)	1837–50	Several local medical societies founded (Maughs).
	1850	*Missouri State Medical Association* founded.
New Hampshire (Putnam)	1791	*New Hampshire Medical Society* founded.
	1806–48	Several district societies founded, some on a stable basis.
New Jersey (Rogers)	1766	*Medical Society of New Jersey* founded, suspended 1775–81 and 1795–1807, when reorganized on a stable basis.
	1790	Local society founded; suspended before 1807.
	1816–1850's	Numerous local societies founded, some on a stable basis.
New York (Walsh)	after mid-1700's	A series of New York City societies founded.

[1] This information was kindly provided by Laura D. S. Harrell, Research Assistant of the State of Mississippi Department of Archives and History, in a letter of October 31, 1969.

State	Date	Medical Society
	1806	*Medical Society of the State of New York* founded.
	1806	Numerous county societies founded throughout the state, many on a stable basis. Additional local societies founded throughout period before Civil War (*Toner*).
North Carolina (Royster, 1949)	1799	First state society founded, suspended in 1804.
	1849	*Medical Society of the State of North Carolina* founded.
Ohio (Paterson)	1812	Legislature incorporated district and state medical societies several times through 1824, but societies never formed on a continuing basis; laws repealed in 1833.
	1835	State society founded.
	1846	*Ohio State Medical Association* founded, merged with other state society in 1851 (Shira, 1941).
	1847–1850's	Numerous local medical societies formed throughout state, several on a stable basis.
Pennsylvania (Radbill)	1765	Philadelphia Medical Society founded, but merged with American Philosophical Society in 1768.
	1770	Local medical society founded in Philadelphia, disbanded in 1792.
	1787	College of Physicians founded in Philadelphia on a stable basis.
	1789	Philadelphia Medical Society founded, suspended in 1846, but revived sporadically for next two decades.
	1821	Numerous other local medical societies founded after this time, some on a stable basis (Petry, *Toner*).
	1848	*Pennsylvania Medical Society* founded (Petry).
Rhode Island (History of Rhode Island Medical Society)	1812	*Rhode Island Medical Society* founded.
	1848	Providence local society founded.
South Carolina (Waring)	1789–1808	Charleston and later other local societies founded on a stable basis.
	1848	*South Carolina Medical Association* founded.
	1850's	Several local societies founded.
Tennessee (Hamer)	1830	*Tennessee Medical Association* founded.
	1843–60	Numerous city and county medical societies founded on a stable basis.
Vermont	1804, 1813	Two county societies founded on a stable basis. Other societies founded during first half of century (*Toner*).

State	Date	Medical Society
	1814	*Vermont State Medical Society* founded, suspended activities during 1830's.
Virginia (Warthen)	1820	Medical society formed in Richmond, incorporated in 1824, suspended in 1826.
	1825	Local society founded (Blanton).
	1841	Richmond society reactivated.
	1852	Richmond society reorganized as *Medical Society of Virginia*.
	1840's and 1850's	Numerous local medical societies founded (Blanton).

APPENDIX II MEDICAL LICENSING LEGISLATION IN SELECTED STATES BEFORE THE CIVIL WAR

COMMENT: The following table shows several significant characteristics of medical licensing legislation enacted before the Civil War in states that were widely settled by 1840. The composition of the licensing agency shows the degree to which medical societies were directly involved in the licensing system. The nature of the sanctions imposed on unlicensed practitioners and the kinds of practitioners who were exempted from the licensing requirements provide evidence of the potential effectiveness of the legislation in limiting the number of medical practitioners.[1] Evidence on the actual effectiveness of the legislation, when available, is also presented. The data do not include information on the statutory requirements for obtaining licenses, partly because such information is not readily available for most states and partly because the ineffective sanctions or significant loopholes in most licensing laws made such questions academic rather than practical ones. Minor modifications in licensing legislation have also been omitted.

Several writers in the first half of the nineteenth century attempted to compile lists of all state licensing laws.[2] After careful examination of the lists compiled by Davis and Coventry, the writer has concluded that they are frequently grossly erroneous, except with regard to the laws of the author's own state. In 1878, Stanford Chaille, in his careful study of Louisiana laws, reached the same conclusion about compilations of that time. He stated that anyone obtaining information about laws in other states "should require *copies* of such laws, with *proofs* of their efficiency."[3]

Except where specifically stated to the contrary, the licensing legislation described for each state consists of all relevant licensing legislation enacted in that state before the Civil War.

[1] Graduates of medical schools are not listed here as being exempt from licensing laws (even though they were usually not required to obtain licenses) because a diploma was considered equivalent to a license, and was therefore not properly a form of exemption.

[2] The most important of these are Charles B. Coventry, "History of Medical Legislation in the State of New York," *New York Journal of Medicine* 4 (1845): 159; N. S. Davis, *History of Medical Education and Institutions in the United States* (Chicago: S. C. Griggs, 1851), pp. 94–104.

[3] Stanford E. Chaille, "History of the Laws Regulating the Practice of Medicine . . . ," *New Orleans Medical and Surgical Journal*, n.s. 5 (1878): 923.

State[4]	Date	Establishment, Composition, and Jurisdiction of Licensing Agency	Enforcement, Exemptions, and Penalties
Alabama (Cannon)	1823	Legislature established and elected licensing board. Numerous regional boards added subsequently.	Only licensed physicians could sue for fees.
	1832		Thomsonian practitioners exempted from provisions of act. License not required for practice.
Connecticut (Thoms)	1792	State society incorporated with power to license and appoint licensing committees in each county. In next decade, division of duties between county and state licensing committees modified.	
	1800		Only licensed physicians could sue for fees.
	1810	State examining committee modified to include equal number of members from state society and faculty of Yale medical school, with president of society to cast vote in case of tie.	
	1848–64	Botanical, eclectic, and homeopathic licensing boards established to issue licenses; botanical and eclectic boards merged.	
Delaware (Bird)	1819	State legislature established and appointed county licensing boards.	
	1822	State society empowered to appoint board members.	
	1835		All persons practicing without fees exempted, even though they accepted gratuities for services rendered (Medical Society of Delaware).
	1843		Botanic, Thomsonian and homeopathic practitioners exempted (Medical Society of Delaware).

---

[4] The names in parentheses below the names of the states refer to the sources in Appendix III. Italics indicate general references; other names are listed under the appropriate state.

State	Date	Establishment, Composition, and Jurisdiction of Licensing Agency	Enforcement, Exemptions, and Penalties
District of Columbia (Lamb)	1819	Medical society incorporated with power to license.	Fine for practice without license. Society suspended activities 1831–38, and weak during remainder of the period.
Georgia[5] (Cobb)	1821	Savannah medical society authorized to license (Bassett).	Probably no penalties for practice without license.
	1825	Legislature created state-wide licensing board with power to fill its own vacancies.	Fine and imprisonment for practice without license. Licensing board suspended activities before 1839 (but probably after 1831, when minor changes were made in the law), because 1839 law was enacted "to revive and keep in force" licensing, according to the preamble.
	1839		All penalties for unlicensed practice repealed. Licensing board suspended activities subsequently, because 1847 law was enacted "to revive and keep in force" licensing, according to preamble.
	1847	Legislature re-enacted 1825 law, but created independent Botanico-Medical licensing board to license botanical physicians	Fine and imprisonment for practice without license for regular physicians. Unlicensed botanical physicians could not sue for fees.
Illinois (Zeuch)	1817	Legislature created two districts in state, each empowered to form societies and issue licenses.	Only licensed physicians could sue for fees; "little heed was given to this law."
	1819	Legislature enacted new law, basically similar to previous law; repealed in 1821.	Only licensed physicians could sue for fees.
	1825	Legislature enacted new law to regulate medical practice; repealed in 1826.	
Indiana (Clutter)	1816	Legislature created licensing boards in several districts.	Only licensed physicians could sue for fees.

---

[5] This information was kindly provided by Mrs. Lilla M. Hawes, Director of the Georgia Historical Society, in a letter of March 31, 1970.

State	Date	Establishment, Composition, and Jurisdiction of Licensing Agency	Enforcement, Exemptions, and Penalties
	1818	Legislature incorporated state medical society and granted it sole power to license.	Unlicensed practitioners subject to fine. State medical society never formed, according to 1825 law.
	1825	Legislature created another state medical society with power to establish district licensing boards.	Same penalty as in 1818 law. State medical society never formed, according to 1830 law.
	1830	Legislature empowered existing societies to license.	Only licensed physicians could sue for fees; apothecaries and female midwives exempted.
	after 1830	Local medical society reported in 1852 that all laws were repealed soon after 1830.	
Kentucky (Rawlings)	—	No licensing law before 1860.	
Louisiana (Duffy)	1723	Chief Surgeon of colony and others empowered to license.	Possible death penalty; licensing never enforced.
	1743	French medical authorities empowered to license.	Apparently limited enforcement.
	1770–1803		"During the Spanish domination nearly all doctors and pharmacists apparently sought official permission before setting themselves up in practice."
	1804	New Orleans created licensing board.	Fine for practice without a license; "there is no evidence that legal action was taken against anyone for noncompliance"; board soon defunct.
(Chaillé)	1808	Legislature empowered mayor of New Orleans to appoint physicians to licensing committee, apparently for whole territory.	Probably no penalty for unlicensed practice.
	1816	New act passed in which governor appointed statewide medical examining board. District boards later replaced state-wide board.	Fine and imprisonment as penalties; but law exempted "any inhabitant . . . who on the application of any of his sick neighbors should procure them some alleviation, or administer them any kind of physic."

State	Date	Establishment, Composition, and Jurisdiction of Licensing Agency	Enforcement, Exemptions, and Penalties
	1840		Imprisonment removed as penalty; 1844 and 1846 editorials in medical journal stated that law was "virtually a dead letter"; committee of state medical society made similar observation in 1851.
	1852	All licensing legislation effectively repealed.	
	1861	Physicians required to make affidavit that they have received M.D. degree.	Unlicensed physicians subject to fine and not permitted to sue for fees. Law never enforced.
Maine (Acts of Incorporation)	1821	Medical Society of Maine incorporated with power to license.	No penalties for unlicensed practitioners up to 1824. Probably no regulatory licensing thereafter.
Maryland (*Kett*)	1799	Legislature incorporated state medical society with power to license.	Unlicensed practitioners subject to fine and not permitted to sue for fees. In 1811, Baltimore licensing board unable to secure convictions from magistrates.
	1838		All practitioners permitted to sue for fees.
Massachusetts (Fitz, *Kett*)	1781	Legislature incorporated state medical society with power to license.	License not required for practice.
	1818		Only licensed physicians could sue for fees.
	1835		All practitioners permitted to sue for fees.
	1859	All licensing legislation repealed.	
Michigan (Burr)	1819	Legislature incorporated state and local societies with power to license.	Unlicensed practitioners subject to fine and not allowed to sue for fees.
	1829		Practitioners not members of incorporated medical societies subject to same penalties as unlicensed physicians.
	1838		Unlicensed practitioners no longer subject to fine.

State	Date	Establishment, Composition, and Jurisdiction of Licensing Agency	Enforcement, Exemptions, and Penalties
	1846		All practitioners permitted to sue for fees.
	1851	All licensing legislation repealed.	
Mississippi (Underwood)	1819	Governor empowered to appoint licensing board.	Only licensed physicians could sue for fees.
	1820		Unlicensed practitioners subject to $500 fine.
	1836	Licensing law declared unconstitutional because of unlimited tenure of board members.	
Missouri[6]	—	No licensing legislation enacted before Civil War.	
New Hampshire (Putnam)	1791	Legislature incorporated medical society with power to license.	License not required to practice.
New Jersey (New Jersey, General Assembly)	1772	Supreme Court judges empowered to license (Caldwell).	Fine of £5 for unlicensed practice; persons not receiving payment for services exempted from law (Caldwell). Probably never enforced, because preamble to 1783 law spoke of "many ignorant and unskilful persons" practicing medicine.
	1783	New law enacted empowering Supreme Court justices to license; modified in 1786 to permit representatives of Justices to license.	Fine of £5 for unlicensed practice.
	1816	District societies of state medical society empowered to license; licensing agencies modified several times in later years.	Only licensed physicians could sue for fees.
	1823		Penalty for unlicensed practice changed to $25 fine.

---

[6] This information was kindly provided by Mrs. Elizabeth Comfort, reference librarian of the State Historical Society of Missouri, in letters of January 9 and 16, 1970.

State	Date	Establishment, Composition, and Jurisdiction of Licensing Agency	Enforcement, Exemptions, and Penalties
	1830		Clause added requiring law to "be so construed, as to prevent all irregular bred" practitioners, including "practical botanist, root, or indian doctor." By 1830's, law was a "dead letter" (Pierson).
	1864		All penalties for unlicensed practice repealed.
New York (Coventry, Kett)	1760	Colonial legislature authorized political and judicial officials in New York City and county to issue licenses.	Fine of £5 for practice without a license. Preamble to 1792 law stated "many ignorant and unskillful persons presume to practise physic and surgery within the city and county of New York . . .," suggesting law was ineffective.
	1792	Legislature enacted new law providing for similar board with similar powers.	Only licensed physicians could sue for fees.
	1797	Legislature enacted statewide law requiring qualified physicians to file with local officials.	Fine of $25 for unlicensed practice.
	1806	Legislature created county and state medical societies and empowered them to issue licenses.	Only licensed physicians could sue for fees.
	1807		Fine of $5 per month for unlicensed practice; law exempted all those using domestic roots and herbs.
	1812		Fine increased to $25 per offense.
	1827		Unlicensed practice made misdemeanor subject to fine and imprisonment; exemption on users of domestic roots and herbs repealed.
	1830		Practitioners using domestic roots and herbs exempted again. Only licensed physicians could sue for fees.
	1844		All penalties on unlicensed practice of medicine repealed.

State	Date	Establishment, Composition, and Jurisdiction of Licensing Agency	Enforcement, Exemptions, and Penalties
North Carolina (Warren)	1859	State medical society empowered to elect state licensing board.	Only licensed physicians could sue for fees.
Ohio (Shira, 1939)	1811	Legislature established and elected several district licensing boards.	Only licensed physicians could sue for fees; law apparently ineffective.
	1812	New law created state medical society and empowered it to establish district licensing boards.	Unlicensed physicians subject to fine and not permitted to sue for fees; state society never formed.
	1813	Legislature enacted new law establishing and electing several district licensing boards. Several minor changes in board membership composition in subsequent years.	Fines for unlicensed practitioners (Forman). Apparently, the law was ineffective.
	1833	All licensing legislation repealed.	
Pennsylvania (Alderfer)	—	No licensing legislation enacted before Civil War.	
Rhode Island (History of Rhode Island Medical Society)	1812	Legislature incorporated state medical society with power to license.	License not required to practice.
South Carolina (*Kett*)	1817	Legislature established two licensing boards.	Unlicensed practitioners subject to fine and imprisonment and not permitted to sue for fees.
	1838		Fine and imprisonment eliminated as penalties.
	1845		All practitioners could sue for fees.
Tennessee (Hamer)	1830	Legislature empowered state medical society to elect licensing boards.	License not required to practice.
Vermont (Caverly)	before 1820	Medical societies empowered to license.	License not required to practice.
	1820	Legislature empowered each supreme court judge, with assistance of two or more physicians, to license.	Only licensed physicians or members of legally constituted medical societies could sue for fees.
	1838	All licensing legislation repealed.	
Virginia (Caldwell)	—	No licensing legislation enacted before Civil War.	

APPENDIX III SOURCES OF CITATIONS GIVEN IN APPENDICES I AND II

GENERAL

Louis G. Caldwell, "Early Legislation Regulating the Practice of Medicine," *Illinois Law Review* 18 (1923), 225–44.

Joseph F. Kett, *The Formation of the American Medical Profession* (New Haven: Yale University Press, 1968), pp. 22, 181–84.

J. M. Toner, "Statistics of Regular Medical Associations and Hospitals of the United States," *Transactions of the American Medical Association* 24 (1873), 285–313.

ALABAMA

Douglas L. Cannon, "Alabama's Eighty-Nine Years of Medical Organization," *Journal of the Medical Association of the State of Alabama* 5 (1936), 314–18.

CONNECTICUT

Byron Stookey, "Found! The Record of the 1767 Medical Society in Litchfield," *Connecticut State Medical Journal* 21 (1957), 353.

Herbert Thoms, ed., *Heritage of Connecticut Medicine* (New Haven: 1942).

DELAWARE

W. Edwin Bird, "New Light on the History of Medicine in Delaware," *Delaware State Medical Journal* 22 (1950), 26–28, 32–33.

Medical Society of Delaware, *One Hundred and Fiftieth Annual Session of the Medical Society of Delaware, 1789–1939* (Wilmington: 1939), pp. 42–44.

DISTRICT OF COLUMBIA

John B. Nichols *et al.*, *History of the Medical Society of the District of Columbia*, Part II, 1833–1944 (Washington, D.C.: 1947), pp. 5–6, 10, 14.

D. S. Lamb *et al.*, *History of the Medical Society of the District of Columbia, 1817–1909* (Washington: 1909), pp. 3–7.

GEORGIA

Victor H. Bassett, "Pages from the History of the Georgia Medical Society of Savannah, Georgia," *Journal of the Medical Association of Georgia* 29 (1940), 122–23, 131.

Thomas R. R. Cobb, *A Digest of the Statute Laws of the State of Georgia* (Athens, Ga.: 1851), pp. 886–90.

ILLINOIS
Lucius H. Zeuch, "Early Medical Legislation and Organization in the Illinois County," *Bulletin of the Society of Medical History of Chicago* 4 (1930), 201–13.
Harold M. Camp, "Early Medical Societies," in David J. Davis, ed., *History of Medical Practice in Illinois*, vol. II, 1850–1900 (Chicago: Illinois State Medical Society, 1955), pp. 490–96.

INDIANA
Raymond O. Clutter, "The History of Medical Jurisprudence in the State of Indiana During the Nineteenth Century," *Journal of the Indiana State Medical Association* 42 (1949), 139–40.
G. W. H. Kemper, *A Medical History of the State of Indiana* (Chicago: American Medical Association Press, 1911).

KENTUCKY
Kenneth W. Rawlings, ed., *Medicine and its Development in Kentucky* (Louisville, Ky.: 1940), pp. 67–75, 79.

LOUISIANA
John Duffy, ed., *The Rudolph Matas History of Medicine in Louisiana* (n.p.: Louisiana State University Press, 1958), I, 64–67, 173–84, 327–28.
Mary Louise Marshall, ed., *Rudolph Matas History of the Louisiana State Medical Society*, vol. I (New Orleans, La.: 1957), pp. 13–19.
Stanford E. Chaille, "History of the Laws Regulating the Practice of Medicine, etc. in Louisiana, 1808 to 1878," *New Orleans Medical and Surgical Journal*, n.s., 5 (1878), 909–26.

MAINE
Thomas A. Foster, "Presidential Address," *Journal of the Maine Medical Association* 32 (1941), 162.
Acts of Incorporation, Constitution, By-Laws, etc. of the Medical Society of Maine (Bath, Me.: 1824), pp. 5–6.

MARYLAND
Eugene F. Cordell, *Medical Annals of Maryland* (Baltimore, Md.: 1903), pp. 27, 71–73, 128.

MASSACHUSETTS
Josiah Bartlett, *A Dissertation on the Progress of Medical Science in the Commonwealth of Massachusetts* (Boston: 1810), p. 19.
Walter L. Burrage, *A History of the Massachusetts Medical Society* (n.p.: 1923), pp. 1–2, 71–72, 81–82, 121.
Reginald H. Fitz, "The Rise and Fall of the Licensed Physician in Massachusetts, 1780–1860," *Transactions of the Association of American Physicians* 9 (1894), 1–18.

MICHIGAN
C. B. Burr, ed., *Medical History of Michigan* (Minneapolis: Bruce, 1930), II, 395–401, 444–99.

MISSISSIPPI
Felix J. Underwood and R. N. Whitfield, *Public Health and Medical Licensure in the State of Mississippi, 1798–1937* (Jackson, Miss.: 1938), pp. 135–39.

MISSOURI
E. J. Goodwin, *A History of Medicine in Missouri* (St. Louis: Smith, 1905), p. 117.
G. M. B. Maughs, "Medical Ultraisms," *Transactions of the Missouri State Medical Association,* 23d session (1880), 19.

NEW HAMPSHIRE
Hamilton S. Putnam, *New Hampshire's Medical Society* (Milford, N.H.: 1966), pp. 14, 38–40.

NEW JERSEY
Fred B. Rogers and A. Reasoner Sayre, *The Healing Art: A History of the Medical Society of New Jersey* (Trenton, N.J.: 1966), pp. 19, 43–45, 54, 65–82, 92–93.
William Pierson, "Historical Narrative," *Transactions of the Medical Society of New Jersey, Centennial meeting* (1866), 97.
New Jersey, General Assembly, *Acts,* Eighth session, 1784, pp. 51–52; Eleventh session, 1786, p. 79; Fortieth session, 1816, p. 32; Forty-eighth session, 1823, p. 56; Fifty-fourth session, 1830, p. 24; Eighty-eighth session, 1864, pp. 250–251.

NEW YORK
Charles B. Coventry, "History of Medical Legislation in the State of New York," *New York Journal of Medicine* 4 (1845), 151–61.
James J. Walsh, *History of Medicine in New York* (New York: National Americana Society, 1919), I, 57–60; III, 653–93.

NORTH CAROLINA
Hubert Ashley Royster, "A Century and a Half of Medicine in North Carolina," *North Carolina Medical Journal* 10 (1949), 395–96.
J. Collins Warren, "Medical Societies: Their Organization and the Nature of their Work," *Medical Communications of the Massachusetts Medical Society* 12 (1881), 513–14.

OHIO
Robert G. Paterson, "The Role of the 'District' as a Unit in Organized Medicine in Ohio," *Ohio State Archaeological and Historical Quarterly* 49 (1940), 367–77.
Jonathan Forman, "Organized Medicine in Ohio, 1811 to 1926," *Ohio State Medical Journal* 43 (1947), 170.
Donald D. Shira, "The Pioneer Physicians of Ohio," *Ohio State Archaeological and Historical Quarterly* 48 (1939), 183–8.
Donald D. Shira, "The Organization of the Ohio State Medical Society and Its Relation to the Ohio Medical Convention," *Ohio State Archaeological and Historical Quarterly* 50 (1941), 366–72.

PENNSYLVANIA

Samuel X Radbill, "The Philadelphia Medical Society, 1789–1868," *Transactions and Studies of the College of Physicians of Philadelphia*, Series 4, vol. 20 (1953), 103–23.

Howard Kistler Petry, ed., *A Century of Medicine, 1848–1948: The History of the Medical Society of the State of Pennsylvania* (n.p., 1952), p. 1.

Harold F. Alderfer, "Legislative History of Medical Licensure in Pennsylvania," *Pennsylvania Medical Journal* 64 (1961), 1605.

RHODE ISLAND

The History of the Rhode Island Medical Society and Its Component Societies, 1812–1962 (n.p.: 1966), pp. 5–6, 51–53, 145.

SOUTH CAROLINA

Joseph I. Waring, ed., *A Brief History of the South Carolina Medical Association* (Charleston: 1948), pp. 5, 14, 25, 39, 42.

TENNESSEE

Philip M. Hamer, ed., *The Centennial History of the Tennessee State Medical Association, 1830–1930* (Nashville, Tenn.: 1930), pp. 27–32, 56.

VERMONT

Frederick Clayton Waite, *The Story of a Country Medical College* (Montpelier, Vt.: Vermont Historical Society, 1945), p. 36.

Charles S. Caverly, "History of the Medical Profession in Vermont," in Walter Hill Crockett, ed., *Vermont: The Green Mountain State* (New York: Century History Co., 1923), V, 628.

VIRGINIA

Wyndham B. Blanton, *Medicine in Virginia in the Nineteenth Century* (Richmond: Garrett and Massie, 1933), pp. 91–97.

Harry J. Warthen, "The Richmond Academy of Medicine—1820–1900," *Virginia Medical Monthly* 89 (1962), 559–61.

APPENDIX IV ENUMERATIONS OF
PHYSICIANS, 1850–1900

THE NUMBER of physicians in the United States in the last half of the nineteenth century can be estimated from two enumerations of medical practitioners: the decennial census of the United States beginning with the census of 1850; and a directory of practitioners published privately by R. L. Polk, and issued irregularly from 1886 through the beginning of the twentieth century under various titles.[1] Both enumerations included professionally trained physicians and other practitioners, as well as some practitioners not in active practice.[2] In general, the census enumerations are from five to ten percent larger than those in Polk's directory (Table 1), probably due to the inclusion of more non-professional practitioners in the census enumerations.

TABLE 1
ENUMERATIONS OF PHYSICIANS, 1850–1900

Year	Census	Polk
1850	40,755	
1860	55,055	
1870	64,414	
1880	85,671	
1886		87,521
1890	104,805	100,180
1893		103,090
1896		104,554
1898		115,524
1900	132,002	119,749

SOURCES: U.S. Bureau of the Census, *Historical Statistics of the United States* (Washington, D.C.: 1960), p. 34. R. G. Leland, *Distribution of Physicians in the United States* (Chicago: American Medical Association, 1935), p. 2.

[1] The title for the 1886 edition was *Medical and Surgical Directory of the United States.*
[2] The editor of an 1877 directory of all physicians in the United States claimed that it was "not likely" that all practitioners enumerated by the census were in active practice: Samuel W. Butler, *Medical Register and Directory of the United States* (Philadelphia: 1877), 2nd ed., p. 9.

344

Estimates of the number of practitioners in each of the major sects in 1850 are of dubious utility. Computations made by several physicians in the 1850's for two states and the nation indicate that about ten percent of all practitioners were non-regular physicians or practitioners without any professional training, the latter group being the larger.[3] If these proportions are applied to the 1850 census data, there were about 37,000 regular physicians and 4,000 other practitioners at that time.

Enumerations of each sect made at the end of the century are also problematic, but the greatest amount of data is available for homeopaths. The *Transactions of the American Institute of Homeopathy* listed the membership of its affiliated state societies annually, but these data fluctuated so markedly from year to year that they appear to be unreliable. Other data in King's *History of Homeopathy* enumerated the number of homeopathic physicians in each state in selected years.[4] Comparisons of the number of physicians in each state (in King's *History*) with the number of members of the appropriate state homeopathic medical societies (in the *Transactions*) show that the proportion of homeopaths who belonged to their appropriate state societies varied from twenty to well over one hundred percent, at various times and in various states. Obviously, both sets of data must be viewed with caution. More plausible data were obtained by a homeopath from Polk's 1898 *Medical and Surgical Register*. He found 9,369 physicians listed in the register who claimed they were homeopaths. They comprised about eight percent of all practitioners listed in the register.[5] These data are corroborated by an examination of the number of medical school graduates in each sect in 1890, 1900, and 1903 (Table XV.1): graduates of homeopathic medical schools constituted about eight percent of all graduates in those years.

If the ratios of graduates of medical schools of each sect are also used to estimate the number of eclectic physicians, it can be estimated that eclectics comprised about four percent of all practitioners in the nation in 1900.

In addition to the professionally trained physicians, there were also many other practitioners practicing at the end of the nineteenth century. These included osteopaths, lay healers, venereal disease doctors, and others. It seems reasonable to assume that there were at least 5,000 of them practicing in the nation.

Thus, it may be estimated that in 1900, there were about 110,000 regular physicians, 10,000 homeopaths, 5,000 eclectics, and over 5,000 other practitioners.

[3] Joseph F. Kett, *The Formation of the American Medical Profession* (New Haven: Yale University Press, 1968), pp. 185–86.

[4] William Harvey King, *History of Homoeopathy* (New York: Lewis, 1905), Vol. I.

[5] George B. Peck, "Homoeopathy in the United States," *Hahnemannian Monthly* 35 (1900): 559–60. Peck claimed that homeopaths comprised 12.51 percent of all practitioners listed, but this is patently an error.

INDEX

Acetanilid, 190
Aconite, 187
Addiction, opiate. *See also* Morphine; Opium
—physicians' indifference to, 191–92
—as social problem, 193
Alabama
—medical licensing in, 309n, 333
—medical societies in, 70, 328
—Thomsonism in, 141
Alcohol, beverage
—as soporific, 251, 253
—as tonic and germicide, 194–96
American Institute of Homeopathy. *See also* Homeopathy
—code of ethics, 236
—definition of homeopath, 245
—founded, 231
—and medical education standards, 239
—members: backgrounds of, 235–36; education of, 231
—and research on drugs, 242–43
—specialty sections: and antiseptic surgery, 259; listed, 236–37
American Medical Association (AMA)
—code of ethics: in AMA constitution, 171, 316; and boards of health, 312; on consultations, 83, 171–73, 299–300; debates over, 199–200, 301–4, 314–16; and dogmas, 172; enforcement of, 201, 314–16; and fee splitting, 259; and medical societies, 304–5, 315–16; and non-regular physicians, 170–73, 299–300, 305–6, 310, 321; on patents, 315; on patient's

obligations, 173, 316, 321; revision of, 320–23; and specialization, 211–12; violations of, 308–9, 313–15, 317; *see also* Code of ethics
—and Congress of American Physicians and Surgeons, 215–16
—and county societies, 318–20
—founding of, 114–15, 170, 174, 202
—and House of Delegates, 319
—limitations of, 200, 316–17
—and medical education, 115–20, 283
—and medical schools, 114–15, 120–21, 283–85, 297
—membership, 104, 121, 171, 199, 284, 317–19
—and National Tuberculosis Association, 271
—and non-regular physicians, 170, 232–34, 297, 313, 319
—paid organizer, 319
—political influence of, 317, 320
—and quinine, 188
—reorganization, 201, 284, 318–20, 322
—scientific activities, 199, 214
—and specialists, 212, 214, 230, 318
—and state medical societies: in Massachusetts, 233–34; in New York, 304–5; relations between, 315–17, 319
—and supply of physicians, 108–9
American Medical College Association. *See* Association of American Medical Colleges
American Pharmaceutical Association, 192

American Surgical Association, 257–58
Amputations. *See* Surgery, amputations
Analgesics, 190–94. *See also* Morphine; Opium
Anatomy
—and dissection, 90
—physicians' knowledge of: in colonial period, 26–27; required in surgery, 250
—professional society and journal established in, 291
—study and teaching, 85, 89–90, 102, 289
—validity accepted: by non-regular physicians, 166, 228, 231, 238; by Thomsonians, 149
Anesthesia
—discovery of, 207, 251
—mortality from, 251–53
—in surgery, 251–52, 258
Anthrax, 263
Antipyretics, 187–90. *See also* Bloodletting
Antipyrine, 189–90
Antiseptics, 256–59
Antitoxin, diphtheria. *See* Diphtheria, antitoxin
Apothecaries, 76
Appendicitis, 258
Apprenticeship
—advantages and limitations, 86, 87, 102–3
—AMA regulations, 115, 116–17
—fees, 85, 117
—licensing, 79–80, 87
—and medical schools, 89, 92–93, 97
—preceptors: competence of, 86–87, 102, 117; fees of, 85, 117; and medical schools, 89, 91–93, 286; regulated by AMA, 115–16, 118; role of, in medical education, 85–87
—prevalence: in colonial period, 34–35; in early 19th century, 85, 87
—and subjects studied, 85–86
Arsenic
—criticized by Thomson, 135
—as tonic, 52–53, 194
Association of American Medical Colleges
—membership number and standards, 286, 288
—and non-regular medical schools, 317
—organization of, 285–86, 288
Auscultation, 231, 262

Bacteriology
—and alcohol usage, 195–96
—and discovery of: anthrax bacillus, 263; diphtheria antitoxin, 275; diphtheria bacillus, 273; pathogenic bacilli, 263–64; relationship of germs of infection, 255–56; solid culture medium, 263; tubercle bacillus, 268; vaccination with old bacilli, 263
—influence: on physicians' practices, 279–80; on therapeutics, 266–67
—in medical education, 91, 293
—and microscopic techniques, 264–65
—professional society in, 291n
—reactions to, 280–81; of non-regular physicians, 278–79; of regular physicians, 265–67; of surgeons, 257
—and "spontaneous generation of life" theory, 254–55
Baltimore. *See also* Maryland
—malaria incidence in, 28
—medical school established, 88
—and Thomsonian movement, 141, 143
Beach, Wooster, 217–19
Beck, John B.
—on heroic therapy, 179, 180
—mentioned, 35n, 43n, 53n
Behring, Emil von, 274–75
Berkshire Medical Institution, 105
Bigelow, Henry J.
—on AMA, 200
—on analgesics, 190
—on ether, 251
—on histology, 186
Bigelow, Jacob
—on heroic medicine, 62, 167, 178
—on homeopathy, 167
—on self-limited diseases, 177–78, 181
—on surgery, 61
—mentioned, 179, 186n, 225
Biggs, Hermann M.
—on alcohol, 196
—on antitoxin, 275, 276, 277n
—on physicians and boards of health, 272, 312, 313n
—on tuberculin, 269n, 270n
—on tuberculosis, 267, 268–69, 271n
Billings, John S.
—on AMA, 199, 200n

—on scientific medical societies, 203
—on stratification within medical profession, 202, 205–6, 207
—mentioned, 98n
Bleeding. *See* Bloodletting
Blisters and cantharides
—criticised: by Hahnemann, 153; by homeopaths, 166; by Thomson, 134–35; by Hersey, 149–50
—as a therapeutic, 43, 53–54; in cholera, 59; decline in use, 183; in diphtheria, 61; in diseases of children, 179; in pneumonia, 183
Bloodletting
—administration of, 48–49
—criticised: by Hahnemann, 152–53; by Hersey, 149–50; by homeopaths, 166; by Thomson, 134
—effects of: antipyretic, 45; spurious, 178
—public opposition to, 160, 180
—studied in medical school, 91
—as a therapeutic, 45–49; after Civil War, 182; in cholera, 59; decline in, 181–83; in diphtheria, 61; in diseases of children, 179–80; in yellow fever, 60
Boards of health
—and antitoxin, 277–78
—establishment of, 310–11
—and medical licensing, 308, 311
—opposed by physicians, 272, 312
—officials' qualifications, 312
—and sects, 233, 311–12
Boerhaave, Hermann, 91
Boston. *See also* Massachusetts
—diphtheria diagnosed bacteriologically in, 277
—homeopaths in, 233
—medical societies in, 65, 66, 71, 84, 204, 329
—smallpox inoculation in, 30–31
—Thomsonism in, 141
—mentioned, 88, 237, 239, 296, 326
Boston University School of Medicine
—curriculum, 239
—established, 237
—homeopathic designation eliminated, 296–97
Botanical drugs
—discovery and use, 32–33

—in Thomsonism, 136–37, 148
Botanical practitioners
—as alternative to regular physicians, 128
—described by Thomson, 129–30
—exempted from licensing laws, 76–77
—Thomson's system adopted by, 141–42
Botany
—in apprenticeship, 85
—in medical schools, 89, 91, 127
Bowditch, Henry I.
—on AMA, 199
—on physicians and public health, 311
—mentioned, 201n, 211n
Brickley, George W. L., 219–20
Bryant, William Cullen, 232
Buchan, William
—author of *Domestic Medicine*, 42, 136
—on bloodletting, 45–46
—on cathartics, 49
—on fevers, 42–43
—on teething, 53, 54n
—on yellow fever, 60
Buchanan, Joseph Rhodes, 219, 220

California
—antitoxin distribution, 278
—medical schools: commercial, 292; homeopathic, 237, 238n; state of, 293
—physicians in San Francisco, 205
Calomel (mercury)
—chemical composition of, 50
—criticised: by Hersey, 149–50; by Thomson, 135
—in eclectic medicine, 222
—effects and side effects, 50–51, 178
—public opposition to, 127–28, 160
—as a therapeutic: and Benjamin Rush, 50; in children, 179–80; in cholera, 59; during Civil War, 182; decline in use of, 181–83; in diphtheria, 60; in pneumonia, 183; in 20th century, 183; in venereal diseases, 50; widespread use of, 50–52; in yellow fever, 60
Cantharides. *See* Blisters
Carbolic acid, 256–57
Cathartics and purgatives. *See also* Calomel (mercury)
—criticised: by Hahnemann, 153; by Hersey, 150
—as a therapeutic, 49–52, 183

Cathell, D. W.
—*Book on the Physician Himself*, 187n
—on cleanliness, 279–80
—on codes of ethics, 315, 322–23
—on consultations, 22, 299–300
—on doses of drugs, 186, 187n
—on homeopaths, 22, 298–99, 322–23
—on medical science, 265–66, 267n
—on opium, 191–92
—on quinine, 189
—on specialists, 211
Census of physicians. *See* Enumerations
of physicians
Chapin, Charles V.
—on tuberculosis, 267n, 268n
—mentioned, 311n
Chase, Salmon P., 47
Chemistry
—in apprenticeship, 85
—in medical education, 88–89
—non-sectarian nature of, 228, 238
Chicago. *See also* Illinois
—heroic therapy in, 181
—homeopathic clientele in, 234–35
—homeopathic medical schools in, 242
—hospital dispute, 233
—licensing opposition, 78
—medical schools in, 291, 310
—tutoring of medical students in, 290
—tuberculosis reporting in, 272
Chiropractic, 323n
Chloral hydrate, 194
Chloroform. *See* Anesthesia
Cholera
—bacillus discovered, 264
—epidemics, 58–59, 233
—in fowl, 263
—symptoms of, 266
—therapy for, 51, 59, 181
Cholera infantum, 57, 126
Christian Science, 323n
Chrono-thermalism, 159
Cinchona. *See also* Quinine
—discovered, 28
—exported from South America, 32
—Hahnemann's experiments with, 153
—and quinine, 29, 187, 189
—as a therapeutic: medically valid, 61;
—non-sectarian, 166; problems in use of,
28–29; widespread use of, 53

—and Thomsonians, 148
Cinchonism, 189
Civil War
—heroic therapy in U.S. Army, 182
—surgery in, 252
Clients
—of eclectics, 228–29
—of homeopaths, 234–35, 246
—and physicians' behavior, 7, 12–13
—and rise of: homeopathy, 158–60;
sectarianism, 23; Thomsonism, 128,
159–60
—and stratification within medicine,
14–15, 65, 202
—therapy sought by, 44, 184–85
Clinical methodology, 166, 183, 185
Clinics. *See* Dispensaries, clinics, and
infirmaries
Coal-tars, 189
Cocaine, 193–94
Code of ethics. *See also* American Medical Association, code of ethics
—importance of, 80–81
—and Percival's code, 82
—regulations concerning: consultations,
82–83; secret nostrums, 83–84
—and sanctions for violation, 81
—study in medical schools, 92
College of Physicians and Surgeons
(Columbia University medical school)
—earnings of faculty members, 95
—established, 88
—students' previous education, 113
College of Physicians of Philadelphia
—elite status of, 66, 72
—established, 66
—on Rush's therapies, 50
Colleges (liberal-arts) and universities
—attended by medical students, 113–14
—curriculum, 118
—entrance requirements, 118
—medical schools affiliated with, 88,
237–38, 294
Congress of American Physicians and
Surgeons, 214–16
Connecticut
—licensing: in 18th century, 37, 72–74
333; in 19th century, 105–6, 145, 333;
by state medical society, 74, 333

—medical societies in: local, 67–69, 300, 328, 333; state, 69–70, 74, 328, 333
—smallpox inoculation in, 30
—Thomsonian licensing board in, 145
—typhus epidemic in, 53
Consultations
—between physicians in different sects, 22; barred by codes of ethics, 300, frequent, 302, 313
—as cause of conflict, 22, 83
—regulated in codes of ethics, 82–83, 299–300, 321
Contraria contrariis, 157
Coventry, Charles B.
—on homeopathy, 168
—mentioned, 77n, 108n, 115n, 170, 332, 342
Croup, 45, 272–73
Cullen, William, 91
Curtis, Alva
—founded botanical medical school, 146
—and physio-medicalism, 217, 309
—and Thomson, 146

Davis, Nathan S.
—on AMA, 114, 115n, 116–17, 198–99, 202, 213, 318
—on graduates of medical schools, 127
—on homeopaths, 232
—on licensing boards, 79
—on medical education, 103, 125, 126n
—on medical schools, 96, 97, 112, 114, 115n, 116–17
—on medical societies, 75, 112
—on self-interest, 24
—on specialists, 213–14, 215, 216, 318
—mentioned, 80n, 84n, 106n, 107n, 109, 114n, 121n, 150, 170, 171n, 282n
Delaware, 328, 333
Diarrhea, 57
Dilutions, homeopathic. *See* Homeopathy, drugs
Diphtheria
—antitoxin: and boards of health, 277–78; clinical tests, 275–77; and death rate, 277; discovered, 275; impact on bacteriology, 278; physicians' reaction to, 275, 281; public reaction to, 277–78
—bacillus, 273–75
—diagnosis, 273–76

—incidence, 60, 273–74
—pseudo-, 273–74
—symptoms, 60, 272
—therapy, 60–61, 196, 272, 275–78
Dispensaries, clinics, and infirmaries
—AMA membership of, 284
—and care for the poor, 100
—homeopathic, 236
—of medical schools, 92, 99–100
—specialty, 208
—Thomsonian infirmaries, 142–43
Dissection
—in apprenticeship, 85
—in medical schools, 90, 115–16
District of Columbia
—diphtheria diagnosed bacteriologically in, 277
—Medical Association, 80, 83, 139, 328
—medical licensing in, 334
—Medical Society, 80, 84, 334
—mentioned, 214
Domestic medicine, 33, 136
Douglass, William, 37n
Drake, Daniel
—on consultations, 83
—on fees, 81–82
—on licenses, 106
—on licensing boards, 80
—medical education of, 85–87
—on medical education, 89, 91
—on medical schools, 95–96, 97, 101–2
—on therapeutics, 64
—mentioned, 47–48
Drugs. *See* Botanical drugs; Therapy
Dyes, analine, 264
Dysentery, 57

Earnings of physicians. *See* Fees
Eberle, John, 48, 126
Eclecticism. *See also* Physicians, eclectic; Schools, eclectic medical
—beginnings, 217–18
—therapeutics, 221–25, 228–29
Eclectic Medical Institute
—and bacteriology, 279
—beginnings, 218–21
—and botany (medicinal), 227
—disputes, 219–20
—leadership: by Buchanan, 219–20; by Scudder, 224–25

—prosperity of, 225–26
Edinburgh Medical School, 34, 36
Education, general, 113–14, 118–120
Education, medical. *See also* Anatomy;
  Apprenticeship; Pathology; Physiology; Schools, medical
—AMA and, 108, 114–15, 283, 316–17
—clinical: AMA standards for, 115; in
  apprenticeship, 86; in medical schools,
  88, 92, 115, 282, 290; and preceptors,
  89, 92–93, 102, 125–26
—curriculum: etiology of disease in, 90–
  91; graded, 227, 229, 238–39, 285–86;
  medical science in, 89–90, 289–91;
  microscope in, 262; sciences in, 89;
  treatment of disease in, 91–92
—degree: licensing standards, 286, 288;
  requirements, 89
—elitist and democratic systems compared, 109–12
—European, 34, 110, 209
—growth of, 107
—length of, 89, 282, 286, 288
—non-regular: eclectic, 226–27, 229;
  homeopathic, 238–39, 295–96; similar
  to regular, 238, 297
—practical orientation of, 186, 289
—specialization and, 209
Ehrlich, Paul, 268
Emetics, 43, 49, 52
Empirics, in colonial period, 35–36
Enumerations of physicians
—in 1800, 108
—in 1850, 108, 345
—1850–1900, 344–45
—by sect: eclectic, 226, 345; homeopathic,
  226, 235, 345; regular, 345
Ether. *See* Anesthesia
Etiology of disease, 90–91

Fees
—earnings of physicians: on medical
  school faculties, 94–95; in private
  practice, (ca. 1850) 76 and 95, (ca. 1865)
  205; reduced, 108
—fee bills, conflicts over, 80–82
—public concern over, 138–39
—splitting of, 258
Fever
—defined as disease, 42

—symptoms of, 42–43
—therapies: antipyretics, 43, 187–90;
  bloodletting, 45
Fitz, Reginald H.
—and appendicitis, 258
—on cooperation with homeopaths, 307,
  308n
—mentioned, 36n, 38n, 65n, 66n, 108n,
  141n
Flexner, Abraham
—impact of study of, 294n
—on medical education, 289–90
—on medical licensing, 291, 309, 310n
—on medical schools: advertising by, 292;
  eclectic, 296
Flint, Austin
—on AMA, 283
—on medical ethics, 82, 172, 303
—on medical science, 281n
—on medical societies, 201
—mentioned, 83n, 171n, 173n
Friendly Botanical Societies. *See also*
Thomsonian practitioners
—national conventions of, 141, 143, 146
—national infirmary proposed by, 143
—organization of, 140
—Thomsonian medical school proposed
  by, 143

General Practitioners
—as AMA presidents, 212
—and specialization, 209–12
—training of, 175
Georgia, 70, 328, 334
Graham, Sylvester, 159–60
Gross, Samuel D.
—on specialists and AMA, 214
—on surgery, 252, 253n, 257

Hahnemann Medical College of Philadelphia
—elimination of courses in homeopathy
  by, 297
—founding of, 242
—and Homeopathic Medical College of
  Pennsylvania, 232, 241–42
Hahnemann, Samuel Christian Friedrich
—contributions of, 157–58
—criticised: by homeopaths, 163–64,
  240–41; by regular physicians, 165, 168

—on drug action, 154–57
—on heroic medicine, 152–53, 157
—and homeopathic law: discovery, 153–54; modification, 230; proof, 157
—life, 152, 157
—on medically valid therapies, 158
—and psora theory of, 156
—mentioned, 278
Hammond, William, 182
Harvard University Medical School
—graded curriculum, 285
—and medical licensing, 104–5
—microscopes used at, 262
—organization of, 88
—and previous education of students, 113
Harvey, William, 26–27
Helmuth, William Tod, 237n, 259
Hering, Constantine, 158, 163, 164, 232n
Hersey, Thomas, 148–50
Histology
—impact on therapeutics, 185–86
—in medical education, 91
—non-sectarian nature of, 238
Holmes, Oliver Wendell
—on heroic therapy, 178–79
—on homeopathy, 166
Homeopathic quacks, 162, 231
Homeopathy. See also American Institute of Homeopathy; Hahnemann; Physicians, homeopathic; Schools, homeopathic medical; Societies, homeopathic medical
—adopted by regular physicians, 160–62, 235–36
—criticised: by J. Bigelow, 167; by Holmes, 166; by homeopaths, 163–64, 239–41, 244; by regular physicians, 165–66, 299; as trade-mark, 172
—and drugs: dilutions and provings, 154–56; commercial preparations, 243; conflicts over dilutions, 239–43; rules of action, 154–56
—and indifference of homeopaths, 295, 303
—law of similia similibus curantur: discovered, 153–54; modified by American Institute of Homeopathy, 245
—popular among wealthy clients, 160–61, 234–35

Hospitalism, 254
Hospitals
—AMA representatives from, 284
—antitoxin tested in, 276
—homeopathic, 236, 237
—in medical education, 92, 237, 282, 290
—specialty, 208
—surgery in: and anesthesia, 251–52; increased amount of, 258; infection from, 253–54
Howe, A. J.
—on antiseptic surgery, 259
—on diphtheria, 272, 273n
—on eclectic physicians, 227, 228, 229n
—as eclectic surgeon, 226
—mentioned, 48n, 51n
Hydropathy, 159

Illinois. See also Chicago
—board of health in, 311
—and diphtheria: antitoxin, 278; mortality, 277
—homeopaths in, 235
—medical licensing in, 76, 334
—medical schools regulated by state, 310
—medical societies in, 313–14, 328
—mosquitoes in, 56
—mentioned, 113
Indiana
—medical licensing in, 76, 309, 334–35
—medical societies in, 328, 335
—Thomsonism in, 141
Infection, wound
—cause of, 27, 250, 254, 256
—and hospitalism, 254
—increased incidence of, 253–54
—prevention of, 256–58
Infirmaries. See Dispensaries, clinics, and infirmaries
Influenza, 57
Inoculation, smallpox, 30–32
Institutions
—defined and classified, 11–12
—measurement of, 5
—in sociological theory, 8
—study of, 3–4
International Hahnemann Association, 241
Iowa, 237, 238n

Jacobi, Abraham
—on AMA, 214
—on Congress of American Physicians and Surgeons, 215
—on homeopaths, 302
—on patent medicines, 315
Jahr's Manual, 155
Jalap, 50, 52, 60, 182
Jefferson, Thomas
—on heroic therapy, 44–45
—on nosologies, 42
—on therapeutic effects of nature, 43–44
Jenner, Edward, 31–32, 148, 263
Johns Hopkins University Medical School, 28, 290
Jurisprudence, medical, 92, 103, 238

Kansas
—anesthesia used in hospitals in, 253
—bacteriology in, 265, 279
—board of health in, 311
—heroic therapy decline, 181
—medical licensing in, 307, 309n
—physicians enumerated by sect, 226
Kentucky
—medical licensing in, 335
—medical societies in, 328
—smallpox vaccination in, 31
King, John M.
—on boards of health, 311
—discovery of podophyllin by, 222
—at Eclectic Medical Institute, 225
—on resinoids, 223
Kitasato, S., 275
Klebs, Edwin, 268, 273
Knowledge, medical, 9–10
Koch, Robert
—anthrax bacillus discovered by, 263
—oil immersion lens system used by, 264
—tuberculin claimed as cure for tuberculosis, 269, 270n
—tubercle bacillus discovered by, 268
—mentioned, 275, 278

Laryngoscope, 207, 262
Licensing, medical
—apprenticeship, 79–80, 87
—boards: conflicts over appointments to, 80; 311; joint for all sects, 307–9; separate for each sect, 305–7, 309
—certificates, 86–87, 106

—defined, 20, 72
—diplomas, 97–98, 106–7, 306
—effectiveness, 20, 75–76, 302, 309–310
—enactment: in colonial period, 37–38, 72–74; in early 19th century, 74–76, 332–39; in late 19th century, 305–10
—enforcement: concerning sects, 305–7; 144–45; failure of, 77–78, 144–45, 306, 310
—examinations, 291
—honorific, 72–73
—and medical schools, 104–6, 286, 291
—and medical societies, 80, 104–6, 107
—and physicians, 78–80, 87, 202
—repeal, 107–8, 145–46
—statutes: described, 76–77; by state, before Civil War, 332–39
—and Thomsonian practitioners, 144–45
Lister, Joseph, 255–57, 259
Lloyd, John Uri, 137n, 142n, 221n, 226
Lobelia inflata
—in botanical practice, 136, 142
—in regular physicians' practice, 136, 146–47
—Thomson on, 130, 132, 137
Loeffler, Frederick, 273
Louisiana. *See also* New Orleans
—bacteriology in, 265
—board of health in, 310
—calomel used in, 183
—medical licensing in, 78, 335–36
—medical societies in, 329
—medicinal botanicals in, 33
—physicians in urban areas, 35–36
—surgery in colonial period, 250
—yellow fever in, 59–60

Maine
—medical licensing, 336
—medical societies, 329, 336
—Thomson's practice in, 131
—mentioned, 113
Malaria
—diagnosis, 28–29, 60
—etiology, 56
—and malarial diseases, 188
—prevalence, 56–57
—symptoms, 28, 153
—therapy for: bloodletting, 46, 57; calomel, 57; cinchona, 28–29, 53, 57, 148; heroic, 181; quinine, 29n, 53, 164, 188

Malpractice, 324–25

Martin, Louis, 275

Maryland. *See also* Baltimore
—licensing, medical: enactment, 74, 307, 336; prevalence, 106; unenforceability, 77
—smallpox vaccine agent, 31–32
—and state medical society: founding, 69, 329; as licensing authority, 74, 336; revenue, 80

Maryland, University of, Medical School, 88, 95

Massachusetts. *See also* Boston; Massachusetts Medical Society
—board of health in, 310–11
—diphtheria mortality in, 277
—high school education in, 119
—homeopaths in, 162, 235
—medical licensing in, 38, 74, 336
—physicians, 35, 76
—smallpox vaccination in, 31
—Thomson's practice in, 131
—tuberculosis in, 57

Massachusetts General Hospital
—amputations in, 249, 251–52
—ether first used in, 251
—operations increased in, 258
—therapy in: alcohol, 195; heroic, 183

Massachusetts Medical Society
—and AMA code of ethics, 317
—and Boston physicians, 66, 70
—founding, 65, 329
—and homeopaths as members, 162, 232–33
—and licensing, 74, 84, 104–5, 307–8, 336
—membership policy, 65, 71
—and scientific work, 84
—and subordinate societies of, 69, 329
—therapeutic nihilism criticized in, 179

Materia medica. *See also* Therapy; Therapy, heroic
—definition, 91
—and medical school curriculum, 238n
—study of, 85, 91

Medical. *See appropriate heading, e.g.,* Schools, medical; Sects, medical; *etc.*

Medical Corps, U.S., 292

Mercury. *See* Calomel

Michigan. *See also* Michigan, University of, Medical School

—diphtheria diagnosed bacteriologically in Detroit, 277
—homeopaths' clientele in Detroit, 235
—licensing laws in, 306, 336–37
—medical societies in, 329, 336
—state medical society and temperance question, 196
—mentioned, 234n

Michigan, University of, Medical School
—admission of students of non-regular physicians to, 234
faculty, 285
—homeopathic medical school in, 237, 238n, 301
—previous education of students at, 113

Microscope, 91, 261, 262, 264

Midwives. *See also* Obstetrics
—in colonial period, 35–37
—exempted from licensing laws, 76
—fees of, 138
—number of, 109

Minnesota, 56, 237, 238n

Mississippi
—and AMA code of ethics, 317
—homeopaths in, 161, 235
—licensing in, 78, 337
—physicians, 108
—smallpox vaccine used in, 31
—state medical society, 329
—Thomsonism in, 141

Missouri
—cholera epidemic in St. Louis, 51, 58–59
—diphtheria diagnosed bacteriologically in St. Louis, 277
—licensing in, 337
—medical societies in, 70, 329
—physicians enumerated by sect, 226

Morphine, 53, 191–92. *See also* Addiction, opiate; Opium

Mosquitoes, 56. *See also* Malaria

National Board of Health, 311

National Conference of State Medical Examining and Licensing Boards, 286

National Eclectic Medical Association, 224, 226–28

National Tuberculosis Association, 271

Nebraska, 237, 238n

Neuralgia, 191

New Guide to Health by Samuel Thomson, 129, 131, 136–39

New Hampshire
—and botanical physicians, 129–30
—licensing in, 74, 337
—smallpox inoculation regulations, 30
—state medical society in, 69, 74, 329, 337
—Thomson's practice in, 131
—mentioned, 113
New Jersey
—bacteriology opposed in, 265
—bloodletting in, 181
—homeopaths in, 235
—medical licensing in, 38, 106, 337–38
—medical societies in, 69–70, 106, 329, 337
New Orleans. *See also* Louisiana
—diphtheria diagnosed bacteriologically in, 277
—homeopaths in, 161
—medical societies in, 329
—physicians, 35
—yellow fever in, 59–60
New York Academy of Medicine
—as elite medical society, 203
—formation of, 169–70
—fund raising program, 313n
—and homeopaths, 169–70, 233, 313
—and medical school clinics, 99–100
New York City. *See also* New York State
—cholera epidemics in, 58
—and diphtheria: diagnosed bacteriologically, 277; incidence, 273–74
—eye infirmary in, 208
—and Free Academy graduates, 120
—heroic therapy, 181–82
—homeopaths in, 158, 162, 236
—medical licensing in, 38, 338
—medical societies, 204, 329
—national medical convention held in, 114
—sectarian conflict over hospital privileges in, 233
—smallpox vaccination in, 31
—Thomson's visit to, 133
—tuberculosis: diagnosed through bacteriology in, 271; mortality, 267; reporting, 272
New York Homeopathic Medical College
—elimination of homeopathy courses, 297
—founding of, 232
—hospital affiliation, 237, 313n

—microscopes used in, 262
—name changed to New York Medical College, 297
—surgery in, 237n, 259
New York Medical and Surgical Society
—and heroic therapy, 45
—members, 162, 203, 205
—mentioned, 204
New York, Medical Society of the County of (*originally*, Medical Society of the State of New York)
—homeopaths in, 162, 169, 303
—listed, 204
—low prestige of, 203
—as predecessor of Medical Society of the State of New York: fee bill, 45–46; members, 70; prestige, 66–67; reorganization, 71
New York, Medical Society of the State of
—code of ethics, 83, 301–5
—committee on specialization, 210
—established, 75, 330
—expelled from AMA, 304
—and New York State Medical Association, 305, 322
—organized national medical convention, 114
New York State. *See also* New York City
—bacteriology opposed in, 265
—eclectics in, 226
—empirics in, 35–36
—homeopathic hospitals and medical schools in, 237
—and medical licensing: enacted, 38, 75, 338; enforced, 77–78, 144, 169; prevalent, 106; repealed, 145
—medical societies in, 75, 329–30, 338
—public health supported in, 312
—smallpox inoculation regulated in, 30
—Thomsonism in, 141, 144–45
—tuberculosis in, 57
New York State Medical Association. *See* New York, Medical Society of the State of
New York Thomsonian Medical Society, 142, 144–45
Nitre, 52, 149
Nitrous oxide. *See* Anesthesia
North Carolina
—homeopaths in, 235

—medical licensing in, 74, 309n, 339
—medical societies in, 74, 330, 339
Nosologies, 42, 91

Obstetrics and midwifery
—in medical education, 92, 209
—non-sectarian, 228, 238
—and specialization, 209
—and Thomson, 133–34
Ohio
—diphtheria diagnosed bacteriologically
  in Cincinnati, 277
—education of physicians in, 103
—homeopathy in Cleveland, 235
—medical licensing: and board of health,
  311; enacted, 75–76, 306, 339; impractical, 78, 306; repealed, 76, 145
—medical schools: eclectic, in Cincinnati,
  218–21, 225–26; homeopathic, in Cleveland, 232, 237, 238n
—medical societies: and AMA code of
  ethics violation, 315; elite, 203; formed,
  69, 330
—smallpox vaccination in, 31
—Thomsonism in, 141, 145
Ophthalmology, 92, 209, 236
Ophthalmoscope, 207–8, 262
Opium. See also Addiction, opiate; Morphine
—criticised: by Hersey, 149; by Thomson,
  130, 135
—ineffectively regulated, 193
—popularity of, 188
—supply and substitutes, 193–94
—as a therapeutic: in early 19th century,
  44, 53, 59; in late 19th century, 191–92
Organon, of Hahnemann, 163
Osler, William
—on bloodletting, 182
—on preceptors, 286
—on sects: and cooperation in medical
  licensing, 307; decline, 325–26; and
  medical education, 298
—on tuberculosis, 267
—mentioned, 190n
Osteopathy, 323n

Park, William Hallock
—on antitoxin, 275, 276, 277n
—and diphtheria incidence study, 273–74

Pasteur, Louis
—discovered anthrax vaccination, 263
—on spontaneous generation, 254–55
—mentioned, 273
Patent medicines
—as alternative to regular medicine,
  158–59
—origin of, 33
—use of opium in, 193
—used by regular physicians, 84, 314–15;
  prohibited in codes of ethics, 83–84
Pathology
—cellular, 261–62
—ignored by physicians, 262
—in medical education, 90–91, 289
—professional society and journal
  establishment in, 291
Pennsylvania. See also Philadelphia
—epidemic of bilious fever in, 47
—medical licensing in, 73–74, 339
—medical societies in, 330
—Thomsonism in, 131, 141
—and tuberculosis program adoption by
  state, 271
Pennsylvania, University of, Medical
  School
—founded, 88
—length of term at, 283
—previous education of students at, 113
—and Thomson, 134
Percival, Thomas, 82, 173
Percussion, 231, 262
Pharmacology
—criticised by Hahnemann, 153
—in medical education, 85, 91, 102
—standards of, 54
Philadelphia. See also Pennsylvania
—and diphtheria: diagnosed bacteriologically, 277
—medical schools in: chronothermalist,
  159; eclectic, 227; homeopathic, 241–42,
  297; tutoring for, 290
—medical societies: elite, 66, 72; fee
  bill of, 82; and homeopaths, 169, 322
—and Thomson's visit, 134
—and tuberculosis reporting, 272
—yellow fever epidemic in, 50, 59
Physicians, eclectic. See also Eclecticism
—admission to regular medical: schools,
  234; societies, 313, 322

—backgrounds of, 229
—and bacteriology, 279
—clients, 221, 224, 228–29
—education of, 221, 226, 228–29
—enumerations of, 226, 345
—ethical standards of, 227–28
—relations with other sects, 305–9, 311–12
—and surgery, 259
—and therapy: botanical, 221–23; heroic, 221, 223–24; nondescript, 224; specific medication, 225
Physicians, homeopathic. *See also* Homeopathy
—and boards of health, 311–12
—clientele of, 221, 234–35, 246
—criticised heroic medicine, 161, 166, 168
—early American, 158, 160–162
—education of, 162, 232, 235–39; and conflict over therapeutics, 241–42; and neglect of homeopathy, 295–96; in regular medical schools, 234–35, 242, 295
—enumerations of, 226, 235, 302, 345
—and homeopathy principles, 163–64, 239–45, 295, 303
—in hospitals, 233, 236–37
—and medical licensing boards, 305–9
—and medical science: accepted, 166, 230–31, 246; in bacteriology, 278–79; in surgery, 259
—medical societies: conflicts in, 239–41; formation of, 162, 231; number of, 236
—and regular medical societies: codes of ethics, 171–73, 299–305, 300n, 321–23; expulsion from, 169, 172, 233–34; membership in, 233, 303, 313–14, 322
—and regular physicians: consultations, between, 299–300, 302–4; homeopaths criticised, 165, 167–68; homeopaths ostracised, 169–73, 232–33, 298–302
—and regular therapies, 243–45
—specialization of, 236–37, 295
—women as, 300n–301n
Physiology
—in medical education, 85, 89–90
—non-sectarian nature of, 149–50, 166, 228, 238
—professional society and journal, 291
—quality of teaching in, 102, 289

Physio-medicalism, 217, 309
Pills, 52n
Pneumonia
—prevalence of, 57
—therapy for, 45, 183, 195
Podophyllin, 222–23
Preceptors. *See* Apprenticeship, preceptors
Profession, definition of, 8
Prophylaxis, medical, 9
Provings of homeopathic drugs, 154–55
Psychiatric medicine, 10n
Public health, 278, 310–13
Puerperal fever, 45, 47
Purgatives. *See* Cathartics
Pus, laudable, 253

Quacks
—defined, 24
—homeopathic, 231
Quinine. *See also* Cinchona
—discovered, 29, 187
—therapeutic use of: by homeopaths, 164–66; in malaria, 29, 53; as tonic, 187–89, 194, 244; in yellow fever, 60

Reed, Charles
—on AMA code of ethics, 315–16
—on cooperation with non-regular physicians, 306, 313–14
—on decline of sectarianism, 325
—mentioned, 309n, 317n, 318
Resinoids, 222–23
Rhode Island
—medical licensing in, 74, 339
—state medical society: and AMA code of ethics, 317; granted licensing privileges, 74, 339; organized, 69, 330
—tuberculosis mortality in Providence, 268n
Romayne, Nicholas, 78–79
Roux, Pierre, 273, 275
Rush, Benjamin
—medical system of, 91
—on practicing medicine, 34
—and therapy for in yellow fever, 50
—mentioned, 52

Sanitaria, 271, 278
Schools, botanical medical, 146, 217

Schools, eclectic medical. *See also*
Eclectic Medical Institute
—enumerated: in 1850–1920, 287; in
1894, 226
—and graded curriculum, 229, 239
—quality of, 226–27
—students in, 226, 229, 287
—suspended, 224, 296
Schools, homeopathic medical
—accredited by AMA, 297
—conflicts in, over homeopathic law,
241–42
—enumerated, 236, 296; in 1850–1920, 287
—established, 232
—and graded curriculum, 238–39, 285
—homeopathic designation removed
from, 296–97
—and hospital affiliation, 237
—quality of, 237–39
—regular textbooks used in, 238n
—students' referral by homeopaths, 295
—suspended, 295–96
—and university affiliation, 237–38, 301
Schools, medical. *See also* Education,
medical; Students, medical
—and AMA: expulsion of, 283–85; meetings, 114–15, 121; standards for,
115–21
—and apprenticeship: compared, 102–4;
disregarded, 97; relations, 89, 92–93,
286
—association of, 285–86, 288
—charters of, 88
—contribution to medicine, 100, 103–4
—criticised: by Hersey, 149–50; by physicians, 101–2
—curriculum: in early 19th century,
88–93; in late 19th century, 288–90, 293
—degrees: equivalent to licenses, 97–98;
prestige, 106–7; requirements for, 89,
92, 96–97, 286, 288
—dispensaries, 92, 97
—expenses: European and American,
compared, 109–110; pre-Civil War,
94–95, 110–11; rural, 98; for scientific
equipment, 293
—faculty: cliques, 203; competition for
positions, 96, 293; earnings, 94–95, 293;
number required, 89; quality of, 102,
290, 293; relations with physicians in

community, 95–96; specialists, 212;
visiting, 98–99
—and graded curriculum, 227, 238–39,
285–86
—and hospitals: affiliated with, 92, 237,
282; relations between, 290
—licensing requirements, 291, 310
—and medical societies' criticism, 99–100,
104–8
—number: declined, 294; in 1850–1920,
287; growth after Civil War, 286–87,
291; by region, 93; in 1770–1860, 93
—proprietary: commercialism of, 291–92;
declined, 292–94, established, 88
—rural, 96, 98–99
—stratification of, 282, 288, 290–92
—and students: competed for, 96–97; fees
for, 94, 291; of non-regular physicians,
232, 234, 295; number of, 98, 287; in
rural areas, 98–99
—terms' length and number, 89, 92, 97,
116, 282, 283, 288
—university affiliations: increased, 294;
jointly with homeopathic schools, 237–
38; to obtain charters, 88
Sciences, medical. *See also* Bacteriology
—impact: on malpractice, 324–25; on
sectarianism, 323, 325–26
—non-sectarian nature of, 166, 228, 238
—study in medical schools, 89–90, 103,
289–91, 293
Scudder, John M.
—on bacteriology, 279
—on eclectic sect, 227, 228
—on eclectic therapeutics, 223
—on heroic therapy, 49n, 51n, 54
—life of, 224
—on medical licensing laws, 306
—on specific medication, 224–25
—mentioned, 229n, 234, 245n, 313
Sects, medical
—defined, 21–23
—demise of, 323, 325–26
—hypothesis concerning, 22–23
Self-limited diseases, 177–79
Seton, 53, 129, 253
Sewage disposal, 55, 278
Sims, J. Marion
—on AMA code of ethics, 200, 314

—on contribution of AMA to medical education, 283
—on diarrhea, 57
—on heroic therapy, 62
—on his medical knowledge after graduation, 126
—on his preceptor, 102
—mentioned, 284n
Smallpox
—bloodletting in, 45
—diagnosis of, 30
—incidence of, 30–31, 61
—inoculation in, 29–31
—vaccination in, 31–32
Smith, James, 31–32
Social mobility of physicians, 112–14, 229, 292
Societies, eclectic medical, 226. See also National Eclectic Medical Association
Societies, elite medical
—formation of, 65–67, 71–72, 202–4
—and professional cliques, 203
—and specialists, 212
—stratification of, 204
Societies, homeopathic. See also American Institute of Homeopathy
—conflicts over therapies, 239–41
—early American, 162
—number of, 236
—ostracised by regular physicians, 302
Societies, medical. See also American Medical Association; American Medical Association code of ethics; Licensing, medical; Societies, elite medical; Societies, scientific medical; Societies, specialty medical
—and AMA organization, 114–15
—exclusive (defined), 15–16
—growth, 70–71; in 1846–1874, 198
—inclusive (defined), 16–17, 318–20
—and licensing, 77–80, 104–7
—local: formed, 64–68, 71, 327–31; hypothesis concerning, 18; membership as indicator of professional status, 201; reorganized, 318–19; stratified, 204
—and malpractice suits, 324–25
—opposition to reporting of tuberculosis, 272
—organizational overlap, 318
—regulation of members' behavior: through codes of ethics, 82–84; through

fee bills, 80–82; hypothesis concerning, 17–18
—scientific activities of, 84
—state: formed, 68–71, 327–31; reorganized, 319
Societies, scientific medical, 84, 202–3.
Societies, specialty medical
—contributed to specialty development, 208
—excluded from AMA, 320
—formed, 212–16
—impractical among homeopaths, 236
South America
—cinchona bark discovered in, 28
—medicinal drugs exported from, 32–33
South Carolina
—homeopaths in, 235
—medical licensing in, 145, 309, 339
—medical societies in, 70, 145, 330
—surgery in Charlestown, 250
Specialization, medical
—and AMA, 215–16, 318, 320
—in AMA code of ethics, 211–12, 258–59
—and attitudes toward consultations with non-regular physicians, 303
—dominance in organized medicine, 210–12
—eclectic, 229
—education in Europe, 209
—and general practitioners, 209–212
—homeopathic, 236–37, 245
—hypothesis concerning development of, 14
—prerequisites for development of, 207–8
—profitability of, 208–9
Steam baths, 132, 136, 142
Sternberg, George M.
—on discovery of tubercle bacillus, 268
—on malpractice, 324
Stratification of physicians
—basis of, 204–7
—hypothesis concerning, 14
—and medical societies, 201–4
Streptococcus, 273
Strychnine, 194
Students, medical
—backgrounds of, 110–11, 113–14, 120, 229
—enumerated: in 1769–1868, 98; in 1850–1920, 287
—female, 227, 300n–301n

—increases in number, 286, 291
—self-selection, 120, 292
—stratification, 282
Surgeons. *See also* Surgery
—and AMA presidency, 212
—and fee splitting, 258–59
—non-regular, 236, 259
—number of, 252, 258
—prestige of, 260
—specialization among, 258
Surgery. *See also* Anesthesia; Infection, wound
—amputations, 28, 249–252
—and anesthesia, 250–52
—antiseptic, 255–58
—in Civil War, 252
—in colonial period, 27–28, 250
—in early 19th century, 61, 250–51
—growth of, 209, 250, 252, 258
—healing of wounds caused by, 253–54
—and homeopaths, 166, 231, 236, 259
—mortality from, 249, 251–52
—non-sectarian nature of, 228, 238
—study of, 91
—and Thomsonians, 149
Sydenham, Thomas, 91

Tartar emetic and antimony
—criticised: by Hersey, 149; by Thomson, 135
—therapeutic use of, 52, 182
Teething, 22, 53–54
Temperance movement, 196
Tennessee
—medical licensing in, 339
—medical societies in, 70, 330, 339
—Thomsonism in, 141
Texas, 309n
Textbooks, medical
—medical schools encouraged writing of, 100
—regular, used in homeopathic schools, 238n
—on therapeutics, 181, 192, 195
Therapeutic nihilism
—advocated: by J. Bigelow, 177–78; by Holmes, 178–79; by Jefferson, 43–44; by Wood, 183–84
—homeopathy as manifestation of, 167
—physicians unwilling to accept, 180–81, 184–85

Therapy. *See also* Eclecticism; Homeopathy; Therapeutic nihilism; Therapy, heroic
—and bacteriology, 266–67
—as basis of conflicts, 64, 228, 238
—medically valid: antitoxin, 275; cinchona (quinine) as, 28–29; defined, 9–10; hypothesis concerning acceptance of, 13; surgery as, 27–28; vaccination as, 29–32
—medically invalid: defined, 9–10
—palliative: hypothesis concerning use of, 13; patients' desire for, 184–85; use by homeopaths, 243–45; use by physicians, 43, 185
—study in medical education, 89, 91–92, 289
—symptomatic basis of, 43
Therapy, heroic
—acceptance by patients, 44
—criticised: by J. Bigelow, 167, 178; by Hahnemann, 152–53; by Hersey, 149–50; by Holmes, 178–79; by homeopaths, 166; by Sims, 62; by Thomson, 134–35
—demise of, 181–83
—effects, 54, 179–80
—elements: bloodletting, 45–49; cantharides, 53; cathartics and purgatives, 49–52; emetics, 52; tonics, 52
—public opposition to, 54, 127–28
—used: by botanical practitioners, 142; by eclectic physicians, 221, 223, 225; by regular physicians, 59–62, 127
Thermometer, 42, 262
Thomsonian movement. *See also* Curtis, Alva; Hersey, Thomas; Thomsonian practitioners; Thomson, John; Thomson, Samuel
—class composition, 141, 159–60
—diversity within, 148, 150
—fragmentation of, 146, 217
—institutionalization of, 142–43
—leaders, 144–45, 160
—and licensing repeal, 145–46
—popularity: in Boston, 141; in midwest, 141; in south, 141
Thomsonian practitioners. *See also* Thomsonian movement
—infirmaries, 142, 143
—licensing, 144–45

—medical schools: established, 146; opposed by Thomson, 142; sought, 143
—social origins of, 141
—societies of, 142, 144
—and their successors, 217
—therapies of, 142
Thomson, John, 144–46
Thomson, Samuel
—agents and competitors, 140–42, 146
—and eclecticism, 218
—heroic therapy criticized by, 134–35, 187n
—licensing repeal sought by, 145
—life of, 128–31, 142
—lobelia used by, 130
—on midwifery, 133–34, 138–39
—and movement's fragmentation, 146
—and *New Guide to Health*: popularity of, 136–38; price of, 139–40; publication and sales of, 131; title of, 129–30
—on putrid meat, 133
—and regular physicians, 138–39, 144, 147–48
—system: developed, 131–33; of empirical nature, 150; lacking novelty, 136–37
—Thomsonian medical schools and infirmaries opposed by, 143, 151
—mentioned, 129n–35n, 137n–40n, 142n–45n, 151n, 218n
Tonics
—alcohol used as, 194–96
—arsenic used as, 52–53
—defined, 52, 194
—quinine used as, 188
—strychnine used as, 194
Trudeau, Edward, 269n, 270, 271n
Tuberculin, 269, 270
Tuberculosis
—alcohol as therapy for, 195
—bacillus, 268–69
—belief in hereditary nature of, 268
—diagnosis, 270–71
—prevalence, 57, 267, 268n
—and public health measures, 271–72
—sanitarium treatment for, 272, 278
—and tuberculin, 269, 270n, 271
Typhoid
—alcohol used in, 195
—bacillus discovered, 264
—in early 19th century, 61
—mistaken for malaria, 28–29

—and public health, 278
Typhus, 53

Universities. *See* Colleges

Vaccination
—accepted: by Hahnemann, 157; by homeopaths, 166; by public, 31–32; by Thomsonians, 148
—neglected, 61
—term as used by Pasteur, 263–64
Venesection. *See* Bloodletting
Veratrum viride, 187
Vermont
—medical licensing, 339
—medical societies in, 69, 330–31, 339
—mentioned, 113
Vesalius, Andreas, 26
Virchow, Rudolph, 269
Virginia
—botanicals trade, 33
—and colonial physicians, 34, 35
—medical licensing in, 74, 309n, 339
—medical societies in, 70, 331
—and smallpox: inoculation regulated, 30; vaccine agent appointed, 32
—Thomsonians and, 141

Warren, J. Collins
—on AMA, 199, 200
—on surgery without anesthesia, 251n
—mentioned, 84n, 254n
Washington, D.C. *See* District of Columbia
Washington, George
—on smallpox, 31
—treatment of, during terminal illness, 54–55
Waterhouse, Benjamin, 31
Whiskey. *See* Alcohol
Wilder, Alexander
—on bacteriology, 279
—on eclecticism, 221
—mentioned, 169n, 224n, 226n, 308
Wisconsin, 56

Yale University Medical School, 98n, 105, 333
Yellow fever, 50, 59–60
Yersin, Alexandre, 273, 275